Dementia Care

Marie Boltz • James E. Galvin

Editors

Dementia Care

An Evidence-Based Approach

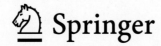

Springer

Editors
Marie Boltz
William F. Connell School of Nursing
Boston College
Chestnut Hill, MA, USA

James E. Galvin
Professor and Associate
  Dean for Clinical Research
Charles E. Schmidt College of Medicine
Florida Atlantic University
Boca Raton, FL, USA

ISBN 978-3-319-18376-3   ISBN 978-3-319-18377-0   (eBook)
DOI 10.1007/978-3-319-18377-0

Library of Congress Control Number: 2015941313

Springer Cham Heidelberg New York Dordrecht London

Printed on acid-free paper

Springer International Publishing AG Switzerland is part of Springer Science+Business Media (www.springer.com)

Preface

Most of us know someone who has dementia or who is affected by it in some way. The number of people living with dementia in the United States is almost six million, with worldwide estimates of 35.6 million. This number is expected to double globally by 2030 and more than triple by 2050 [1]. As one of the major causes of disability and dependency among older people worldwide, it is overwhelming not only for the people who have it but also for their caregivers and families. Furthermore, dementia presents diagnostic and treatment challenges to the clinician, as well as complex conundrums for the researcher and policy maker.

The National Alzheimer's Plan [2] identifies the following goals: the prevention and early detection of Alzheimer's disease, effective treatment, support of people with dementia and their families, and efficient and coordinated care delivery. Consistent with these goals, the purpose of this book is to describe the evidence-based practices that support the patient and family across the trajectory of the dementia clinical course. We also offer the perspective of the patient and family, as their views and experiences ideally shape clinical decisions and program development.

The first section of the book is ***Dementia Prevention, Detection, and Early Support.*** As the population ages at an unprecedented rate, effective strategies to promote cognitive functioning and health are imperative. The chapter, **Prevention of Dementia**, describes the pathological changes that occur with cognitive decline and the risk factors linked to the occurrence of Alzheimer's disease. The efficacy of preventive measures including diet, nutritional interventions and dietary supplements, modification of cardiovascular risk (including physical activity and lifestyle modifications), cognitive engagement, and pharmacologic strategies is presented. Early detection is important in order to secure targeted treatment, prevent avoidable complications, initiate planning for future needs, and mobilize support and resources to the patient and family. The chapter, **Detection of Dementia**, describes the elements and benefits of a comprehensive mental status as well as common barriers to implementation. Assessment methods and use of currently available biomarkers to improve detection of dementia are discussed. Memory clinics and care management offer services and supports during, the initial phases of care delivery and onward. The chapter, **Memory Clinics and Care Management Programs**, reviews memory clinics from a historical perspective and describes its attributes, population serviced, staffing, and outcomes, as well as gives a review of care management models. A diagnosis of dementia often brings with it feelings of loss, social stigma, and uncertainty, placing major demands on the coping abilities for the individual. The chapter, **Early Stage Dementia: Maximizing Self-Direction and Health**, presents strategies to support the person's integrity and autonomy. Diagnostic disclosure, legal and financial planning, supporting functional independence, and maximizing dementia-specific resources are some of the approaches discussed.

The second section of the book is *Clinical Management of Dementia*. No treatments are currently available to cure the progressive course of dementia. There are, however, interventions designed to manage symptoms and promote safety, while maximizing the sense of well-being in the person with dementia. The chapter, **Challenges and Opportunities in Primary and Specialty Memory Care to Provide Best Practice Care**, examines the challenges to recognizing, diagnosing, and treating dementia in both primary and specialty care and offers strategies, including collaborative care delivered by an interdisciplinary teams. The chapter, **Treatment of Dementia: Pharmacological Approaches**, discusses current and promising pharmacologic approaches to managing the cognitive, functional, and behavioral aspects of Alzheimer's disease. The chapter, **Treatment of Dementia: Non-pharmacological Approaches**, describes the behavioral symptoms common in persons with dementia, their impact, origins, and triggers, and assessment. Non-pharmacological interventions, including sensory stimulation, cognitive stimulation and training, emotion-oriented interventions, physical activity and exercise, and behavioral education and training interventions, are presented. These interdisciplinary interventions are consistent with the International Association of Gerontology and Geriatrics, the Center for Medicare and Medicaid (CMS), and the National Alzheimer Project Act (NAPA) advocacy for the use of non-pharmacologic interventions as first-line treatment in the management of behavioral symptoms [3–5].

Persons with dementia have reported loss of driving as catastrophic, leading to feelings of extreme loss of independence and social isolation. The chapter, **Community Mobility in the Person with Dementia**, describes the implications of driving in the medically at risk and offers the state of the science on screening assessments and the role of the driving rehabilitation specialist. The concept of supportive transportation for the person with cognitive impairment who is transitioning from driver to passenger is also discussed.

The third section of the book is entitled *Toward Person-centered Community-based Dementia Care*. Expert dementia care recognizes that the patient and family are the unit of care, and the needs and well-being of the person with dementia and the family caregiver are often interwoven. Further, people with dementia and their caregivers have substantive and unique insights into their condition and life and thus should direct their care. The chapter, **Experience and Perspective of the Person with Dementia**, emphasizes the retained sense of self, well-being, and purpose in the interpersonal worlds of the person with dementia. The authors describe tools and approaches that affirm the individual's self-hood, self-esteem, and quality of life. The chapter, **Home-based Dementia Care Interventions**, provides a systematic review of the extant research on home-based interventions that are designed to improve the quality of life of individuals living with dementia. The authors describe interventions such as caregiver education about dementia, behavior management, activity engagement and case management, describing their merit, as well as opportunities to advancement in this area. The chapter, **Experience and Perspective of the Family Caregiver of the Person with Dementia**, examines the realities of dementia caregiving, from six perspectives of the family member. These perspectives are physical care, lifestyle changes, emotional and psychological needs of the ill person and their carers, relational changes, pragmatic (legal and financial) dimensions, and finally ethical decision-making dilemmas. Then the chapter, **Interventions to Support Caregiver Well-Being**, describes role-related changes in family caregivers and presents interventions including those that focus on improving caregiver health (psychological and physical), offer respite, and provide post-caregiving support.

The fourth section of the book, ***Dementia Continuing Care***, addresses the needs of persons with dementia and their family at various stages of health and in different settings. The chapter, **Transitions in Care for the Person with Dementia**, describes best practices and programs for the person with dementia in periods of transition, including an admission to the hospital and relocation to and within long-term care. The chapter, **Dementia Palliative Care**, discusses how to provide generalist palliative care services, emphasizing symptom management and psychosocial support of patients and families. The chapter, **Hospice Dementia Care**, offers a robust description of the hospice referral and eligibility requirements, the pathobiology and neuropathology, clinical management including symptom control, and bereavement care. Ethical challenges and the support of caregivers are also discussed. Finally, The chapter, **Challenges in Dementia Care Policy**, offers **recommendations on how** various public and private agencies might approach developing dementia-capable systems. Public education, early detection of dementia, worker dementia competency, quality assurance programs, and development of dementia-friendly communities are all discussed as key elements of a dementia-capable system.

The more information, we have the greater is our capacity to help persons with dementia and their family members to take and maintain control of their lives. We hope that this book provides a valuable resource for the student, the clinician, the administrator, the researcher, and the educator in their individual efforts toward that goal.

Chestnut Hill, MA, USA   Marie Boltz
Boca Raton, FL, USA   James E. Galvin

References

1. Alzheimer's Association. Alzheimer's disease facts and figures. 2014. Available at: http://www.alz.org/downloads/Facts_Figures_2014.pdf
2. National plan to address Alzheimer's disease: 2014 Update. http://aspe.hhs.gov/daltcp/napa/NatlPlan2014.pdf

3. Tolson D, Rolland Y, Andrieu S, Aquino J-P, Beard J, Benetos A, et al. International Association of Gerontology and Geriatrics: a global agenda for clinical research and quality of care in nursing homes. J Am Med Dir Assoc. 2011; 12(3):184–9.
4. Workgroup on NAPA's scientific agenda for a national initiative on Alzheimer's disease. Alzheimers Dement J Alzheimers Assoc. 2012; 8(4):357–71.
5. Mitka M. CMS seeks to reduce antipsychotic use in nursing home residents with dementia. JAMA J Am Med Assoc. 2012; 308(2):119, 121.

Acknowledgments

We would like to thank the following for their contributions and support of this book:

- The expert authors, clinicians, educators, and researchers who are recognized for their expertise as well as their dedication and passion to the field of aging and dementia
- Springer Science + Business Media for recognizing dementia care as a critical focus for their publication
- Project Coordinator, Susan Westendorf, for her tremendous guidance, organization, and patience
- Persons with dementia and their family members who inspire us to learn more and do more to become better clinicians, researchers, and administrators.

Marie Boltz
James E. Galvin

Contents

Introduction: Principles of Dementia Care 1
Marie Boltz and James E. Galvin

Part I Dementia Prevention, Detection, and Early Support

Prevention of Dementia 9
Nicole Haynes, Alon Seifan, and Richard S. Isaacson

Detection of Dementia 33
James E. Galvin

Memory Clinics and Care Management Programs 45
Yael R. Zweig

Early Stage Dementia: Maximizing Self-Direction and Health 61
Valerie T. Cotter and Julie Teixeira

Part II Clinical Management of Dementia

Treatment of Dementia: Pharmacological Approaches 73
Nicole J. Brandt and Daniel Z. Mansour

Treatment of Dementia: Non-pharmacological Approaches 97
Elizabeth Galik

**Experience and Perspective of the Primary Care Physician
and Memory Care Specialist** 113
Catherine A. Alder, Michael A. LaMantia,
Mary Guerriero Austrom, and Malaz A. Boustani

**Community Mobility and Dementia: The Role for Health
Care Professionals** 123
Nina M. Silverstein, Anne E. Dickerson, and Elin Schold Davis

**Part III Toward Person-Centered Community-Based
Dementia Care**

Experiences and Perspectives of Persons with Dementia 151
Abhilash K. Desai, F. Galliano Desai, Susan McFadden,
and G.T. Grossberg

Home-Based Interventions Targeting Persons with Dementia:
What Is the Evidence and Where Do We Go from Here? 167
Laura N. Gitlin, Nancy A. Hodgson, and Scott Seung W. Choi

Experiences and Perspectives of Family Caregivers
of the Person with Dementia 189
Jan McGillick and Maggie Murphy-White

Interventions to Support Caregiver Well-Being 215
Meredeth A. Rowe, Jerrica Farias, and Marie Boltz

Part IV Dementia Continuing Care

Transitions in Care for the Person with Dementia 233
Marie Boltz

Dementia Palliative Care 247
Abraham A. Brody

Hospice Dementia Care 261
Richard E. Powers and Heather L. Herrington

Challenges in Dementia Care Policy 299
Jane Tilly and Kate Gordon

Index 313

Contributors

Catherine A. Alder, JD, MSW, LSW Aging Brain Care, Eskenazi Health, Indianapolis, IN, USA

Mary Guerriero Austrom, PhD Department of Psychiatry, Indiana University School of Medicine (IUSM), Indianapolis, IN, USA

Outreach, Recruitment and Education Core, Indiana Alzheimer's Disease Center, Indiana University School of Medicine (IUSM), Indianapolis, IN, USA

Office for Diversity and Inclusion, Indiana University School of Medicine (IUSM), Indianapolis, IN, USA

Marie Boltz, PhD, RN, GNP-BC, FGSA, FAAN William F. Connell School of Nursing, Boston College, Chestnut Hill, MA, USA

Malaz A. Boustani, MD, MPH Indiana University Center for Aging Research, Indianapolis, IN, USA

Regenstrief Institute, Inc., Indianapolis, IN, USA

Center for Health Innovation and Implementation Science, Indiana University School of Medicine (IUSM), Indianapolis, IN, USA

Nicole J. Brandt, PharmD, MBA, CGP, BCPP, FASCP School of Pharmacy, Geriatric Pharmacotherapy, Pharmacy Practice and Science University of Maryland, Baltimore, MD, USA

Clinical and Educational Programs of Peter Lamy Center Drug Therapy and Aging, Baltimore, MD, USA

Abraham A. Brody, RN, PhD, GNP-BC Hartford Institute for Geriatric Nursing, NYU College of Nursing, New York, NY, USA

Scott Seung W. Choi, MA, RN School of Nursing, Johns Hopkins University, Baltimore, MD, USA

Valerie T. Cotter, DrNP, AGPCNP-BC, FAANP University of Pennsylvania School of Nursing, Philadelphia, PA, USA

Elin Schold Davis American Occupational Therapy Association, Bethesda, MD, USA

F. Galliano Desai, PhD Idaho Memory and Aging Center, PLLC, Boise, ID, USA

Abhilash K. Desai, MD Department of Neurology and Psychiatry, Saint Louis University School of Medicine, St. Louis, MO, USA

Idahot Memory and Aging Center, P.L.L.C., Boise, ID, USA

Anne E. Dickerson, PhD, OTR/L, FAOTA East Carolina University, Greenville, NC, USA

Jerrica Farias, RN, MSN University of South Florida College of Nursing, Tampa, FL, USA

Elizabeth Galik, PhD, CRNP University of Maryland School of Nursing, Baltimore, MD, USA

James E. Galvin, MD, MPH Professor and Associate Dean for Clinical Research, Charles E. Schmidt College of Medicine, Florida Atlantic University, Boca Raton, FL, USA

Laura N. Gitlin, PhD Department of Community Public Health, School of Nursing, Johns Hopkins University, Baltimore, MD, USA

Division of Geriatrics and Gerontology, Department of Psychiatry, School of Medicine, Johns Hopkins University, Baltimore, MD, USA

Center for Innovative Care in Aging, Johns Hopkins University, Baltimore, MD, USA

Kate Gordon, MSW Splaine Consulting, Columbia, MD, USA

G.T. Grossberg, MD Department of Neurology and Psychiatry, Saint Louis University School of Medicine, St. Louis, MO, USA

Nicole Haynes, BS Department of Neurology, Weill Cornell Medical College, New York, NY, USA

Heather L. Herrington, MD Department of Medicine, University of Alabama at Birmingham, Birmingham, AL, USA

Nancy A. Hodgson, PhD, RN Center for Innovative Care in Aging, Johns Hopkins University, Baltimore, MD, USA

Department of Acute and Chronic Care, School of Nursing, Johns Hopkins University, Baltimore, MD, USA

Richard S. Isaacson, MD Department of Neurology, Weill Cornell Medical College, New York, NY, USA

Michael A. LaMantia, MD, MPH Indiana University Center for Aging Research, Indianapolis, IN, USA

Regenstrief Institute, Inc., Indianapolis, IN, USA

Daniel Z. Mansour, PharmD School of Pharmacy, Geriatric Pharmacotherapy, Pharmacy Practice and Science University of Maryland, Baltimore, MD, USA

Susan McFadden, PhD Fox Valley Memory Project, Appleton, WI, USA

Jan McGillick Dolan Memory Care Homes, Chesterfield, MO, USA

Maggie Murphy-White Dardenne Prairie, MO, USA

Richard E. Powers Division of Neuropathology, Department of Pathology and Psychiatry, UAB School of Medicine, Birmingham, AL, USA
Post-Traumatic Stress Disorder Program, Veterans Administration Hospital, Birmingham, AL, USA

Meredeth A. Rowe, PhD, RN, FAAN, FGSA University of South Florida College of Nursing, Tampa, FL, USA

Alon Seifan, MD, MS Department of Neurology, Weill Cornell Medical College, New York, NY, USA

Nina M. Silverstein, PhD University of Massachusetts Boston, Boston, MA, USA

Julie Teixeira, BFA, MA Alzheimer's Association Delaware Valley Chapter, Philadelphia, PA, USA

Jane Tilly, DrPH U.S. Administration for Community Living, Washington, DC, USA

Yael R. Zweig, MSN, ANP-BC, GNP-BC Department of Geriatrics, New York University Langone Medical Center, New York, NY, USA

Introduction: Principles of Dementia Care

Marie Boltz and James E. Galvin

It is estimated that every 4 s there is a new case of dementia in the world [1] and once every 67 s someone in the United States develops Alzheimer's Disease [2]. Approximately 5.6 million Americans live with Alzheimer's disease or other form of dementia. Although Alzheimer's disease is not a normal part of aging, the risk of developing the illness rises with advanced age; the prevalence of Alzheimer's disease doubles every 5 years beyond age 65. Over the next 20 years, as the number of people older than 65 almost doubles and over 85 almost quadruples, the incidence, morbidity and mortality rates for Alzheimer's disease will increase dramatically [2].

The major criterion for a diagnosis of dementia is an impairment of two or more core mental functions. These functions include memory, language skills, visual perception, and the ability to focus and pay attention. They also include cognitive skills such as the ability to reason and solve problems. The loss of brain function is severe enough to interfere with everyday functioning [3]. Alzheimer's disease, the most common form of dementia, is accountable for approximately 60–70 % of cases. Vascular dementia, dementia with Lewy bodies, and a group of diseases that contribute to frontotemporal dementia comprise other causes. Mixed forms of dementia often co-exist [4]. The World Health Organization and Alzheimer's International describes the common symptoms of dementia categorized within three stages of dementia, as described in Table 1 [5]. Not all persons experience all these symptoms and some may progress more quickly, others more slowly in their disease progression.

Currently, there is no cure or treatment to significantly alter the course of dementia, although numerous new therapies are being investigated in various stages of clinical trials. There is, however, much that can be offered to support and improve the lives of people with dementia and their caregivers and families. Several principles deserve consideration when delivering care, developing programs, or conducting research.

M. Boltz, PhD, RN, GNP-BC, FGSA, FAAN (✉)
William F. Connell School of Nursing, Boston College, Mahoney Hall, 140 Commonwealth Avenue, Chestnut Hill, MA 02467, USA
e-mail: boltzm@bc.edu

J.E. Galvin, MD, MPH
Professor and Associate Dean for Clinical Research, Charles E. Schmidt College of Medicine, Florida Atlantic University, Boca Raton, FL, USA

Dementia Is a Public Health Imperative

Although it is one of the leading causes of disability in later life, dementia is one of the most poorly understood and under-detected conditions. Lack of awareness and understanding contribute to stigmatization and social isolation, both for the patient and family members. As a result, there is often delayed detection and lack

Table 1 Stages of dementia

Early stage (1st year or 2)	Middle stage (2nd to 4th or 5th years)	Late stage (5th year onward)
Symptoms may be overlooked or attributed to normal aging	More obvious and restrictive limitations. Unable to live alone without considerable support	Total or almost total dependence
• Forgets things that recently happened	• More forgetful of recent events and people names	• Unable to recognize relatives, friends and familiar objects
• Shows difficulty with communication, especially word-finding	• Has difficulty with speech and comprehension	• Usually unaware of time and place
• Experiences difficulty managing finances	• Has difficulty managing personal care	• Needs extensive help with personal care, often incontinent of bowel and bladder
• Becomes lost in familiar places	• May get lost at home	• May be unable to eat without assistance, may have difficulty in swallowing
• Loses track of the time, including time of day, season, year	• Has difficulty comprehending time, date, events, place	• May have mobility loss, may be unable to walk
• May gave difficulty with household tasks or hobbies	• Unable to successfully prepare food, cook, clean or shop	• May not find his/her way around the house
• Mood and behavior changes may include: – Less physical activity and motivation – Mood swings – Uncharacteristic anger	Behavioral changes may include: repeated questions, calling out, wandering, unsafe exiting, sleep disturbances, refusal of care, aggression, hallucinations	• Behavior changes may escalate and include aggression and nonverbal manifestations of distress

Adapted from: Alzheimer's Disease International and World Health Organization Dementia: A Public Health Priority

of access to treatment and social support. Delays negatively impact patient mood, health function, and diminish family resilience. The resultant morbidity and care dependency increases societal costs. Thus efforts to increase public awareness and detect dementia in early stages are a public health priority [5].

Dementia Care and Support Is About Knowing the Person

Kitwood's concept of personhood illuminates the image of the person with dementia as someone who is able to experience emotions, both positive and negative, as well as the ability to share these emotions to those who are able and willing to be fully present and attentive [6]. The dignity of the person with dementia is supported when his/her value as a human being is upheld.

This can come about when the person is "known." An understanding of the life of the person as well as values, accomplishments, and preferences, promotes meaningful communication and supports efforts to develop an individualized plan of care [7]. Instead of a mere emphasis on the pathology of the disease, the focus shifts to maximizing the person's capabilities and looking for opportunities to promote quality in everyday life. This "enabling" approach can replace passivity and boredom with active engagement in meaningful activity and connection with others [8].

Dementia Is a Family Matter

The majority of persons with dementia in the US (estimated at 70–80 %) live in the community [9]. For nearly 75 % of these individuals, care that is critical to their quality of life is provided by family caregivers [2]. For every person with dementia, it is estimated that nearly three family and other unpaid caregivers provide over 17 billion hours of care for a total cost valued at over $200 billion [10]. The main functions provided by the 1.1 family caregivers are those related to care provision and care management. Care provision includes hands-on care, dressing, assisting with finances and other daily activities; care management includes arranging for care and services [11]. Educational programs and information on treatment options can impact their ability to continue in their roles of care provider or care manager. Further, family caregivers are a critical resource, serving as advocates, representing the views and preferences of the patient when they are no longer able. Thus, opportunities should be seized to engage them in care –related decision-making, program planning, and policies [5, 12].

As the approximately 1.1 million caregivers, struggle to meet the care needs of their family member, they face compromises to their time, finances, quality of life, and even productivity in the work place [2]. Even those family members not directly providing care are affected by dementia. Dementia—capable care considers how the needs of the person with dementia impact the family as a whole and vice versa. Family caregivers are referred to as the "invisible second patients," because they have their own needs for guidance and support [9]. Thus, essential components of the dementia family care plan are the measures to alleviate caregiver anxiety, burden and strain. In summary, efforts should be made to strengthen family caregiver effectiveness while simultaneously alleviating their physical, psychological and financial burden.

Dementia Requires Diligent Clinical Care

Dementia is primarily a disease of old age and it often coexists with other conditions associated with aging. Evidence suggests that among people with dementia there is a high prevalence of comorbid medical conditions [13–16]. Certain comorbid medical conditions, such as diabetes, may exacerbate the progression of cognitive decline in dementia [17]. Moreover, the presence of dementia may adversely affect and complicate the clinical care of other conditions and be a key factor in how patients' needs are anticipated and specialist and emergency services are used [18, 19]. Consequently, there is a need for consistent primary care follow-up, education of patient/caregivers about management of chronic conditions and health maintenance [19].

Dementia: Friendly Environments Improve Quality of Life and Care

The physical and social environment affects the sense of well-being, function and even health of the person with dementia [20]. The environment should compensate for reduced sensory, cognitive and motor ability. Independence should be supported while providing safety and security; obstacles, barriers, poor lighting, glare and hazards should be removed. Color contrast can help the person with dementia identify important items such as doorways, toilets, and sinks. Privacy and dignity are also important goals; the need to have time and space alone continues to be important to persons with dementia.

A simple, familiar, uncluttered environment offers a sense of security. Adult day care and residential facilities should include a home-like setting which allows the person with dementia to use existing skills to continue the tasks of daily living. Personal possessions help create a familiar environment and can be a source of joy for people with dementia. They communicate much about a person especially if the person is no longer able to do so, and can be a topic of conversation for staff and family members [21–24].

The Workforce Requires Dementia: Specific Competencies

Multiple health care and social service workers interface with the person with dementia and family. They include primary and specialty clinicians, community care workers, social workers, nurses, nurse practitioners, rehabilitation staff, allied health professionals, personal assistants, domiciliary and personal care assistants, and staff in mental health services, rehabilitation services, long term care and palliative care services. Basic knowledge and skills for those working with dementia and their families include: the types and presentation of dementia, communication techniques, family dynamics and support, person-centered care, function-focused approaches and community resources. Experiential learning that supports examination of one's own biases and values can promote insights and empathy. Additional competencies for clinicians include detection and treatment of dementia, cognitive and functional assessment, pharmacologic considerations, and prevention and detection of complications such as delirium [12, 25, 26]. A strong emphasis on interdisciplinary collaboration is also essential. Finally, ways of engaging with the person with dementia and the family as a partner in care has been frequently shown to improve health outcomes [12].

Summary and Conclusion

For persons with dementia and their families, every day brings challenges. The principles described here have at their core the principle value of alleviating their suffering and promoting their quality of life. Although those who are committed to this value face their own challenges, the work is rewarding and full of possibilities for personal and professional growth.

References

1. Alzheimer's Disease International and the World Health Organization. Dementia: a public health priority; 2012.
2. Alzheimer's Association. Alzheimer's disease facts and figures. Alzheimers Dement. 2014;10(2).
3. World Health Organization. International statistical classification of diseases and related health problems, 10th revision. Geneva: World Health Organization; 1992.
4. National Institute of Health. The dementias: hope through research. National Institute Of Neurological

Disorders and Stroke and National Institute on Aging. http://www.ninds.nih.gov/disorders/dementias/the-dementias.pdf
5. Alzheimer's Disease International and World Health Organization. (2012). Dementia: a public health priority. Accessed at: http://www.who.int/mental_health/publications/dementia_report_2012/en/.
6. Kitwood T. Dementia reconsidered—the person comes first. Buckingham: Open University Press; 1997.
7. Bano B, Benbow S, Read K. Dementia and spirituality: a perfume always remembered. In: Gilbert P, editor. Spirituality and mental health. Brighton: Pavilion Publishers; 2011.
8. Radden J, Fordyce J. Into the darkness: losing identity with dementia. In: Hughes J, Louw S, Sabat S, editors. Dementia—mind, meaning and the person. Oxford: Oxford University Press; 2006.
9. Brodaty H, Donkin M. Family caregivers of people with dementia. Dialogues Clin Neurosci. 2009;11(2):217–28.
10. Zhao Y, Kuo T-C, Weir S, Kramer M, Ash A. Healthcare costs and utilization for medicare beneficiaries with Alzheimer's. BMC Health Serv Res. 2008;8(1):108.
11. Archbold PG. Impact of parent caring on women. Paper presented at XII International Congress of Gerontology, Hamburg, West Germany; 1981.
12. Boltz, M., Chippendale, T., Resnick, B., & Galvin, J. (in press). Testing family centered, function-focused care in hospitalized persons with dementia. *Neurodegenerative Disease Management*.
13. Doraiswamy PM, Leon J, Cummings JL, Marin D, Neumann PJ. Prevalence and impact of medical comorbidity in Alzheimer's disease. J Gerontol A Biol Sci Med Sci. 2002;57:M173–7.
14. Kuo TC, Zhao Y, Weir S, Kramer MS, Ash AS. Implications of comorbidity on costs for patients with Alzheimer disease. Med Care. 2008;46:839–46.
15. Schubert CC, Boustani M, Callahan CM, Perkins AJ, Carney CP, Fox C, Unverzagt F, Hui S, Hendrie HC. Comorbidity profile of dementia patients in primary care: are they sicker? J Am Geriatr Soc. 2006;54:104–9.
16. Bunn F, Burn AM, Goodman C, Rait G, Norton S, Robinson L, Schoeman J, Brayne C. Comorbidity and dementia: a scoping review of the literature. BMC Med. 2014;12:192.
17. Biessels GJ, Staekenborg S, Brunner E, Brayne C, Scheltens P. Risk of dementia in diabetes mellitus: a systematic review. Lancet Neurol. 2006;5:64–74.
18. Whitmer RA, Karter AJ, Yaffe K, Quesenberry CP, Selby JV. Hypoglycemic episodes and risk of dementia in older patients with type 2 diabetes mellitus. JAMA. 2009;301:1565–72.
19. Keenan TD, Goldacre R, Goldacre MJ. Associations between age-related macular degeneration, Alzheimer disease, and dementia: record linkage study of hospital admissions. JAMA Ophthalmol. 2014;132:63–8.
20. Lawton MP, Nahemo L. Ecology and the aging process. In: Eisdorfer C, Lawton MP, editors. Psychology

of adult development and aging. Washington, DC: American Psychological Association; 1973.

21. Brush J, Fleder H, Calkins M. Using the environment to support communication and foster independence in people with Dementia: a review of case studies in long term care settings. Kirtland, OH: I.D.E.A.S. Inc.; 2012.

22. Calkins M. Home modifications for people with dementia. MAX: Max Hum Potent. 2006;13(4):4.

23. Brush J, Calkins M, Bruce C, Sanford J. Environment and communication assessment toolkit for Dementia care. Baltimore, MD: Health Professions Press; 2012.

24. Brawley E. Design Innovations for ageing and Alzheimer's: creating caring environments. Hoboken, NJ: Wiley; 2006.

25. Galvin JE, Kuntemeier B, Al-Hammadi N, Germino J, Murphy-White M, McGillick J. Dementia-friendly hospitals: care not crisis: an educational program designed to improve the care of the hospitalized patient with Dementia. Alzheimer Dis Assoc Disord. 2010;24(4):372–9.

26. Brody AA, Galvin JE. A review of interprofessional dissemination and education interventions for recognizing and managing dementia. Gerontol Geriatr Educ. 2013;34:225–56.

Part I

Dementia Prevention, Detection, and Early Support

Prevention of Dementia

Nicole Haynes, Alon Seifan,
and Richard S. Isaacson

Introduction

While we have made great strides toward achieving measurable gains in dementia prevention, efforts to prevent cognitive decline and dementia have failed to show consistent results. The significance of researching preventative measures stems from the impeding dementia epidemic that affects individuals, society, and global healthcare. As the older population continues to advance in age, both cognitive decline and dementia become increasingly prevalent and apparent. Accompanying advancing age is a decline of cognitive abilities including perceptual speed, reasoning, episodic memory and working memory [1]. Cognitive decline covers a vast array of symptoms, and may occur due to a variety of causes, ranging from mild, stable symptoms observed with normal aging, to progressive symptoms as seen in dementia.

As previously discussed throughout this book, dementia is characterized by the gradual loss of cognitive abilities, in multiple domains, severe enough to interfere with daily living [2]. Alzheimer's Disease (AD), the most common form of dementia, occurs in approximately 10 %

N. Haynes, BS • A. Seifan, MD, MS
R.S. Isaacson, MD (✉)
Department of Neurology, Weill Cornell Medical
College, New York, NY, USA
e-mail: rii9004@med.cornell.edu

of persons older than 65 years old and up to 50 % of those older than 85 years old [3]. The risk of dementia nearly doubles with every 5 years of age. The US Medicare economic cost of caring for people with dementia in 2008 was 91 billion dollars, and is predicted to double by 2015. By 2050, it is expected that the amount of people diagnosed with AD will triple, leaving a great impact on global healthcare and families alike [4].

Over the years, countless modifiable and non-modifiable risk factors have been brought to light, suggesting a high potential for research of both non-pharmaceutical and pharmaceutical strategies for AD therapeutics. While this global problem of dementia is often associated with the elderly, many of the pathologic changes associated with AD may occur decades before symptom onset, leaving ample time for preventative measures [5]. Earlier identification of at-risk individuals could lead to faster diagnoses, better stratification of patients, higher levels of enrollment in clinical trials and ultimately to more effective preventative treatments [4]. Preclinical Alzheimer's disease is the state of being cognitively normal but testing positive for the presence of cerebral amyloid [6]. Future dementia prevention trials focusing on patients with preclinical Alzheimer's disease will need to screen out up to 80 % of potential participants, but the cost of scanning all potential participants for the presence of amyloid would be prohibitive. The use of non-invasive screening measures including web-based programs will become increasingly important to reduce the number who need to be scanned, prior to enrollment in these trials [7]. Several risk indices are available for this purpose. Researchers have identified at least 11 AD risk factors and four protective factors for AD (age, sex, education, body mass index, diabetes, depression, serum cholesterol, traumatic brain injury, smoking, alcohol intake, social engagement, physical activity, cognitive activity, fish intake, and pesticide exposure) [8]. Studies with emphasis on genotype, lifestyle, and nutritional intake may serve to be an important consideration for neurodegenerative diagnosis and disease modification. As such, health authorities should focus on identifying high-risk individuals at an early stage, when intervention is more likely to help [9].

It should also be noted that because adult brain structure is primarily established in early life and young adulthood, childhood factors such as socioeconomic status and early life brain growth could also influence AD risk. Learning disabilities may predispose to atypical phenotypes of AD [10]. Interactions between these and other inter-related factors are difficult to detect. The adult life mechanisms, by which early life factors exert influence on AD risk, remain unknown. Early life brain development could render different brain regions selectively vulnerable to the onset, accumulation, or spread of AD-related pathology during late-life.

While in past years the concept of dementia prevention has been perceived by many clinicians as impossible, in 2014 a group of 109 scientists from 36 countries signed a statement detailing how dementia (including AD) can be prevented [9]. While there is no one "magic" pill, or definitive single way to prevent dementia, the most recent projects have found that if indeed the known modifiable risk factors for AD are in the causal pathway to dementia, then one out of every three cases could potentially be prevented by addressing those factors [11]. It is currently unclear which specific interventions would be most effective, in which patients and during which life stages. Although the entire life course is relevant to dementia prevention, this review focuses on only those risk factors which are modifiable and which have been demonstrated in adults or the elderly.

Understanding Cognitive Decline

Normal cognition requires complex neural networks localized in different parts of the brain such as the medial temporal lobes including the hippocampus and the entorhinal cortex and the fronto-parietal cortices [12]. Memory, attention, executive function, perception, language and psychomotor function are key components [13]. In relation to neurodegeneration, impairment of any of these components has a pathological substrate in a corresponding brain area, culpable for its processing. Different pathological changes correlate to the various form of dementia. Provided that AD is the most prevalent neurodegenerative disease associated with dementia, it is the most studied and pertinent focus for many clinical trials. In practice, dementia due to coincident disease (mixed pathology) is more common than dementia due to pure AD [14]. In AD, deposition of amyloid beta protein ($A\beta$) aggregates and accumulation of tau protein in areas of the brain, such as the hippocampus and the entorhinal cortex, are associated with early-disease related changes in AD. These two proteins and their respective signaling pathways are thought to influence rate-limiting steps in AD pathology. The $A\beta$ and tau aggregates gradually become widespread plaques and tangles in the brain of AD patients. Years of accumulation result in decreased synaptic function and neuronal atrophy, likely a significant driving force behind the cognitive deficit [12]. Oxidative damage, excessive glutaminergic activity, energy failure, inflammation and apoptosis seem to be significant contributors to neuronal loss and progressive cognitive dysfunction [15–19]. The order in which these pathologic features occur is still being debated. Degeneration of certain brain regions results indeficiencies in neurotransmitters that serve essential roles in neuronal circuits dealing with cognition (e.g., degeneration of the basal forebrain is associated with decrements in acetylcholine-mediated neuronal activity involved in memory).

Distinguished genetic, clinical, and environmental risk factors have been directly linked to the occurrence of AD. Appearance of dementia later in life is believed to be a result of the combination of age-related changes in the brain, predominantly vascular changes, AD, and α-synuclein pathology [5]. Vascular risk factors like hypertension (HTN) and diabetes mellitus (DM) appeal to the interest of the public perspective on health due to their global prevalence, ease of administered treatment, and affiliation to diseases with similar risk factors. The magnitude of these risk factors appears to be directly proportional to the observed prevalence and intensity associated with the disease.

Evidence also suggests abnormalities in glucose metabolism, mitochondrial function and oxidative stress are an invariant feature of AD and may occur decades before the onset of clinical symptoms (during the "pre-clinical AD" stage) in both genetic and non-genetic AD forms [5]. As one example, the presence of the apolipoprotein E ε4 allele (ApoE4) is a well-studied genetic risk factor for late onset AD. In ApoE4-positive younger adults, cerebral glucose hypometabolism has been observed in asymptomatic individuals in the temporal, parietal, posterior cingulate, and prefrontal lobes decades before the expected development of AD (average age of 30.7) [20]. Mitochondrial dysfunction may also be a key link in AD pathogenesis. While it is not entirely clear whether amyloid and tau may lead to mitochondrial dysfunction, there is well-grounded scientific rationale that mitochondrial dysfunction may more likely lead to glucose hypometabolism, and has been seen early in the brains of patients at risk for developing AD [21]. Mitochondrial dysfunction may lead to most of the mechanisms thought to impair brain function in AD, including oxidative stress, apoptosis, and inhibition of protein degradation and autophagy, potentially leading to the accumulation of amyloid and tau. Other changes such as alterations in calcium homeostasis also precede clinical symptoms, and abnormal glucose metabolism, mitochondrial dysfunction and oxidative stress may promote plaques, tangles and calcium abnormalities that accompany AD [22]. Therapies targeting mitochondrial function, glucose hypometabolism, and their associated distinctive metabolic requirements, are under active investigation. This 'mitocentric' view of the pathogenesis of AD offers some key theory behind why a myriad of the interventions discussed below may be practical options toward lowering dementia risk, while also being generally low in risk [23].

Diet

The first suggestion that diet could offer protection against cognitive decline and dementia came from the Mediterranean region. A high dietary intake of fruit, whole grains, legumes, fish, and vegetables resulted in a lower occurrence of cognitive decline and brain-related diseases. Since then, several studies have investigated the "Mediterranean diet" (also referred to as MeDi) as well as other dietary patterns [24]. At least five high-quality, prospective cohort studies examining the MeDi with longitudinal cognitive follow-up of at least 1 year support the idea that among cognitively normal individuals, higher adherence to the MeDi is associated with a reduced risk of mild cognitive impairment (MCI), a dementia prodromal stage, and AD [25]. Randomized trials show that healthful diets can even show effects on cardiovascular disease markers and cognitive performance in as little as 4 weeks. A 4-week, low-saturated fat/low-glycemic index diet, compared to a high-saturated fat/high-glycemic index diet, modified cerebrospinal fluid (CSF) biomarkers and improved delayed visual memory for normal adults and adults with MCI [26]. A diet with high anti-oxidative capacity (fatty fish, rapeseed oil, oat, barley and rye foods, bread supplemented with guar gum, soybeans and dry almonds), compared to a control, healthful diet devoid of the "active" components, significantly improved cardiovascular risk variables and also resulted in improved performance tests of selective attention and also auditory verbal learning [27]. A recent study found that normal subjects with higher adherence to the MeDi diet had less cortical thinning in the same brain regions as clinical AD patients [28]. These data suggested a protective effect against tissue loss, and suggest that the MeDi diet may play a role in the prevention of AD.

In general, a healthy diet is attributed to having sufficient mineral, vitamin, and other elemental component intake, necessary for basic cellular functioning. These elements could reduce the risk of dementia and cognitive decline by interfering with pro-inflammatory responses in the brain [29]. Examples include neurodegenerative protection in the form of high supply of natural fish oil, vitamins, and polyphenols [4, 19].

Several scores and outcome scales have been created to assess adherence to the Mediterranean diet [30]. In a recent prospective cohort study, a higher Mediterranean diet score was associated with better cognition. In this same cohort, a dose-response effect of Mediterranean diet was suggested based on the progressive lower risk for developing dementia or MCI in the middle and the upper score tertile when compared with the bottom tertile (21 % and 47 % risk reduction, respectively) [31, 32]. Another prospective cohort demonstrated that high adherence to the Mediterranean diet was associated with better cognitive output and episodic memory test results over time, but did not show any protective effect for the development of AD [33].

Variable information regarding education, geographic location, exercise and less prevalent cardiovascular risk factors are reason for current debate over the final impact of the Mediterranean diet on cognition. Regardless of these discrepancies, it is generally assumed that early introduction of a healthy diet is beneficial for cognition and for various cardiovascular risks associated with contributing to the occurrence of AD and cognitive decline [24]. While there is insufficient randomized prospective data to prove the efficacy of Mediterranean diet vs. other dietary patterns, the Mediterranean diet still exemplifies the most commonly recommended potentially beneficial diet to overall brain health.

Gu and colleagues [34] proposed a different approach to the evaluation of diet and the risk for cognitive decline/AD. Provided the potential for low prevalence of Mediterranean diet in local communities, statistical analyses assessed nutrients and dietary patterns in order to compartmentalize diet elements associated with lower risk of AD development. Resulting data illustrated that greater intake of nuts, fish, poultry, fruits, and cruciferous and leafy vegetables associated with a lower risk of AD, and a negative correlation with red meat, high-fat dairy, and butter intake. Overall, previous results suggest a diet rich in fruits, vegetables, legumes, fish, nuts, and grains to be healthiest [1, 2, 4]. Regardless of these recommendations, the effect that an individual dietary component has on others remains in question.

Diet interventions may affect individuals in different ways, specifically with respect to APOE4 allele carrier status [35]. In Yoruba populations in Nigeria, there is no association between APOE4 status and AD, as compared to genetically similar populations with a Western lifestyle and diet [36]. In older individuals, CRP levels are associated with cognitive decline only in APOE4 negative individuals [37]. Consumption of fatty fish more than twice per week was associated with a reduction in risk of dementia and AD only in APOE4 negative subjects [38, 39]. Saturated fat intake was associated with an increased risk for dementia 20 years later, but only among the APOE4 carriers [40].

Nutritional Interventions and Dietary Supplements

Evidence on nutritional interventions for cognitive decline and dementia is in a constant state of growth. While the content below is a fairly broad and up-to-date summary for dementia, a recent initiative, begun by the Alzheimer's Drug Discovery Foundation, called Cognitive Vitality attempts to update the evidence for many of the topics below on an ongoing basis. For more information about this initiative visit: http://www.alzdiscovery.org/cognitive-vitality/nutrition-natural-products-and-supplements.

Garlic

Garlic is high in antioxidants and organosulfurs. An extract preparation has been associated with decreased cholesterol levels and blood pressure. Additionally, it is thought that garlic may be doubly beneficial in that it lowers cardiovascular risk factors and their impact on AD development as well as supplying antioxidants capable of counteracting the ongoing neurodegenerative process. It has been shown in animal models that garlic can reduce homocysteine [41]. In vitro studies demonstrated that garlic extract can inhibit Aβ and caspase- enzymes that promote the deposition of amyloid [42].

Budoff and coworkers [43] demonstrated garlic to be able to decrease levels of homocysteine in humans, however it is unclear if this result was independent of the concurrent statin therapy the subjects were receiving.

Gingko Biloba

Flavonoids and terpenes contained in gingko biloba have been linked to pleiotropic actions that can affect inflammation and oxidative processes in the human body [44]. It is approved in some European countries for the treatment of cerebrovascular insufficiency and cognitive decline, although in the US it is sold as a supplement [1]. Short term supplementation has provided conflicting results, with some studies showing marginal improvement in cognition while others fail to reproduce any significant effect [19, 45]. One small randomized clinical trial (RCT) showed that gingko extract was associated with marginal improvement in the clinical dementia rating scale (CDR) when adjusting for medication adherence [46]. However, the clinical significance of this marginal improvement in cognitive testing in conjunction with a higher incidence of cerebrovascular events in the treatment arm could have confounded the results. While there has been a lot of uncertainty around the effect of ginkgo biloba in AD treatment and prevention, definitive research has shown that this is not effective for the prevention of AD [47]. In fact, there are now several studies that show that this supplement is not effective in prevention of dementia nor cognitive decline, in general. While low doses are generally safe, most clinicians are hesitant to recommend it for use. However, a meta-analysis [48] on nine trials

using standardized formulation in the treatment of dementia showed statistically significant improvement in cognitive scales with no significant benefit in activities of daily living performance. The high variability of study designs hampers the generalization of these results.

Alcohol

Some observational studies have shown that low to moderate alcohol consumption may lower the risk of dementia [49, 50]. There is speculation that alcohol exerts its benefit though lipid profile improvement, although the content of flavonoids in red wine could also contribute [15, 51]. A recent meta-analysis of 23 observational studies demonstrated that alcohol in small amounts can be protective against dementia and AD but did not impact the rate of cognitive decline or the incidence of vascular dementia [49]. Inconsistent results of the analysis prevent a firm conclusion to be made on the applicability of the findings. In another study, moderate alcohol consumption was linked with resistance to the effects of Aβ, which could reduce risks of developing dementia and cognitive decline [52]. Considering the evidence, many clinicians would support moderate alcohol intake (1 drink in women, 1–2 drinks in men) for the potential risk reduction of dementia over time. Neafsey and Collins concluded that this amount may reduce the risk of dementia and cognitive decline [53], although further studies are warranted. Most clinicians advise against consumption of more than two servings per day, as this may lead to significant health consequences. In the United States, a "standard" drink contains about 0.6 fluid ounces or 14 g of "pure" alcohol. Typical servings of alcohol are as follows: 12 oz beer = 8–9 oz malt liquor = 5 oz wine = 3–4 oz fortified wine (e.g., sherry or port) = 1.5 oz hard liquor (i.e., "a shot").

Caffeine

Since ancient times, caffeine has been a great resource. Its popularity has granted it status as the more popular and most consumed behaviorally acting substance around the world [54]. Caffeine is an antagonist of adenosine receptors A_1 and A_{2A}, although it can also interact with other enzymes and receptors like $GABA_A$ or $5'$ nucleotidase at higher levels [55]. In animal models, antagonist of A_{2A} receptors like caffeine decreased the levels in cerebrospinal fluid and serum of $A\beta$ peptides and counteracted its noxious effects at the neuronal levels [56, 57]. Inhibition of phosphodiesterase is thought to be a potential mechanism to convey neuroprotection [58]. The activation of A_{2A} receptors has been associated with long term potentiation in striatal and hippocampal synapses essential for memory processing. The excessive or insufficient activation of these receptors results in aberrant synaptic functioning [58–60]. Caffeine can act as normalizer of aberrant memory performance rather than enhancing this process, especially in conditions with excessive endogenous adenosine stimulation such as fatigue and stress [58, 61].

In humans, caffeine reaches a peak in plasma 45–120 min after oral ingestion and has a half-life that ranges from 2.5 to 4.5 h [55]. Caffeine facilitates learning on tasks in which information is presented passively, but it has not proven effective for those tasks that involve intentional learning. The caffeine effect on memory tasks seems to have an inverted U shape curve, showing improvement during mild to moderate complexity tasks but impaired performance for high complexity tasks [13]. Caffeine confers a boost for cognitive performance among fatigued individuals and it might also improve cognitive functioning with chronic consumption, although its acute effect is more evident in non-usual consumers [62, 63]. The effects of caffeine appear to vary across the age span. Administration of caffeine in the older population is more effective for improving attention, psychomotor performance, and cognitive functioning, possibly offsetting the decline associated with age. A large part of these effects may be explained by counteracting age-related, decreased arousal [64, 65].

The relationship between AD and caffeine has been more difficult to understand. A retrospective cohort study suggested that caffeine intake at midlife has protective effects against the subsequent development of AD [66]. In prospective

studies, Ritchie et al. showed a protective effect of caffeine in women consuming more than three cups of coffee per day [67] and van Gelder and colleagues showed that men also benefited from caffeine intake. In his prospective cohort, men who drank more than three coffee cups per day showed slower cognitive decline when compared with those drinking less than three cups per day and non-coffee drinkers [68]. Another prospective cohort analysis showed that cognitive performance was strongly associated with caffeine intake, with no gender differences in its protective effects. However, caffeine intake was also strongly associated with age, IQ, and social class, thus education confounding effects could not be ruled out [69]. Finally, Boxtel and coworkers were not able to reproduce any of the above mentioned findings, and demonstrated no associations between long time caffeine intake and cognitive performance [70]. Provided the variability of the studies and results of clinical outcomes, it is difficult to strongly recommend caffeine intake as an effective measure against cognitive decline; nevertheless, it seems safe to say that caffeine can provide a boost in cognitive ability and has been shown to be protective in some populations.

B Vitamins

B Vitamins are organic compounds acquired through dietary intake. They are known for their major roles in cell metabolism and are associated with protective roles in cognition. Vitamin B1 (thiamine) and Vitamin B2 (riboflavin) are found in a variety of foods, such as whole grain cereals, organ meats, milk and vegetables. Vitamin B6 (pyridoxine) and Vitamin B12 (cobalamin) are typically from poultry, seafood, meat, and eggs, and often in enriched cereals. The major source of folates is the green leafy vegetables [71]. Thiamine, riboflavin, and niacin function in major biochemical pathways in the metabolism of glucose, amino acids, and fatty acids, while the coenzymes of vitamin B12, folate and vitamin B6 interact together in the metabolism of homocysteine, a risk factor for vascular disease and dementia [72, 73]. Investigating the anti-oxidant and anti-inflammatory properties of these vitamins, along with their contribution to nucleotide synthesis and nerve functions, is important in the context of cognition [71]. Interaction between vitamin B12, folate, and pyridoxine could prove influential to some effects in cognitive decline. These vitamins are key determinants of homocysteine levels, of which, high levels can be destructive due to neurotoxic and vasotoxic effects on brain vasculature and normal cognitive functioning [74–76]. Other studies have shown folate levels associated with varying degrees of cognitive decline independent of the homocysteine and vitamin B levels [76–78]. To further clarify the interaction of B vitamins and folate supplementation, future studies should control for homocysteine levels. Trials of combined vitamin supplementation are difficult to interpret because of various covariates that make it challenging to isolate an effect [71, 79]. The strongest evidence to date studied the effect of a combination of B vitamins on cognitive functioning and clinical decline in MCI patients with elevated homocysteine. In this double-blind study, MCI patients (ages seventy and above) with high homocysteine levels receiving 0.8 mg of folic acid, 0.5 mg of vitamin B12, and 20 mg of vitamin B6 each day show improved cognitive test scores on the Mini Mental State Examination (MMSE) and a category fluency test. In this RCT, this specific B vitamin combination appeared to slow cognitive and clinical decline in people with MCI, as well as slow atrophy of the hippocampus. Further studies are warranted to determine whether these vitamins may slow or prevent the progression from MCI to AD, or delay or prevent the onset of MCI [80].

Vitamin B1 (Thiamine)

Animal models have shown that rats with low thiamine diet have impaired cognitive performance compared to controls fed with adequate thiamine supplementation [81], and repetitive episodes of thiamine deficiency can cause worsening of cognitive performance and severe brain damage [82, 83]. Thiamine deficiency has been associated with blood brain barrier (BBB) dysfunction

and intracellular edema in animal models, revealing pathological changes that could derail the normal functioning of the brain [71].

In a non-randomized controlled trial (RCT), Meador and colleagues [84] found that older individuals supplemented 3–8 g/day of oral thiamine showed significant improvement in the ADAS in the initial months with slowing of the cognitive decline rate during 11–13 months after the trial stopped. The small sample and open design are concerns in this trial. Mimori and colleagues [85] showed that higher blood levels of thiamine after supplementation with an oral form were associated with improvement in scores on the MMSE in an open design trial. Low thiamine levels have not been consistently associated with higher prevalence of AD [71], and there is currently not enough evidence at this point to recommend thiamine supplementation for the prevention of cognitive decline [2, 79, 86].

Vitamin B2 (Riboflavin)

Godwin and colleagues showed that individuals at the bottom decile of riboflavin dietary intake had worse cognitive performance in some domains compared to the upper deciles [87], and Lee and coworkers [88] found that MMSE scores increased as riboflavin intake increased in women but not in men. Nevertheless, low riboflavin serum levels have not been linked with the presence of AD. There is no RCT specifically designed to assess the effects of riboflavin in cognitive decline or dementia. Riboflavin supplementation is not recommended for AD prevention [2, 79, 86, 89].

Vitamin B6 (Pyridoxine)

In rodents, the supplementation of pyridoxine did not improve cognition or learning functions. Low pyridoxine was associated with worse motor skills when analyzing the linear dose-response relationship [71]. In high-dose supplementation trials in humans [71], pyridoxine was associated with improved long-term memory, but threats to validity make conclusions based on these trials uncertain. Mizrahi et al. found an association of low pyridoxine dietary intake with AD, however, the recall bias for dietary exposure among patients with dementia limits interpretation of this data [90]. Currently, there is evidence to support the use of pyridoxine in combination with folic acid and vitamin B12 for the prevention of cognitive decline in those MCI patients with elevated homocysteine [2, 79, 80, 86, 91].

Vitamin B12 (Cobalamin)

In rats with nucleus basalis magnocellularis lesions (mimicking a hypocholinergic state), cobalamin showed no effect on movements and did not improve memory [92]. In observational studies, high methylmalonic acid level, a more specific marker for vitamin B12 deficiency, was associated with faster rates of cognitive decline, especially in APOEε4 carries R [93]. The administration of cobalamin was associated with improvement on a 12-word list learning test at 15 min, and a trend was found for improvement on other cognitive measures in a RCT of cognitively impaired individuals with B12 deficiency [94, 95]. In uncontrolled trials, there is conflicting evidence on the effects of cobalamin supplementation in normal and cognitively impaired patients. In most of the studies where cobalamin supplementation was associated with cognitive improvement, the cobalamin was administered via parenteral route. Dietary intake of cobalamin has not been associated to the presence AD in cross sectional studies [71]. The heterogeneity of the trials, cognitive outcomes and populations studied contribute to the inconsistency of the findings. The supplementation of cobalamin alone for the prevention of cognitive decline is not supported at this point, however there is evidence to support the use of B12 in combination with folic acid and pyridoxine for the prevention of cognitive decline in those patients with elevated homocysteine [2, 79, 80, 86, 91]. Additionally, vitamin B12 levels are part of the workup for reversible causes of dementia as well as other neurological diseases and deficiencies should be a target of clinical intervention.

Folate

In amyloid precursor protein (APP) mutant mice model, Kruman and colleagues [96] showed that the amount of deposition of Aβ amyloid did not differ among folate-deficient mice vs. a control group. However, the *cornus amonis* (CA) 3 region of the hippocampus in folate-deficient mice had at least 20 % fewer neurons compared to controls, suggesting susceptibility of this region to folate deficiency independent of Aβ production or deposition. Thought to be at increased susceptibility to oxidative damage, ApoE deficient mice were fed a folate-free diet in one group and folate-supplemented diet in the other one. The folate-supplemented group showed significant decrement in the amount of oxidative by-products when challenged with iron, an oxidizing substance [71, 97]. These results suggest that the oxidative potential of ApoE deficiency could be alleviated with folate supplementation. In a diet-induced hyperhomocysteinemia rat model, investigators evaluated the impact of folate supplementation on the homocysteine-induced endothelial dysfunction [88]. Folate supplementation showed reduced endothelial nitric oxide synthetase activity and glucose transporter protein-1 activity, suggesting that folate supplementation could offset the oxidative potential of homocysteine at the endothelial level.

In regards to dietary intake of folate and the presence of AD, observational studies have shown conflicting data. Tucker et al. investigated the association of dietary intake and several vitamins and found that high dietary folate offered independent protection against cognitive decline [78]. In a study conducted by Morris et al., a faster rate of cognitive decline in a cohort of aging individuals was linked with high levels of folate from food or supplements [98]. Despite these conflicting findings, most of the cross-sectional and case-controls studies suggest that lower levels of serum folate or higher prevalence of folate deficiency is found in patients with AD [71].

In human studies, one RCT showed cognitive benefit of folate supplementation in demented, cognitively impaired and normal subjects, but no clinical benefit was reported [71]. Fioravanti and coworkers showed that folate supplementation improved cognitive scores in aged patients with cognitive impairment and low folate levels.

Of interest, initial cognitive status did not correlate with initial folate levels [99]. Bryan and colleagues studied women of all ages without cognitive impairment and reported that folate supplementation improved cognition in the older women. Unfortunately, the dietary intake of these women could potentially be an interaction that was not controlled for, since dietary intake of folate and other vitamins was correlated with speed of processing, recall and recognition and verbal ability [100]. In a small sample, Sommer and colleagues showed that very high doses of folate supplementation (20 mg/day) could be associated with worsening cognitive function [101]. While recent systematic reviews and meta-analyses do not support the use of folate with or without vitamin B supplements for the prevention of cognitive decline in the short term, the use of B12, folic acid and pyridoxine for the prevention of cognitive decline in those patients with elevated homocysteine may be recommended [2, 79, 80, 86, 91, 102]. Long-term administration of folate supplements to healthy and cognitively impaired individuals has yet to be systematically studied.

Vitamin C and E

The protective factors of antioxidants is the proposed mechanism of action of vitamin C for the prevention of cognitive decline. It has been observed that higher levels of ascorbic acid (vitamin C) are associated with better cognitive performance in a cohort study [103]. Vitamin E is considered a powerful antioxidant available in oily food. In adults over 65 year of age, individuals in the upper tercile of vitamin E consumption (data obtained by a food questionnaire) showed better cognitive performance than the lower tercile [104]. Wengreen et al. studied the dietary intake of vitamin C and E in individuals older than 65 followed on average for 7 years and found that the higher intake of vitamin E and C was associated with higher MMSE scores, and that low intake of these vitamins and carotene was associated with a higher rate of decline in MMSE [105]. However, trials examining the combination of vitamins E and C supplementation have not consistently demonstrated significant improvements, and currently, there is no evidence to support the prescription of vitamin C, and conflicting evidence regarding vitamin E, with a recent study suggesting that 2000 I.U. slows functional decline in mild to moderate AD [91, 106, 107].

Chromium

Insulin resistance and secondary hyperinsulinemia are associated with metabolic syndrome. The receptor for insulin transport across the BBB becomes saturated with the flush of plasmatic insulin, thus creating a hypoinsulinimic state in the brain. Hypoinsulinemia is associated with increased rate of Aβ aggregation. Peripheral hyperinsulinemia has also been associated with worse cognitive performance among AD and non-AD patients [108]. Inside the brain, abnormal distributions of transition metals can potentially serve as diagnostic markers for neurodegenerative diseases, including AD [109]. Chromium, an essential trace mineral used in insulin receptor signaling, is thought to amplify the insulin action [110]. Improved insulin resistance in diabetic patients has been shown at doses of 200–1,000 mcg [111, 112]. Krikorian and colleagues [110] randomly assigned 26 patients to receive chromium supplementation vs. placebo and followed them for 12 weeks with examination on multiple cognitive tests. No effects were seen on fasting insulin or fasting glucose, but a reduced rate of intrusion errors was found in the active group. Functional magnetic resonance imaging (fMRI) data showed that individuals in the active arm had increased activation in multiple regions of the brain including the thalamus and the frontal cortex; however, areas of activation did not correspond to improved cognitive performance. These findings suggest that chromium may have functions independent of its effects on metabolism and should be further explored. Chromium supplementation shows promising results, but not enough to unequivocally determine an association with AD or cognitive decline

[79]. In order to strengthen current evidence, a better-designed study using a greater sample size should be undertaken.

Polyphenolic Compounds (Flavonoids)

Polyphenols are the most prevalent component in our daily foods, and represent the major portion of the phytochemicals found in plants. Polyphenols have received special attention because of their antioxidant capacity and ability to debilitate the pathological process seen in neurodegenerative disorders, such as AD [113]. Aβ mediated neurodegeneration is one of the most well studied hypothesis underlying AD causation. Several phenolic compounds, such as wine-related myricetin (MYR), curcumin, nordihydroguaiaretic acid (NDGA) and rosmarinic acid (RA), have shown to possess strong anti-Aβ aggregation properties in vitro and in vivo [51]. Flavonoids, a subclass of polyphenols, are a group of phytochemicals thought to have important antioxidative, anti-viral and anti-carcinogenic properties [71]. They are ubiquitous in vegetables and they provide the plant with its color that attracts pollinators and repels insect attacks [15]. They are found in high concentrations in berries, onions, dark chocolate, broccoli, apples, tea, red wine, purple grape juice, soybean, and tomatoes [114]. Below we will discuss the more conspicuous members of the phenolic family that have been studied to date.

Berries

Berries are thought to be rich in antioxidants and their consumption is hypothesized to provide neuroprotection against the oxidative and inflammatory process associated with aging. Strawberries, blueberries, blackberries, cranberries and raspberries are fruits with high antioxidant capacity due to the high content of anti-inflammatory anthocyanins and/or proanthocyanidins (flavonoid compounds) [71, 115, 116].

Anthocyanins can cross the BBB and block 5′-deiodinase activity and stimulate T3 transport into rat brains [117]. Histopathology and cognitive test results suggest a protective effect in blueberry-fed rats, compared with controls. Blueberry extract was associated with increased precursor cells (increased neurogenesis) in the dentate gyrus in rats that also performed better on cognitive testing [118]. In animal experiments, strawberry extract supplementation has been associated with improved biochemical markers in the brain suggestive of neuroprotection; however, an association with cognitive performance has not been reported [71]. In vitro studies suggest that various berry extracts can protect the deleterious effects of Aβ-induced oxidative damage [119]. A weekly minimum of two servings of blueberries and/or strawberries was linked with decreased rates of cognitive decline [5]. Randomized, prospective human studies are lacking to recommend berries extracts for the prevention of cognitive decline; nevertheless, inclusion of berries in the diet has a theoretical benefit and is recommended as part of a balanced diet.

Curcumin

Hamaguchi and colleagues showed that RA, CUR and MYR inhibit the aggregation of Aβ monomers to Aβ oligomers and from oligomers to Aβ deposition [51]. Curcumin is a potent antioxidant and an effective anti-inflammatory compound. Curcumin can inhibit the formation of Aβ oligomers and fibrils, bind plaque, and reduce plaque burden [120]. In another animal model of dementia, curcumin (20 mg/kg p.o. daily for 14 days) successfully attenuated Streptozotocin STZ-induced memory deficits. Higher levels of brain AChE activity and oxidative stress were observed in STZ-treated animals, which were significantly attenuated by curcumin [121]. Other animal studies raise the possibility that curcumin may act as a metal chelator, have anti-apoptotic or immunomodulator properties, or promote neurogenesis [12].

Poor bioavailability of curcumin is one of the main challenges faced in human studies [122]. In a pilot study, a small RCT evaluated the pharmacokinetics and effects of curcumin supplementation in humans [123]. The preliminary results showed promising MMSE changes without major side effects, but the short period of follow up and lack of cognitive decline in the placebo group limit interpretation of the data. The risks associated with the administration of curcumin are uncertain and further studies are warranted in regard to safety and efficacy. In the trial by Baum et al. [123] gastric, neurological and pulmonary symptoms were reported at an equal rate among patients taking placebo and those on active treatment. While there is no clinical trial evidence for AD prevention, studies have been performed in the area of AD treatment [123, 124]. A more recent study by Ringman and colleagues found that curcumin was generally well-tolerated in a group of mild to moderate AD patients, although there was no clinical or biochemical effect over 24 weeks. The study helped us to understand why curcumin was not effective, and that was most likely related to the body not being able to absorb the curcumin, and limitations in bioavailability likely led to the lack of effectiveness [53]. The risk:benefit ratio of curcumin supplementation should be discussed in detail with patients and caregivers.

Resveretrol

Resveratrol is an antioxidant that is most commonly known for being found in wine (from grapes) but it is also found in a variety of food sources like blueberries, peanuts, and cocoa powder. However, the highest concentration is specifically contained in red grapes (in their skin) and as such high in red wine. The problem with resveratrol is that the actual amount in these sources is quite low—a person would have to drink several hundred glasses of red wine in order to get the same amount that is contained in one capsule of a resveratrol supplement. In these supplements, while some of the actual resveratrol

may come from red grape skin, most commonly it is derived from Japanese knotweed. While studies in animals have shown that resveratrol may delay age-related cognitive decline, data are more limited when it comes to humans with AD, as well as for prevention. One recent study of 23 people without memory loss who took 200 mg per day found that supplementation improved memory function, as well as a host of metabolic markers, including glucose metabolism, and decreased body fat [125]. Using neuroimaging studies, researchers also found the function of the memory centers of the brain also improved. Further research is necessary to clarify the relationship between resveratrol and AD prevention and treatment, yet in the meantime, some individuals may choose to try it for more optimal brain and body health.

Docosahexaenoic Acid

Docosahexaenoic Acid (DHA) is a long-chain 22-carbon omega-3 polyunsaturated fatty acid with six double bonds. It is found abundantly in marine algae, fatty fish, and fish oil [12]. While there have been various discrepancies, many studies have shown that people with more of these fatty acids in their blood are less likely to develop AD [126]. The main proposed mechanism of action of DHA, in the context of cognitive decline, is the preservation of debrin, a vital component for the adequate synaptic function. Other pleiotropic mechanisms in which DHA can affect the progression of cognitive decline are anti-inflammatory activity, neuroprotection, neurogenesis, antioxidant, metabolic enhancer and weak amyloid aggregation inhibitor [12].

In animal models, depleting DHA from the system was associated with cognitive impairment, but replacing DHA prevented pathological changes similar to those seen in AD [127, 128]. A small trial of DHA in MCI and AD groups was associated with a slower rate of cognitive decline [129, 130]. A recent randomized, double-blind, placebo-controlled study with 485 subjects (aged 55 and older) called the "Memory Improvement with Docosahexaenoic Acid Study" (MIDAS) aimed at evaluating the effects of 900 mg/day of algae-based DHA in healthy older adults with age-related cognitive decline [129, 130]. The study found that DHA taken over the course of 6 months improved memory and learning in healthy, older adults with mild memory complaints.

Recent systematic reviews of RCT and observational studies published for DHA supplementation have failed to identify unequivocal evidence suggestive of a protective effect of DHA on cognitive decline [79, 86, 91], although the association of DHA with slower cognitive decline seems to be somewhat consistent across studies [2]. Collectively, while data suggest that DHA supplementation does not help AD patients overall, further studies are warranted to clarify but could lead to delayed cognitive decline [131, 132]. Early supplementation as well as the long-term effects of DHA warrants further investigation.

Cardiovascular Risk Profile

Although age is the single most important risk factor for the development of dementia, cardiovascular risk factors appear strongly associated with cognitive decline and dementia, and carry the great advantage of being modifiable. Traditional risk factors like hypertension, diabetes, dyslipidemia, and smoking are believed to convey risk for vascular disease. Vascular disease is associated with cerebral hypoperfusion, oxidative stress, neurodegeneration and cognitive decline [133]. The clinical expression of vascular disease can manifest as either mild cognitive symptoms or as full-blown dementia that may be attributable to an AD process, mixed AD/vascular pathology, or vascular disease alone [134]. There is general agreement that the pure cases of AD account for less than 20 % of all the cases, and that AD with various components of vascular disease are much more common than AD alone [135–137]. The amount of AD pathology necessary to produce clinical dementia seems to be less when concurring with the presence of vascular risk factors [134]. The cumulative presence of

vascular disease has a biological gradient in the severity of cognitive decline moderated by covariates like age, gender and race [138–140]. This is difficult to disentangle, as it would be unethical to perform a RCT to evaluate the effects of controlling for risk factors in some, but not other subjects.

There is uncertainty regarding secondary prophylaxis with treatment of cardiovascular risk factors. Heterogeneous definitions of MCI and varying methodologies in conversion studies confounds our understanding of the impact of these risk factors on the progression of MCI to dementia. Even with a stable and reproducible definition of MCI, no strong association has been found with the presence of cardiovascular risk factors [141]. To date, no strategy has been successful to halt the progression of MCI to dementia [135]. As mentioned above, general recommendations to engage in a healthy life should be applied to patients with MCI.

Hypertension and Hypercholesterolemia

It seems that a life-time exposure to cardiovascular risk factors can be associated with higher odds of dementia, suggestive of a time period where exposure is more fundamental for subsequent risk. The interaction of the risk exposure and time of onset varies according to each risk factor. As an example, evidence has shown that higher levels of systolic pressure in midlife are associated with higher risk of dementia later in life, but lower levels of systolic pressure later in life can also be associated with dementia [142]. The same effect has been described for cholesterol levels [143]. Nevertheless, diminished vascular integrity of the blood-brain barrier is characteristic of hypertension, and results in protein extravasation into brain tissue. As such, this can lead to cell damage or death, a reduction in synaptic function, and may directly contribute to the beta amyloid accumulation seen in AD pathology [144].

In primary prevention trials of cardiovascular disease, conflicting evidence exists about the effect of controlling risk factors on the incidence of dementia. While treatment of hypertension with calcium channels blockers and ACE inhibitors showed reduction in all cardiovascular outcomes and halved the risk to develop AD [145], other trials using diuretics and beta-blockers or angiotensin receptors blockers, did not reproduce the findings [146, 147]. A Cochrane review including 14 clinical trials which tested nimodipine in patients with AD and/or cerebrovascular dementia found statistically significant benefits at 12 weeks, on clinical global impression and cognitive function, in the treatment of patients with features of dementia due to Alzheimer's disease, cerebrovascular disease, or mixed Alzheimer's and cerebrovascular disease [148]. Other meta-analyses have not found a significant effect in the treatment of hypertension with the subsequent risk of developing AD [79, 149, 150]. The SPRINT (Systolic Blood Pressure Intervention Trial) Study, to be completed in 2018, may help to determine whether antihypertensive treatment can prevent cognitive decline (NCT01206062).

Trials and meta-analysis investigating the effects of cholesterol lowering medications (statins) have failed to demonstrate protective effects of statins on the subsequent risk of developing AD [79, 151–153]. Effect of statins may depend on baseline cholesterol, stage of AD, and ApoE4 carrier status [154]. Studies may have been underpowered, too short, too late in the lifespan, or affected by selective dropout of participants with cognitive impairment. Also of note, polymorphisms affecting individual response to statins (KIF6 gene, HMGCR isoforms) have yet to be been taken into account. Cardiovascular risk factors should be aggressively treated in populations with or without cognitive decline to reduce cardiovascular mortality.

Diabetes and Insulin Resistance

Several investigators have claimed that insulin resistance is a risk factor for cognitive decline [135]. Insulin facilitates cognition when given concomitantly with glucose to support metabolism and may play a role in overcoming the decreased utilization and transport of glucose in AD patients [155]. Defects in insulin signaling are associated with increased deposition of Aβ and tau hypophosphorylation. Insulin-degrading enzyme (IDE) is a protease involved in the degradation of insulin and Aβ. In patients with hyperinsulinemia, insulin can saturate IDE and subsequently increase the AB serum levels [156] Patients with diabetes have lower hippocampal and prefrontal volumes when compared with non-diabetic controls [157]. The progression of dementia in patients with stroke and diabetes was more prominent when compared to patients without stroke and diabetes [158]. Diagnosed and undiagnosed diabetes have been associated with lower MMSE scores in a population-based sample [159]. Although diabetes has been strongly associated with the presence of AD [160–162], less is known about its treatment and the effects on dementia incidence [159, 163]. The treatment of diabetes should be a priority in all patients for its multiple deleterious consequences.

Smoking

Initial observational studies suggested that smoking could be associated with lower risk for developing Alzheimer disease in carriers of APOEε4 [164, 165]. Former smokers had a decreased risk for developing dementia with increasing numbers of pack-per-year smoked. This was suggestive of a dose-effect relationship of higher exposure to nicotine and a lower incidence of dementia [164, 166]. The interaction between APOEε4 status and smoking exposure has been a matter of debate and remains unclear. Nevertheless, it is generally accepted that smokers have higher risk of developing dementia and that there is a dose-effect gradient with higher odds for heavier smokers [167]. Additionally, smoking can accelerate atrophy and degenerative changes resulting from neuronal loss [168, 169]. In a recent meta-analysis of prospective studies, Anstey et al. showed that current smokers had an increased risk of Alzheimer's disease compared with former smokers at baseline. Current smokers also shower greater decline in cognitive abilities, but the groups were not different regarding risk of vascular dementia or other dementias. The authors concluded that elderly smokers have increased risks of dementia and cognitive decline [170]. A recent systematic review found low quality evidence to unequivocally support the association of tobacco use and dementia, although it was categorized as a risk factor [79]. There is no question that all smokers should be encouraged to quit. In the case of patients with cognitive decline and dementia, it should be further emphasized.

Physical Exercise

Interventional studies have demonstrated that people who become physically active can improve their cognition and can slow down the rate of decline as early as 4 months after the intervention [171, 172]. Physical exercise is thought to exert its protective effects on cognition through the improvement of cardiovascular disease, as well as by decreasing amyloid throughout the brain (e.g., frontal lobes and hippocampus) [4, 173]. Additionally, exercise stimulates production of brain neurotrophic factors that are used in repair processes [4, 173]. In observational studies, there appears to be a lower prevalence of dementia in people who exercise regularly compared with those who do not [174, 175]. Promoting exercise should be part of a holistic strategy to promote healthy lifestyles in patients and should be advised in patients with cognitive decline or AD, unless contraindicated or impractical. Tailoring of both physical activity type and routine, to the patient's needs and capacities, is advisable.

In summary, it would be unethical to advise against treating cardiovascular risk factors in the absence of evidence toward preventing cognitive decline or dementia. The development of cerebrovascular disease is a well-known consequence of uncontrolled risk factors and the incidence of stroke is strongly associated with cognitive problem or dementia [176–179]. It is safe to say that

addressing the cardiovascular profile should be a priority in patients with cognitive dysfunction, dementia, or those at risk of developing either.

Cognitive Engagement

Subjects with preclinical Alzheimer's disease who have higher levels of education demonstrate lower levels of functional connectivity by FDG-PET in areas affected by Alzheimer's disease, suggesting that there is indeed a compensatory role of education to maintain cognitive performance in preclinical AD [180]. The term "cognitive reserve" has been applied in the literature to describe this general idea that the greater number of neurons or advance neuropsychological competence (intelligence) can protect an individual from developing clinically evident cognitive decline or dementia [181]. A more comprehensive definition of cognitive reserve involves neuro computational flexibility, where the end goal is adaption. It suggests that high brain-reserve individuals have a larger repertoire of strategies to resolve complex tasks as well as redundant neuronal networks to carry out the same activities. As such, in the case of a particular network malfunction, other networks can be used to conduct the same strategy or, if not possible, other strategies can be used to solve the same tasks [182]. Environmental enrichment has been associated with neurotrophic and nerve growth factors, increased synaptogenesis, and synaptic plasticity [181].

Cognitive Training

Cohort studies assessing the association of mental activities and the incidence of dementia have shown that engaging in highly complex mental activities is a protective factor against the development of dementia, with a dose-dependent effect observed in some studies [183, 184]. A systematic review of observational studies evaluated 22 population-based cohorts and showed that education attainment, cognitive lifestyle activities and occupational complexity conferred protection against the subsequent development of dementia [185]. An older trial found that individuals who received cognitive training had a favorable influence on everyday coping and on memory performance [186].

The ACTIVE trial published in 2002 was a major study in this field that randomized 2,832 patients to 4 groups, three interventions arms: 10-session group training for memory (verbal episodic memory; n=711), or reasoning (ability to solve problems that follow a serial pattern; n=705), or speed of processing (visual search and identification; n=712); or a no-contact control group (n=704). The results showed significant improvement in 87 % of processing speed, 74 % of reasoning, and 26 % of memory-trained participants, and demonstrated reliable cognitive improvement immediately after the intervention period. Booster training significantly enhanced training gains in processing speed and reasoning interventions (speed booster, 92 %; no booster, 68 %; reasoning booster, 72 %; no booster, 49 %), which were maintained at the second year of follow-up. No training effects on everyday functioning were detected in the second year of follow up [187]. A 5-year follow up of the same population showed improved cognitive abilities, specific to the abilities trained, that persisted after the intervention was stopped compared with the control group [188].

A computer-based cognitive training RCT with a focus on improving aural language processing, was linked to improvement in targeted cognition and non-trained cognitive function in the active group compared to controls [189]. In individuals with MCI, unimodal memory training might not be enough [190, 191]. A small study indicated that multimodal intervention might be more effective in patients with MCI [192]. Encouraging results have come with using the multi-domain cognitive training approach in patients with dementia [190]. However, longer follow-up is needed to investigate whether the effects of cognitive training are sustained. Based on previous results, it seems advisable for individuals at risk for developing dementia to engage in cognitive training programs as part of a formal multimodal therapeutic approach.

Social Engagement

It has been well documented that individuals with reduced social networks are at greater risk for developing cognitive decline compared to those who have broader social interactions. Activities that exposed the individual to interact with others and create bonds are considered protective against cognitive decline [4]. A few critics have challenged the notion that this is a predictive association, suggesting that retraction from social networks might precede the onset of cognitive symptoms during midlife, and could be a sign of premature non-cognition symptoms of neurodegeneration [193]. Other difficulties in isolating social engagement effects on the risk of dementia, have been the multiple covariates associated with both such as exercise and cognitive reserve. It seems reasonable to advise engagement in social activities as tolerated to promote healthy aging.

Management of Depression

One of the reversible causes of cognitive impairment that all aged adults with cognitive complaints should be assessed for is depression. It can be difficult to isolate depression from dementia, since patients with dementia have a higher prevalence of depression than non-demented populations, and sometimes depression could be a prodromal sign of dementia [4]. A recent meta-analysis of observational studies showed that depression doubles the risk of developing dementia in later life. Findings of increased risk were robust to sensitivity analyses. Interval between diagnoses of depression and AD was positively related to increased risk of developing AD, suggesting that rather than a prodrome, depression might be a risk factor for AD [194]. Even if the overall evidence quality is low [79], patients with cognitive complaints should be screened for depression and treated when indicated. New-onset depression in an adult with no prior history could be one of the earliest signs of brain changes due to AD. By contrast, lifelong depression in someone with cognitive complaints is a risk factor for dementia with Lewy Bodies.

Pharmacological Strategies

Hormones

Hipoccampal atrophy is a major pathological change seen in patients with MCI or AD. Shrinkage of the hippocampus can start in early adulthood and accelerate with age; losses of 0.3–2.1 % per year are reported, with slower rate of progression reported in women compared with men [195, 196]. The apparent slower degeneration in women in early adulthood reverses in the post menopause stage, with greater odds of dementia for women when compared with men [197]. As a result, multiple studies evaluating the role of estrogens and other gonadal hormones as neuroprotectectors have taken place.

Estrogens are known to influence verbal fluency and memory, performance on spatial tasks, and fine motor skills [198]. They can mediate neuroprotection provided their ability to mediate the oxidative processes in the brain, besides altering the potassium conductance, apoptosis and transcriptional factors regulation [197]. The aging process is associated with decreased memory abilities, focusing attention efficiently, and the speed of processing information. However, women tend to have smaller hippocampal volumes, decreased glucose metabolism in areas concerned with cognition, and greater age-adjusted prevalence of dementia [199]. Observational studies have suggested that memory problems are often associated with menopause, although healthy post-menopausal women do not have significant memory problems, as measured by standard psychological testing [200, 201]. Blood levels of estrogenic hormones are not consistently associated with differential cognitive performance [202]. Another explanation for the excess of AD cases in women seen in observational designs has been attributed to longer survival of women compared to men [203].

Several clinical trials and longitudinal studies have attempted to solve this puzzle. Researchers observing a longitudinal cohort reported an association with hormone replacement therapy (HTR) and better performance on psychological testing [204] although another group with a different cohort failed to reproduce this claim [205]. Two recent metanalyses found a 29–34 % risk reduction for women using HRT vs. non-users [202, 206]. The Women's Health Initiative Memory Study (WHIMS) used a sample from a large, population-based prospective cohort to enroll in a RCT to test the hypothesis that HRT with estrogen with progestin could reduce the risk of MCI or dementia. They enrolled 4,532 patients, who were randomized to active and control arms, and followed up around 13 months. The study failed to show that estrogen in combination with progesterone offers protective effects against cognitive decline in the form of MCI or probable dementia. On the contrary, they found an elevated risk of developing either MCI or dementia in patients using the HRT, nearly doubling the risk for those not using it [3]. This is the largest and best-structured RCT to test the hypothesis behind the possible cognitive benefits provided by hormonal supplements. The possibility of hormonal replacement at earlier stages of gonadal hormone withdrawal in peri menopausal women has not been explored, and some believe that larger periods of estrogen deprivation can lead to irreversible damage to some brain structures [203, 207, 208]. This remains to be settled with future RCT specifically designed to test this hypothesis. Currently, there is no evidence to recommend hormonal supplementation in postmenopausal women to prevent or treat cognitive decline [2, 79].

The role of dehydroepiandrosterone (DHEA) has also been explored in the context of cognitive decline. They are the most abundant circulating hormones in young adults and the major precursors of androgens and estrogens in the central nervous system [209], especially in the postmenopausal stage in aged individuals where the gonadal production of sex hormones drops [210]. Some observational studies have suggested that the DHEA drop seen with aging may account for some of the cognitive difficulties associated with age, partially due to the unopposed deleterious effect of cortisol on the oxidative stress balance

[16, 211]. Although DHEA supplementation may be an appealing as a way to prevent cognitive decline, human results have failed to prove significant improvement in chronic supplementation of the hormones, and few have shown negative effects. As theorized with HRT, the timing of supplementation is thought important and future trials should explore early supplementation after the drop of "youthful" levels of the hormones [212]. The age-associated decrement in enzymatic activity necessary to convert the hormones into their active metabolites, as well as individuals with advanced disease, is another explanation for the lack of results. There is no evidence at this point to recommend the supplementation of DHEA for the prevention or treatment of cognitive decline.

Piracetam and Piracetam-like Drugs

Piracetam are nootropic compounds ("nootrope" comes from ancient Greek meaning "for or toward the mind") [213]. The mechanisms of action of these medications are related to their effects as GABA-mimetic, antioxidants, modulators of intracellular calcium as well as facilitators of cholinergic transmission in the hippocampal area [214]. Due to their facilitation of cognitive processes, some members of this family are known as cognitive enhancers.

Piracetam is the most studied cognitive enhancer compound. It has been used to evaluate protection against cognitive decline in numerous clinical settings such as traumatic brain injury, cerebrovascular insufficiency, cardiac bypass, cognitive deficit and MCI with promising results [214]. Part of its efficacy can be attributed to the offset of depressive symptoms. Conflicting evidence has been produced by meta-analysis [215, 216] and thus far, no large-scale trial has demonstrated the effects of this compound in patients with MCI and dementia [215, 216]. Oxiracetam, aniracetam and pramiracetam are less studied nootropic compounds. Overall, the level of evidence currently available is not enough to systematically recommend Piracetam or any nootropic drugs for the prevention of cognitive decline.

Conclusions

Effective strategies to prevent cognitive decline in the context of normal aging, mild cognitive impairment and dementia are imperative to face the oncoming epidemic of dementia and cognitive disease in our society. Evidence-based recommendations are imperative to avoid unnecessary expenses and the creation of false expectation in patients and their families. Methodological difficulties and biases have intertwined with several good-intentioned trials. Existing studies have provided some clues into the puzzle of prevention of cognitive decline, yet it is rare that the evidence is unquestionable. The issue of studying a complex process like cognition represents challenges that researchers must be aware of. The presence of multiple factors and covariates that can bias the results presents a major hurdle in the design stage as well as in the statistical analysis, especially in small sample studies. However, from a practical clinical perspective, a good rule of thumb would be to keep expectations metered, and to always balance existing evidence with safety, as low-risk interventions are of paramount importance.

When evaluating diet components, the major difficulty is in isolating the effect that a nutrient or diet component has on cognition or the evolution of dementia. The fact that isolated vitamins, minerals and other components have failed to demonstrate a reliable association does not mean that the intake of these is not beneficial. There is a possibility that the combination of multiple components is what makes the difference. Additionally, trying to adhere to healthy lifestyle recommendations including a diet rich in essential nutrients, smoking abstinence, regular exercise as well as adequate cardiovascular profile is by all means a goal in any patient. Challenging the brain with new information and new experiences seems to be advisable, especially in those who already have early cognitive complains.

References

1. Brown LA, Riby LM, Reay JL. Supplementing cognitive aging: a selective review of the effects of ginkgo biloba and a number of everyday nutritional substances. Exp Aging Res. 2010;36:105–22.
2. Daviglus ML, et al. National institutes of health state-of-the-science conference statement: preventing Alzheimer disease and cognitive decline. Ann Intern Med. 2010;153:176–81.
3. Shumaker SA, et al. Estrogen plus progestin and the incidence of dementia and mild cognitive impairment in postmenopausal women: the women's health initiative memory study: a randomized controlled trial. JAMA. 2003;289:2651–62.
4. Middleton LE, Yaffe K. Promising strategies for the prevention of dementia. Arch Neurol. 2009;66:1210–5.
5. Oboudiyat C, et al. Alzheimer's disease. Semin Neurol. 2013;33(4):313–29.
6. Sperling RA, Aisen PS, Beckett LA, et al. Toward defining the preclinical stages of Alzheimer's disease: recommendations from the National Institute on Aging-Alzheimer's Association workgroups on diagnostic guidelines for Alzheimer's disease. Alzheimers Dement. 2011;7:280–92.
7. Williams JW, Plassman BL, Burke J, Benjamin S. Preventing Alzheimer's disease and cognitive decline. Evid Rep Technol Assess (Full Rep). 2010:1–727.
8. Anstey KJ, Cherbuin N, Herath PM, et al. A self-report risk index to predict occurrence of dementia in three independent cohorts of older adults: the ANU-ADRI. PLoS One. 2014;9, e86141.
9. Smith AD, Yaffe K. Dementia (including Alzheimer's disease) can be prevented: statement supported by international experts. J Alzheimers Dis. 2014;38(4):699–703.
10. Miller ZA, Mandelli ML, Rankin KP, et al. Handedness and language learning disability differentially distribute in progressive aphasia variants. Brain. 2013;136(Pt 11):3461–73.
11. Norton S, Matthews FE, Barnes DE, et al. Potential for primary prevention of Alzheimer's disease: an analysis of population-based data. Lancet Neuro. 2014;13(8):788–94.
12. Frautschy SA, Cole GM. Why pleiotropic interventions are needed for Alzheimer's disease. Mol Neurobiol. 2010;41:392–409.
13. Nehlig A. Is caffeine a cognitive enhancer? J Alzheimers Dis. 2010;20 Suppl 1:S85–94.
14. Schneider JA, Arvanitakis Z, Bang W, Bennett DA. Mixed brain pathologies account for most dementia cases in community-dwelling older persons. Neurology. 2007;69:2197–204.
15. Prasain JK, Carlson SH, Wyss JM. Flavonoids and age-related disease: risk, benefits and critical windows. Maturitas. 2010;66:163–71.
16. Miller DB, O'Callaghan JP. Aging, stress and the hippocampus. Ageing Res Rev. 2005;4:123–40.
17. Glade MJ. Oxidative stress and cognitive longevity. Nutrition. 2010;26:595–603.
18. Akiyama H, et al. Inflammation and Alzheimer's disease. Neurobiol Aging. 2000;21:383–421.
19. Tapsell LC, et al. Health benefits of herbs and spices: the past, the present, the future. Med J Aust. 2006;185:S4–24.
20. Reiman EM, Chen K, Alexander GE, et al. Functional brain abnormalities in young adults at genetic risk for late-onset alzheimer's dementia. Proc Natl Acad Sci USA. 2004;101(1):284–9.
21. Silva DF, Selfridge JE, Lu J, Lezi E, Cardoso SM, Swerdlow RH. Mitochondrial abnormalities in Alzheimer's disease: possible targets for therapeutic intervention. Adv Pharmacol. 2012;64:83–126.
22. Supnet C, Bezprozvanny I. The dysregulation of intracellular calcium in Alzheimer disease. Cell Calcium. 2010;47(2):183–9.
23. Gibson GE, Shi Q. A mitocentric view of Alzheimer's disease suggests multi-faceted treatments. J Alzheimers Dis. 2010;20 Suppl 2:S591–607.
24. Feart C, Samieri C, Barberger-Gateau P. Mediterranean diet and cognitive function in older adults. Curr Opin Clin Nutr Metab Care. 2010;13:14–8.
25. Singh B, Parsaik AK, Mielke MM, et al. Association of Mediterranean diet with mild cognitive impairment and Alzheimer's disease: a systematic review and meta-analysis. J Alzheimers Dis. 2014;39:271–82.
26. Bayer-Carter JL, Green PS, Montine TJ, et al. Diet intervention and cerebrospinal fluid biomarkers in amnestic mild cognitive impairment. Arch Neurol. 2011;68:743–52.
27. Nilsson A, Tovar J, Johansson M, Radeborg K, Bjorck I. A diet based on multiple functional concepts improves cognitive performance in healthy subjects. Nutr Metab (Lond). 2013;10:49.
28. Mosconi L, Murray J, Tsui WH, et al. Mediterranean diet and magnetic resonance imaging-assessed brain atrophy in cognitively normal individuals at risk for Alzheimer's disease. J Prev Alzheimers Dis. 2014;1(1):23–32.
29. Vitali C, Wellington CL, Calabresi L. HDL and cholesterol handling in the brain. Cardiovasc Res. 2014;103(3):405–13.
30. Kourlaba G, Polychronopoulos E, Zampelas A, Lionis C, Panagiotakos DB. Development of a diet index for older adults and its relation to cardiovascular disease risk factors: the elderly dietary index. J Am Diet Assoc. 2009;109:1022–30.
31. Scarmeas N, Stern Y, Tang MX, Mayeux R, Luchsinger JA. Mediterranean diet and risk for Alzheimer's disease. Ann Neurol. 2006;59:912–21.
32. Scarmeas N, et al. Mediterranean diet and mild cognitive impairment. Arch Neurol. 2009;66:216–25.

33. Feart C, et al. Adherence to a Mediterranean diet, cognitive decline, and risk of dementia. JAMA. 2009;302:638–48.
34. Gu Y, Nieves JW, Stern Y, Luchsinger JA, Scarmeas N. Food combination and Alzheimer disease risk: a protective diet. Arch Neurol. 2010;67:699–706.
35. Padilla CR, Isaacson RS. Genetics of dementia. Continuum (Minneap Minn). 2011;17(2 Neurogenetics):326–42.
36. Gureje O, Ogunniyi A, Baiyewu O, et al. APOE epsilon4 is not associated with Alzheimer's disease in elderly Nigerians. Ann Neurol. 2006;59:182–5.
37. Lima TA, Adler AL, Minett T, Matthews FE, Brayne C, Marioni RE. C-reactive protein, APOE genotype and longitudinal cognitive change in an older population. Age Ageing. 2014;43(2):289–92.
38. Huang TL, Zandi PP, Tucker KL, et al. Benefits of fatty fish on dementia risk are stronger for those without APOE epsilon4. Neurology. 2005;65:1409–14.
39. Barberger-Gateau P, Raffaitin C, Letenneur L, et al. Dietary patterns and risk of dementia: the Three-City cohort study. Neurology. 2007;69:1921–30.
40. Laitinen MH, Ngandu T, Rovio S, et al. Fat intake at midlife and risk of dementia and Alzheimer's disease: a population-based study. Dement Geriatr Cogn Disord. 2006;22:99–107.
41. Borek C. Garlic reduces dementia and heart-disease risk. J Nutr. 2006;136:810S–2.
42. Peng Q, Buz'Zard AR, Lau BH. Neuroprotective effect of garlic compounds in amyloid-beta peptide-induced apoptosis in vitro. Med Sci Monit. 2002;8:BR328–37.
43. Budoff MJ, et al. Inhibiting progression of coronary calcification using aged garlic extract in patients receiving statin therapy: a preliminary study. Prev Med. 2004;39:985–91.
44. Gold PE, Cahill L, Wenk GL. The lowdown on Ginkgo biloba. Sci Am. 2003;288:86–91.
45. Oken BS, Storzbach DM, Kaye JA. The efficacy of Ginkgo biloba on cognitive function in Alzheimer disease. Arch Neurol. 1998;55:1409–15.
46. Dodge HH, Zitzelberger T, Oken BS, Howieson D, Kaye J. A randomized placebo-controlled trial of Ginkgo biloba for the prevention of cognitive decline. Neurology. 2008;70:1809–17.
47. Vellas B, Coley N, Ousset PJ, Berrut G, Dartigues JF, Dubois B, Grandjean H, Pasquier F, Piette F, et al. Long-term use of standardised Ginkgo biloba extract for the prevention of Alzheimer's disease (GuidAge): a randomised placebo-controlled trial. Lancet Neurol. 2012;11:851–9.
48. Weinmann S, Roll S, Schwarzbach C, Vauth C, Willich SN. Effects of Ginkgo biloba in dementia: systematic review and meta-analysis. BMC Geriatr. 2010;10:14.
49. Peters R, Peters J, Warner J, Beckett N, Bulpitt C. Alcohol, dementia and cognitive decline in the elderly: a systematic review. Age Ageing. 2008;37:505–12.
50. Orgogozo JM, et al. Wine consumption and dementia in the elderly: a prospective community study in the Bordeaux area. Rev Neurol (Paris). 1997;153:185–92.
51. Hamaguchi T, Ono K, Murase A, Yamada M. Phenolic compounds prevent Alzheimer's pathology through different effects on the amyloid-beta aggregation pathway. Am J Pathol. 2009;175:2557–65.
52. Mitchell RM, Neafsey EJ, Collins MA. Essential involvement of the NMDA receptor in ethanol preconditioning-dependent neuroprotection from amyloid-betain vitro. J Neurochem. 2009;111(2):580–8.
53. Ringman JM, Frautschy SA, Teng E, et al. Oral curcumin for Alzheimer's disease: tolerability and efficacy in a 24-week randomized, double blind, placebo-controlled study. Alzheimers Res Ther. 2012;4:43.
54. Koppelstaetter F, et al. Caffeine and cognition in functional magnetic resonance imaging. J Alzheimers Dis. 2010;20 Suppl 1:S71–84.
55. Fredholm BB, Battig K, Holmen J, Nehlig A, Zvartau EE. Actions of caffeine in the brain with special reference to factors that contribute to its widespread use. Pharmacol Rev. 1999;51:83–133.
56. Dall'Igna OP, Porciuncula LO, Souza DO, Cunha RA, Lara DR. Neuroprotection by caffeine and adenosine A2A receptor blockade of beta-amyloid neurotoxicity. Br J Pharmacol. 2003;138:1207–9.
57. Arendash GW, et al. Caffeine protects Alzheimer's mice against cognitive impairment and reduces brain beta-amyloid production. Neuroscience. 2006;142:941–52.
58. Cunha RA, Agostinho PM. Chronic caffeine consumption prevents memory disturbance in different animal models of memory decline. J Alzheimers Dis. 2010;20 Suppl 1:S95–116.
59. Huang CC, Liang YC, Hsu KS. A role for extracellular adenosine in time-dependent reversal of long-term potentiation by low-frequency stimulation at hippocampal CA1 synapses. J Neurosci. 1999;19:9728–38.
60. d'Alcantara P, Ledent C, Swillens S, Schiffmann SN. Inactivation of adenosine A2A receptor impairs long term potentiation in the accumbens nucleus without altering basal synaptic transmission. Neuroscience. 2001;107:455–64.
61. Lieberman HR, Tharion WJ, Shukitt-Hale B, Speckman KL, Tulley R. Effects of caffeine, sleep loss, and stress on cognitive performance and mood during U.S. Navy SEAL training. Sea-Air-Land. Psychopharmacology (Berl). 2002;164:250–61.
62. Smith AP. Caffeine, cognitive failures and health in a non-working community sample. Hum Psychopharmacol. 2009;24:29–34.

63. Rees K, Allen D, Lader M. The influences of age and caffeine on psychomotor and cognitive function. Psychopharmacology (Berl). 1999;145:181–8.

64. Jarvis MJ. Does caffeine intake enhance absolute levels of cognitive performance? Psychopharmacology (Berl). 1993;110:45–52.

65. Lorist MM, Snel J, Mulder G, Kok A. Aging, caffeine, and information processing: an event-related potential analysis. Electroencephalogr Clin Neurophysiol. 1995;96:453–67.

66. Eskelinen MH, Ngandu T, Tuomilehto J, Soininen H, Kivipelto M. Midlife coffee and tea drinking and the risk of late-life dementia: a population-based CAIDE study. J Alzheimers Dis. 2009;16:85–91.

67. Ritchie K, et al. The neuroprotective effects of caffeine: a prospective population study (the Three City study). Neurology. 2007;69:536–45.

68. van Gelder BM, et al. Coffee consumption is inversely associated with cognitive decline in elderly European men: the FINE study. Eur J Clin Nutr. 2007;61:226–32.

69. Corley J, et al. Caffeine consumption and cognitive function at age 70: the Lothian Birth Cohort 1936 study. Psychosom Med. 2010;72:206–14.

70. van Boxtel MP, Schmitt JA, Bosma H, Jolles J. The effects of habitual caffeine use on cognitive change: a longitudinal perspective. Pharmacol Biochem Behav. 2003;75:921–7.

71. Balk E, et al. B vitamins and berries and age-related neurodegenerative disorders. Evid Rep Technol Assess (Full Rep). 2006;164:1–161.

72. Riggs KM, Spiro 3rd A, Tucker K, Rush D. Relations of vitamin B-12, vitamin B-6, folate, and homocysteine to cognitive performance in the normative aging study. Am J Clin Nutr. 1996;63:306–14.

73. Wang HX, et al. Vitamin B(12) and folate in relation to the development of Alzheimer's disease. Neurology. 2001;56:1188–94.

74. Seshadri S, et al. Plasma homocysteine as a risk factor for dementia and Alzheimer's disease. N Engl J Med. 2002;346:476–83.

75. Garcia A, Zanibbi K. Homocysteine and cognitive function in elderly people. CMAJ. 2004;171:897–904.

76. Ravaglia G, et al. Homocysteine and folate as risk factors for dementia and Alzheimer disease. Am J Clin Nutr. 2005;82:636–43.

77. Kado DM, et al. Homocysteine versus the vitamins folate, B6, and B12 as predictors of cognitive function and decline in older high-functioning adults: MacArthur studies of successful aging. Am J Med. 2005;118:161–7.

78. Tucker KL, Qiao N, Scott T, Rosenberg I, Spiro 3rd A. High homocysteine and low B vitamins predict cognitive decline in aging men: the veterans affairs normative aging study. Am J Clin Nutr. 2005;82:627–35.

79. Plassman BL, Williams Jr JW, Burke JR, Holsinger T, Benjamin S. Systematic review: factors associated with risk for and possible prevention of cognitive decline in later life. Ann Intern Med. 2010;153: 182–93.

80. Douaud G, Refsum H, de Jager CA, et al. Preventing Alzheimer's disease-related gray matter atrophy by B-vitamin treatment. Proc Natl Acad Sci USA. 2013;110:9523–8.

81. Terasawa M, Nakahara T, Tsukada N, Sugawara A, Itokawa Y. The relationship between thiamine deficiency and performance of a learning task in rats. Metab Brain Dis. 1999;14:137–48.

82. Jolicoeur FB, Rondeau DB, Barbeau A, Wayner MJ. Comparison of neurobehavioral effects induced by various experimental models of ataxia in the rat. Neurobehav Toxicol. 1979;1 Suppl 1:175–8.

83. Ciccia RM, Langlais PJ. An examination of the synergistic interaction of ethanol and thiamine deficiency in the development of neurological signs and long-term cognitive and memory impairments. Alcohol Clin Exp Res. 2000;24:622–34.

84. Meador K, et al. Preliminary findings of high-dose thiamine in dementia of Alzheimer's type. J Geriatr Psychiatry Neurol. 1993;6:222–9.

85. Mimori Y, Katsuoka H, Nakamura S. Thiamine therapy in Alzheimer's disease. Metab Brain Dis. 1996;11:89–94.

86. Jia X, McNeill G, Avenell A. Does taking vitamin, mineral and fatty acid supplements prevent cognitive decline? A systematic review of randomized controlled trials. J Hum Nutr Diet. 2008;21:317–36.

87. Goodwin JS, Goodwin JM, Garry PJ. Association between nutritional status and cognitive functioning in a healthy elderly population. JAMA. 1983;249:2917–21.

88. Lee H, Kim HJ, Kim JM, Chang N. Effects of dietary folic acid supplementation on cerebrovascular endothelial dysfunction in rats with induced hyperhomocysteinemia. Brain Res. 2004;996:139–47.

89. Scileppi KP, Blass JP, Baker HG. Circulating vitamins in Alzheimer's dementia as compared with other dementias. J Am Geriatr Soc. 1984;32:709–11.

90. Mizrahi EH, et al. Plasma total homocysteine levels, dietary vitamin B6 and folate intake in AD and healthy aging. J Nutr Health Aging. 2003;7:160–5.

91. Dangour AD, et al. B-vitamins and fatty acids in the prevention and treatment of Alzheimer's disease and dementia: a systematic review. J Alzheimers Dis. 2010;22:205–24.

92. Masuda Y, Kokubu T, Yamashita M, Ikeda H, Inoue S. EGG phosphatidylcholine combined with vitamin B12 improved memory impairment following lesioning of nucleus basalis in rats. Life Sci. 1998;62:813–22.

93. Tangney CC, Tang Y, Evans DA, Morris MC. Biochemical indicators of vitamin B12 and folate insufficiency and cognitive decline. Neurology. 2009;72:361–7.

94. Kwok T, et al. Randomized trial of the effect of supplementation on the cognitive function of older people with subnormal cobalamin levels. Int J Geriatr Psychiatry. 1998;13:611–6.

95. Hvas AM, Juul S, Lauritzen L, Nexo E, Ellegaard J. No effect of vitamin B-12 treatment on cognitive function and depression: a randomized placebo controlled study. J Affect Disord. 2004;81:269–73.
96. Kruman II, et al. Folic acid deficiency and homocysteine impair DNA repair in hippocampal neurons and sensitize them to amyloid toxicity in experimental models of Alzheimer's disease. J Neurosci. 2002;22:1752–62.
97. Mattson MP, Chan SL, Duan W. Modification of brain aging and neurodegenerative disorders by genes, diet, and behavior. Physiol Rev. 2002;82:637–72.
98. Morris MC, et al. Dietary folate and vitamin B12 intake and cognitive decline among community-dwelling older persons. Arch Neurol. 2005;62:641–5.
99. Fioravanti M, et al. Low folate levels in the cognitive decline of elderly patients and the efficacy of folate as a treatment for improving memory deficits. Arch Gerontol Geriatr. 1998;26:1–13.
100. Bryan J, Calvaresi E, Hughes D. Short-term folate, vitamin B-12 or vitamin B-6 supplementation slightly affects memory performance but not mood in women of various ages. J Nutr. 2002;132:1345–56.
101. Sommer BR, Hoff AL, Costa M. Folic acid supplementation in dementia: a preliminary report. J Geriatr Psychiatry Neurol. 2003;16:156–9.
102. Wald DS, Kasturiratne A, Simmonds M. Effect of folic acid, with or without other B vitamins, on cognitive decline: meta-analysis of randomized trials. Am J Med. 2010;123(6):522–7. e522.
103. Perrig WJ, Perrig P, Stahelin HB. The relation between antioxidants and memory performance in the old and very old. J Am Geriatr Soc. 1997;45:718–24.
104. Morris MC, Evans DA, Bienias JL, Tangney CC, Wilson RS. Vitamin E and cognitive decline in older persons. Arch Neurol. 2002;59:1125–32.
105. Wengreen HJ, et al. Antioxidant intake and cognitive function of elderly men and women: the Cache county study. J Nutr Health Aging. 2007;11:230–7.
106. Dangour AD, Sibson VL, Fletcher AE. Micronutrient supplementation in later life: limited evidence for benefit. J Gerontol A Biol Sci Med Sci. 2004;59:659–73.
107. Dysken MW, Sano M, Asthana S, et al. Effect of vitamin E and memantine on functional decline in Alzheimer disease: the TEAM-AD VA cooperative randomized trial. JAMA. 2014;311(1):33–44.
108. Wallum BJ, et al. Cerebrospinal fluid insulin levels increase during intravenous insulin infusions in man. J Clin Endocrinol Metab. 1987;64:190–4.
109. Akatsu H, et al. Transition metal abnormalities in progressive dementias. Biometals. 2012;25(2):337–50.
110. Krikorian R, Eliassen JC, Boespflug EL, Nash TA, Shidler MD. Improved cognitive-cerebral function in older adults with chromium supplementation. Nutr Neurosci. 2010;13:116–22.
111. Cefalu WT, Wang ZQ, Zhang XH, Baldor LC, Russell JC. Oral chromium picolinate improves carbohydrate and lipid metabolism and enhances skeletal muscle Glut-4 translocation in obese, hyperinsulinemic (JCR-LA corpulent) rats. J Nutr. 2002;132:1107–14.
112. Anderson RA, et al. Elevated intakes of supplemental chromium improve glucose and insulin variables in individuals with type 2 diabetes. Diabetes. 1997;46:1786–91.
113. Malar DS, Devi KP. Dietary polyphenols for treatment of Alzheimer's disease- future research and development. Curr Pharm Biotechnol. 2014;15(4):330–42.
114. Crozier A, Del Rio D, Clifford MN. Bioavailability of dietary flavonoids and phenolic compounds. Mol Aspects Med. 2010;31:446–67.
115. Moyer RA, Hummer KE, Finn CE, Frei B, Wrolstad RE. Anthocyanins, phenolics, and antioxidant capacity in diverse small fruits: vaccinium, rubus, and ribes. J Agric Food Chem. 2002;50:519–25.
116. Halvorsen BL, et al. A systematic screening of total antioxidants in dietary plants. J Nutr. 2002;132:461–71.
117. Saija A, Princi P, D'Amico N, De Pasquale R, Costa G. Effect of Vaccinium myrtillus anthocyanins on triiodothyronine transport into brain in the rat. Pharmacol Res. 1990;22 Suppl 3:59–60.
118. Casadesus G, et al. Modulation of hippocampal plasticity and cognitive behavior by short-term blueberry supplementation in aged rats. Nutr Neurosci. 2004;7:309–16.
119. Joseph JA, Fisher DR, Carey AN. Fruit extracts antagonize Abeta- or DA-induced deficits in Ca2+ flux in M1-transfected COS-7 cells. J Alzheimers Dis. 2004;6:403–11. discussion 443–409.
120. Yang F, et al. Curcumin inhibits formation of amyloid beta oligomers and fibrils, binds plaques, and reduces amyloid in vivo. J Biol Chem. 2005;280:5892–901.
121. Rinwa P, Kaur B, Jaggi AS, Singh N. Involvement of PPAR-gamma in curcumin-mediated beneficial effects in experimental dementia. Naunyn Schmiedebergs Arch Pharmacol. 2010;381:529–39.
122. Lao CD, et al. Dose escalation of a curcuminoid formulation. BMC Complement Altern Med. 2006;6:10.
123. Baum L, et al. Six-month randomized, placebo-controlled, double-blind, pilot clinical trial of curcumin in patients with Alzheimer disease. J Clin Psychopharmacol. 2008;28:110–3.
124. Hamaguchi T, Ono K, Yamada M. REVIEW: curcumin and Alzheimer's disease. CNS Neurosci Ther. 2010;16:285–97.
125. Witte AV, Kerti L, Marquiles DS, Floel A. Effects of resveratrol on memory performance, hippocampal functional connectivity, and glucose metabolism in

healthy older adults. J Neurosci. 2014;34(23): 7862–70.

126. Dacks PA, Shineman DW, Fillit HM. Current evidence for the clinical use of long-chain polyunsaturated n-3 fatty acids to prevent age-related cognitive decline and Alzheimer's disease. J Nutr Health Aging. 2013;17(3):240–51.

127. Oster T, Pillot T. Docosahexaenoic acid and synaptic protection in Alzheimer's disease mice. Biochim Biophys Acta. 2010;1801:791–8.

128. Greiner RS, Moriguchi T, Hutton A, Slotnick BM, Salem Jr N. Rats with low levels of brain docosahexaenoic acid show impaired performance in olfactory-based and spatial learning tasks. Lipids. 1999;34:S239–43.

129. Chiu CC, et al. The effects of omega-3 fatty acids monotherapy in Alzheimer's disease and mild cognitive impairment: a preliminary randomized double-blind placebo-controlled study. Prog Neuropsychopharmacol Biol Psychiatry. 2008;32: 1538–44.

130. Freund-Levi Y, et al. Omega-3 fatty acid treatment in 174 patients with mild to moderate Alzheimer disease: OmegAD study: a randomized double-blind trial. Arch Neurol. 2006;63:1402–8.

131. Quinn JF, et al. Docosahexaenoic acid supplementation and cognitive decline in Alzheimer disease: a randomized trial. JAMA. 2010;304:1903–11.

132. Mahmoudi MJ, et al. Effect of low dose omega-3 poly unsaturated fatty acids on cognitive status among older people: a double-blind randomized placebo-controlled study. J Diabetes Metab Disord. 2014;13(1):34.

133. de la Torre JC. Alzheimer disease as a vascular disorder: nosological evidence. Stroke. 2002;33:1152–62.

134. Snowdon DA, et al. Brain infarction and the clinical expression of Alzheimer disease. The Nun study. JAMA. 1997;277:813–7.

135. Stephan BC, Brayne C. Vascular factors and prevention of dementia. Int Rev Psychiatry. 2008;20:344–56.

136. Kalaria RN. Comparison between Alzheimer's disease and vascular dementia: implications for treatment. Neurol Res. 2003;25:661–4.

137. Fernando MS, Ince PG. Vascular pathologies and cognition in a population-based cohort of elderly people. J Neurol Sci. 2004;226:13–7.

138. Luchsinger JA, et al. Aggregation of vascular risk factors and risk of incident Alzheimer disease. Neurology. 2005;65:545–51.

139. Dartigues JF, Fabrigoule C, Barberger-Gateau P, Orgogozo JM. Memory, aging and risk factors. Lessons from clinical trials and epidemiologic studies. Therapie. 2000;55:503–5.

140. Launer LJ. Regional differences in rates of dementia: MRC-CFAS. Lancet Neurol. 2005;4:694–5.

141. Matthews FE, Stephan BC, McKeith IG, Bond J, Brayne C. Two-year progression from mild cognitive impairment to dementia: to what extent do different definitions agree? J Am Geriatr Soc. 2008;56:1424–33.

142. Skoog I, et al. 15-year longitudinal study of blood pressure and dementia. Lancet. 1996;347:1141–5.

143. Mielke MM, Zandi PP. Hematologic risk factors of vascular disease and their relation to dementia. Dement Geriatr Cogn Disord. 2006;21:335–52.

144. Rocca WA, Petersen RC, Knopman DS, Hebert LE, Evans DA, Hall KS, et al. Trends in the incidence and prevalence of Alzheimer's disease, dementia, and cognitive impairment in the United States. Alzheimers Dement. 2011;7(1):80–93.

145. Forette F, et al. Prevention of dementia in randomised double-blind placebo-controlled systolic hypertension in Europe (Syst-Eur) trial. Lancet. 1998;352:1347–51.

146. Lithell H, et al. The study on cognition and prognosis in the elderly (SCOPE): principal results of a randomized double-blind intervention trial. J Hypertens. 2003;21:875–86.

147. Curb JD, et al. Effect of diuretic-based antihypertensive treatment on cardiovascular disease risk in older diabetic patients with isolated systolic hypertension. Systolic hypertension in the elderly program cooperative research group. JAMA. 1996;276:1886–92.

148. Lopez-Arrieta JM, Birks J. Nimodipine for primary degenerative, mixed and vascular dementia. Cochrane Database Syst Rev. 2002;3, CD000147.

149. McGuinness B, Todd S, Passmore P, Bullock R. The effects of blood pressure lowering on development of cognitive impairment and dementia in patients without apparent prior cerebrovascular disease. Cochrane Database Syst Rev. 2006;19(2), CD004034.

150. McGuinness B, Todd S, Passmore P, Bullock R. Blood pressure lowering in patients without prior cerebrovascular disease for prevention of cognitive impairment and dementia. Cochrane Database Syst Rev. 2009;7(4), CD004034.

151. McGuinness B, Craig D, Bullock R, Passmore P. Statins for the prevention of dementia. Cochrane Database Syst Rev. 2009;15(2), CD003160.

152. Zhou B, Teramukai S, Fukushima M. Prevention and treatment of dementia or Alzheimer's disease by statins: a meta-analysis. Dement Geriatr Cogn Disord. 2007;23:194–201.

153. Agostini JV, et al. Effects of statin use on muscle strength, cognition, and depressive symptoms in older adults. J Am Geriatr Soc. 2007;55:420–5.

154. Sparks DL, Connor DJ, Sabbagh MN, Petersen RB, Lopez J, Browne P. Circulating cholesterol levels, apolipoprotein E genotype and dementia severity influence the benefit of atorvastatin treatment in Alzheimer's disease: results of the Alzheimer's disease cholesterol-lowering treatment (ADCLT) trial. Acta Neurol Scand Suppl. 2006;185:3–7.

155. Rdzak GM, Abdelghany O. Does insulin therapy for Type 1 diabetes mellitus protect against Alzheimer's disease? Pharmacotherapy. 2014;34(12):1317–23.

156. Cook DG, et al. Reduced hippocampal insulin-degrading enzyme in late-onset alzheimer's disease is associated with the apolipoprotein E-epsilon4 allele. Am J Pathol. 2003;162:313–9.

157. Bruehl H, et al. Modifiers of cognitive function and brain structure in middle-aged and elderly individuals with type 2 diabetes mellitus. Brain Res. 2009;1280:186–94.

158. Censori B, et al. Dementia after first stroke. Stroke. 1996;27:1205–10.

159. Bourdel-Marchasson I, et al. Characteristics of undiagnosed diabetes in community-dwelling French elderly: the 3C study. Diabetes Res Clin Pract. 2007;76:257–64.

160. Arvanitakis Z, Wilson RS, Bienias JL, Evans DA, Bennett DA. Diabetes mellitus and risk of Alzheimer disease and decline in cognitive function. Arch Neurol. 2004;61:661–6.

161. Allen KV, Frier BM, Strachan MW. The relationship between type 2 diabetes and cognitive dysfunction: longitudinal studies and their methodological limitations. Eur J Pharmacol. 2004;490:169–75.

162. Yaffe K, et al. Diabetes, impaired fasting glucose, and development of cognitive impairment in older women. Neurology. 2004;63:658–63.

163. Areosa SA, Grimley EV. Effect of the treatment of Type II diabetes mellitus on the development of cognitive impairment and dementia. Cochrane Database Syst Rev. 2002:CD003804.

164. Aggarwal NT, et al. The relation of cigarette smoking to incident Alzheimer's disease in a biracial urban community population. Neuroepidemiology. 2006;26:140–6.

165. Ott A, et al. Smoking and risk of dementia and Alzheimer's disease in a population-based cohort study: the Rotterdam Study. Lancet. 1998;351:1840–3.

166. Merchant C, et al. The influence of smoking on the risk of Alzheimer's disease. Neurology. 1999;52:1408–12.

167. Juan D, et al. A 2-year follow-up study of cigarette smoking and risk of dementia. Eur J Neurol. 2004;11:277–82.

168. Meyer J, Xu G, Thornby J, Chowdhury M, Quach M. Longitudinal analysis of abnormal domains comprising mild cognitive impairment (MCI) during aging. J Neurol Sci. 2002;201:19–25.

169. Fratiglioni L, Wang HX. Smoking and Parkinson's and Alzheimer's disease: review of the epidemiological studies. Behav Brain Res. 2000;113:117–20.

170. Anstey KJ, von Sanden C, Salim A, O'Kearney R. Smoking as a risk factor for dementia and cognitive decline: a meta-analysis of prospective studies. Am J Epidemiol. 2007;166:367–78.

171. Lautenschlager NT, et al. Effect of physical activity on cognitive function in older adults at risk for Alzheimer disease: a randomized trial. JAMA. 2008;300:1027–37.

172. Angevaren M, Aufdemkampe G, Verhaar HJ, Aleman A, Vanhees L. Physical activity and enhanced fitness to improve cognitive function in older people without known cognitive impairment. Cochrane Database Syst Rev. 2008;3, CD005381.

173. Dishman RK, et al. Neurobiology of exercise. Obesity (Silver Spring). 2006;14:345–56.

174. Rockwood K, Middleton L. Physical activity and the maintenance of cognitive function. Alzheimers Dement. 2007;3:S38–44.

175. Ravaglia G, et al. Physical activity and dementia risk in the elderly: findings from a prospective Italian study. Neurology. 2008;70:1786–94.

176. Kirshner HS. Vascular dementia: a review of recent evidence for prevention and treatment. Curr Neurol Neurosci Rep. 2009;9:437–42.

177. Pohjasvaara T, et al. How complex interactions of ischemic brain infarcts, white matter lesions, and atrophy relate to poststroke dementia. Arch Neurol. 2000;57:1295–300.

178. Tatemichi TK, et al. Risk of dementia after stroke in a hospitalized cohort: results of a longitudinal study. Neurology. 1994;44:1885–91.

179. Moroney JT, et al. Risk factors for incident dementia after stroke. Role of hypoxic and ischemic disorders. Stroke. 1996;27:1283–9.

180. Ewers M, Insel PS, Stern Y, Weiner MW. Cognitive reserve associated with FDG-PET in preclinical Alzheimer disease. Neurology. 2013;80:1194–201.

181. Valenzuela MJ. Brain reserve and the prevention of dementia. Curr Opin Psychiatry. 2008;21:296–302.

182. Stern Y. What is cognitive reserve? Theory and research application of the reserve concept. J Int Neuropsychol Soc. 2002;8:448–60.

183. Verghese J, et al. Leisure activities and the risk of dementia in the elderly. N Engl J Med. 2003;348:2508–16.

184. Fratiglioni L, Wang HX, Ericsson K, Maytan M, Winblad B. Influence of social network on occurrence of dementia: a community-based longitudinal study. Lancet. 2000;355:1315–9.

185. Valenzuela MJ, Sachdev P. Brain reserve and dementia: a systematic review. Psychol Med. 2006;36:441–54.

186. Oswald WD, Rupprecht R, Gunzelmann T, Tritt K. The SIMA-project: effects of 1 year cognitive and psychomotor training on cognitive abilities of the elderly. Behav Brain Res. 1996;78:67–72.

187. Ball K, et al. Effects of cognitive training interventions with older adults: a randomized controlled trial. JAMA. 2002;288:2271–81.

188. Willis SL, et al. Long-term effects of cognitive training on everyday functional outcomes in older adults. JAMA. 2006;296:2805–14.

189. Mahncke HW, et al. Memory enhancement in healthy older adults using a brain plasticity-based training program: a randomized, controlled study. Proc Natl Acad Sci USA. 2006;103:12523–8.

190. Gates N, Valenzuela M. Cognitive exercise and its role in cognitive function in older adults. Curr Psychiatry Rep. 2010;12:20–7.

191. Troyer AK, Murphy KJ, Anderson ND, Moscovitch M, Craik FI. Changing everyday memory behaviour in amnestic mild cognitive impairment: a randomised controlled trial. Neuropsychol Rehabil. 2008;18:65–88.

192. Rozzini L, et al. Efficacy of cognitive rehabilitation in patients with mild cognitive impairment treated with cholinesterase inhibitors. Int J Geriatr Psychiatry. 2007;22:356–60.

193. Saczynski JS, et al. The effect of social engagement on incident dementia: the Honolulu-Asia aging study. Am J Epidemiol. 2006;163:433–40.

194. Ownby RL, Crocco E, Acevedo A, John V, Loewenstein D. Depression and risk for Alzheimer disease: systematic review, meta-analysis, and metaregression analysis. Arch Gen Psychiatry. 2006;63:530–8.

195. Tisserand DJ, Visser PJ, van Boxtel MP, Jolles J. The relation between global and limbic brain volumes on MRI and cognitive performance in healthy individuals across the age range. Neurobiol Aging. 2000;21:569–76.

196. Wolf H, et al. Structural correlates of mild cognitive impairment. Neurobiol Aging. 2004;25:913–24.

197. Markou A, Duka T, Prelevic GM. Estrogens and brain function. Hormones (Athens). 2005;4:9–17.

198. Sherwin BB. Estrogenic effects on memory in women. Ann N Y Acad Sci. 1994;743:213–30; discussion 230–211.

199. Murphy DG, et al. Sex differences in human brain morphometry and metabolism: an in vivo quantitative magnetic resonance imaging and positron emission tomography study on the effect of aging. Arch Gen Psychiatry. 1996;53:585–94.

200. Caldwell BM, Watson RI. An evaluation of psychologic effects of sex hormone administration in aged women. I. Results of therapy after six months. J Gerontol. 1952;7:228–44.

201. Portin R, et al. Serum estrogen level, attention, memory and other cognitive functions in middle-aged women. Climacteric. 1999;2:115–23.

202. Yaffe K, Sawaya G, Lieberburg I, Grady D. Estrogen therapy in postmenopausal women: effects on cognitive function and dementia. JAMA. 1998;279: 688–95.

203. Barrett-Connor E, Laughlin GA. Endogenous and exogenous estrogen, cognitive function, and dementia in postmenopausal women: evidence from epidemiologic studies and clinical trials. Semin Reprod Med. 2009;27:275–82.

204. Maki PM, Zonderman AB, Resnick SM. Enhanced verbal memory in nondemented elderly women receiving hormone-replacement therapy. Am J Psychiatry. 2001;158:227–33.

205. Lokkegaard E, et al. The influence of hormone replacement therapy on the aging-related change in cognitive performance. Analysis based on a Danish cohort study. Maturitas. 2002;42:209–18.

206. LeBlanc ES, Janowsky J, Chan BK, Nelson HD. Hormone replacement therapy and cognition: systematic review and meta-analysis. JAMA. 2001;285:1489–99.

207. Matthews K, Cauley J, Yaffe K, Zmuda JM. Estrogen replacement therapy and cognitive decline in older community women. J Am Geriatr Soc. 1999;47: 518–23.

208. Zandi PP, et al. Hormone replacement therapy and incidence of Alzheimer disease in older women: the Cache county study. JAMA. 2002;288:2123–9.

209. Sorwell KG, Urbanski HF. Dehydroepiandrosterone and age-related cognitive decline. Age (Dordr). 2010;32:61–7.

210. Labrie F, et al. DHEA and the intracrine formation of androgens and estrogens in peripheral target tissues: its role during aging. Steroids. 1998;63:322–8.

211. Karishma KK, Herbert J. Dehydroepiandrosterone (DHEA) stimulates neurogenesis in the hippocampus of the rat, promotes survival of newly formed neurons and prevents corticosterone-induced suppression. Eur J Neurosci. 2002;16:445–53.

212. Wolf OT, Kudielka BM, Hellhammer DH, Hellhammer J, Kirschbaum C. Opposing effects of DHEA replacement in elderly subjects on declarative memory and attention after exposure to a laboratory stressor. Psychoneuroendocrinology. 1998;23: 617–29.

213. Giurgea C. The "nootropic" approach to the pharmacology of the integrative activity of the brain. Cond Reflex. 1973;8:108–15.

214. Malykh AG, Sadaie MR. Piracetam and piracetam-like drugs: from basic science to novel clinical applications to CNS disorders. Drugs. 2010;70:287–312.

215. Waegemans T, et al. Clinical efficacy of piracetam in cognitive impairment: a meta-analysis. Dement Geriatr Cogn Disord. 2002;13:217–24.

216. Flicker L, Grimley Evans J. Piracetam for dementia or cognitive impairment. Cochrane Database Syst Rev. 2000:CD001011.

Detection of Dementia

James E. Galvin

Nearly six million Americans live with Alzheimer's disease and related disorders (AD), many with co-morbid medical conditions and depression [1–3]. Between the years 2000 and 2010, the mortality rate for persons with AD increased by 68 % [1]. Over the next 20 years, the number of people over 65 year and 85 year is expected to grow by 62 % and 84 %, respectively [4, 5]. The incidence, morbidity and mortality rates for dementia will thus increase dramatically. With increased longevity and the aging of the population, the societal financial burden of illness and dependency will expand exponentially. AD affects not only patients but also families. Each AD patient is estimated to have 2.9 informal (mostly family) caregivers who are estimated to provide 17.5 billion hours of care annually valued at $216 billion [1]. The burden on unpaid caregivers for individuals with AD costs society in replacement costs and lost wages $374 billion in 2010 and are expected to increase 79 % by 2050 [1]. This same burden also increases the unpaid caregivers own health care cost of $9.1 billion in 2012 [1]. The Affordable Care Act [6]

places emphasis on preventive services, cognitive screening, and quality measures for clinical care while the National Alzheimer Project Act (NAPA) [7] places emphasis on advancing national goals to: (a) raise awareness of AD; (b) better understand the burden of AD on patients, families, providers and health delivery systems; (c) increase research participation in older adults; and (d) translate this acquired knowledge into public health practice in the context of an increasingly diverse older adult population. Thus an accountable way to improve dementia detection, care, and patient- and family-centered outcomes is greatly needed.

Mild Cognitive Impairment (MCI) and AD may have limited detection in the community due to the lack of brief screening tests that detect the earliest signs of impairment. At present, there are no clear recommendations for or against dementia screening from the US Preventive Services Task Force [8]. Many current brief screening measures (i.e., the Mini Mental State Exam or MMSE [9]) have limited ability to detect cognitive impairment in the community [10–12]. The Affordable Care Act [6] includes a Personalized Prevention Plan including screening for cognitive disorders, reimbursable through Medicare. Early detection as a core element, coupled with treatments or preventative actions to reduce the burden of disease [13] and provide benefits to the patient and family (Table 1). Dementia detection may identify individuals in whom a disease has

J.E. Galvin, MD, MPH (✉)
Professor and Associate Dean for Clinical Research,
Charles E. Schmidt College of Medicine, Florida
Atlantic University, Boca Raton, FL, USA
e-mail: James.Galvin@nyumc.org

© Springer International Publishing Switzerland 2016
M. Boltz, J.E. Galvin (eds.), *Dementia Care*, DOI 10.1007/978-3-319-18377-0_3

Table 1 Benefits of early detection of dementia

1. Start currently available symptomatic medications at earliest possible stage—may reduce burden of symptoms
2. Identify patients who would best benefit from disease modifying medications as they become available
3. Patients can participate in clinical trials to test new therapies
4. Allows clinicians to anticipate problems the patients may have adhering to recommended therapy
5. Assisting the patient's caregiver and family in planning for the future—advanced directives, durable power of attorney, long-term care plans
6. Permits input from patient at a stage where they are capable of contributing to their medical, financial, and social decision-making process
7. Early referral to community resources, social services, and support groups
8. Non-pharmacological interventions including those directed at caregivers to reduce stress, alleviate mood, delay nursing home placement and improve well-being

Table 2 Cultural differences in dementia

• The older adult population in the US is becoming more diverse
– In 2006, 81 % of adults age 65+ were Caucasian; by 2050 this is estimated to decrease to 61 %
– Consider cross-cultural differences in case ascertainment, recruitment and retention
• Cultural factors related to case detection, delay in diagnosis, access to care, and poorer outcomes
– Knowledge and awareness of dementia vs. normal aging and perceptions/expectations of care
– Structural obstacles (rural locality, number of specialists, transportation)
– Language barriers
– Differences in symptom presentation
• Psychosocial factors that impact patient-family dyads
– Perceived role of the family in care (a term known as Familism) and cultural identity
– Gender roles
– Expectations about caregiving
– Role of faith and religion
• Cultural factors that account for differences in research participation
– Mistrust of medical institutions and research
– Health beliefs—e.g., that "senility" represents a life stage
– Frequency and types of contacts with medical professionals
– Tuskegee legacy and related phenomena

already begun and who may be experiencing mild clinical symptoms but have not yet sought out medical care. The objective of effective screening is to detect the disease earlier than it would be detected with usual care and begin interventions at a stage when they might be most effective. Additionally, early detection may provide opportunities for modifying risk factors through a combination and diet, exercise and lifestyle recommendations. Dementia screening would be best suited to detect cognitive impairment at the beginning of disease signs, particularly if these screening measures reflect what is known about the symptomatic phase of AD and correlate with the pathologic and biomarker changes associated with AD [12]. In this way treatments (both current and future) can be initiated [14]. Furthermore, early recognition of dementia allows clinicians to anticipate problems the patients may have adhering to recommended therapy and assisting the patient's caregiver and family in planning for future problems resulting from progression of disease [15].

Despite the benefits of early detection, including effective treatment of the disease and its com-plications and enabling the patient (and family) to prepare for the future, dementia is still under-recognized in the community [16, 17]. This is in part due to dismissal by patients and families of early signs of the disease as normal aging, cultural differences in perceptions of aging and dementia (Table 2), denial, lack of time in a busy clinical practice and the lack of time-sensitive, effective screening tools [12]. Given the brief time available to primary care physicians in a standard office visit, sensitive and specific cognitive impairment screening tools that are valid, easy to administer, and minimally time consuming are needed (Table 3) [17, 18].

The challenge with brief instruments is whether it can reliably discriminate normal aging from very mild impairments in a time-efficient manner. A number of brief performance-based

Table 3 Desirable attributes of a brief instrument to detect dementia

- Predictive of early dementia
- Inexpensive
- High face validity
- Reliable, sensitive and specific
- Brief
- Easy to administer and score
- Socially acceptable
- Culturally sensitive

dementia screening measures are already in use, but may be (1) unable to detect or quantify change from previous levels of function; (2) insensitive to subtle changes in high functioning individuals (i.e., ceiling effects) who may score well within the normal range throughout the early stages of dementia; (3) unable to discern decline in individuals with poorer lifelong abilities; and (4) culturally insensitive thereby underestimating abilities of underrepresented minority groups. Informant-based assessments are less likely to have floor or ceiling effects and may be more valid in assessing individuals regardless of age, gender, language, race or educational level [19–23]. However, reliable informants may not always be available, may minimize symptoms, have cognitive impairment of their own, or may have secondary motivations. The Alzheimer Association [13] and the National Guideline Clearinghouse [24] recommends the combined use of an informant interview with a performance measurement to detect dementia most efficiently. Dementia screening requires a consideration of the population-at-risk and the sensitivity and specificity of the instruments used [11]. A large number of false positive individuals might expend limited health care dollars; a large number of individuals receiving false negatives would be denied treatment and miss opportunities to participate in clinical research. Thus, a staged dementia screening approach would make the most sense clinically and economically. It is also important to consider whether patients are willing to be screened for dementia. Studies have reported a willingness of patients to be screened

if there are perceived benefits to being screened and if the clinician can offer treatments for problems when detected [24, 25].

A last consideration is the potential use of biological markers (biomarkers) to complement interview and performance-based evaluations and improve dementia detection [26, 27]. Criteria for an ideal biomarker of AD have been proposed by a consensus group on molecular and biochemical markers of AD; *"The ideal biomarker for AD should detect a fundamental feature of neuropathology and be validated in neuropathologically-confirmed cases; it should have a diagnostic sensitivity >80 % for detecting AD and a specificity of >80 % for distinguishing other dementias; it should be reliable, reproducible, non-invasive, simple to perform, and inexpensive"* [28]. Beyond these criteria for early and accurate diagnosis, it would be especially useful if the biomarker could capture the beneficial effect of disease modifying therapy [29], predict conversion from MCI to Alzheimer's disease, correspond closely to available clinical detections methods and thus provide an opportunity for early intervention or prevention [26]. Biomarkers of disease may provide important avenues of research to enhance the diagnosis of individuals with early AD and could assist in the identification of those individuals at risk for developing AD. The pathology of AD provides a number of potential sources of biomarkers. Characteristic histological changes including neurofibrillary tangles and amyloid plaques remain the hallmarks of the disease [30]. Early neurofibrillary tangles and amyloid plaque pathology are estimated to start decades before the symptoms [27]; in the evolution, clinical symptoms closely relate to NFTs, neurodegeneration, and synapse loss [31, 32]. Because the pathology begins decades before clinical symptoms, measurements of amyloid, tau and associated neurochemical and neurophysiological alterations provide a potential pool of biological markers of disease presence and progression [33–37]. Pathologic evidence of disease can be obtained from biomarkers such as MRI measurements of atrophy [38] or surface deformation

[39], glucose hypometabolism on FDG-PET [40], CSF measurements of amyloid and tau [41–43] or PET imaging with amyloid ligands [44]. Some biological biomarkers offer the opportunity to look at specific pathological features of AD neuropathology, although they may not be sensitive to disease progression (i.e., CSF Aβ42), while others (i.e., FDG-PET) strongly correlate with disease progression but may not be specific for AD [26]. Although biomarkers can increase the diagnostic likelihood that AD is present; biomarkers may be invasive, uncomfortable, expensive, and not be readily available to rural areas, underserved communities, underinsured individuals or developing countries sometimes making them impractical for broad use.

The Mental Status Examination

The elements of a comprehensive mental status examination include observational, cognitive and neuropsychiatric assessments. The initial contact with the patient affords the opportunity to assess whether a cognitive, attention, or language disorder is present. Questioning of an informant may bring to light changes in cognition, function and behavior that the patient either is not aware of or denies. While informant interviews may provide a more reliable way to determine cognitive and functional change in dementia patients, informants are not always attendant in clinical practice. Brief office visits such as annual check-ups, often without the presence of informants, may not uncover very mild symptoms of dementia. Self-rating scales for dementia have not gained common use because of the perception that dementia patients lack insight and deny cognitive problems even in mild forms of dementia [45–47]. Dementia patients are not thought to be reliable reporters of cognitive symptoms due to the unawareness of cognitive deficits (cognitive anosognosia) [45–47], leading to discrepancies between self-ratings and informant ratings or between self-rating and objective performance [48]. Awareness of deficits may vary greatly across individuals with some patients offering

reliable accounts of memory changes and others failing to appreciate their decline. Denial of cognitive deficits does not correlate with age of dementia onset, duration of illness or education and is negatively correlated with depression [45] but does correlate with dementia severity [49]. However, dementia patients are asked to self-rate a number of physical and psychological symptoms. One study assessed physical, psychological and social health of dementia patients, 75 % of whom had MMSE scores <16 [50]. There was reasonable agreement between patient and informant rating for physical health, but poor agreement for psychological and social well-being. Dementia patients are also asked to self-rate presence of depressive symptoms [51] and quality of life [52]. Most patients are able to complete these assessments and, dementia patients were not only able to rate their own quality of life but were able to give reasonable estimates of the caregiver's rating of quality of life [52].

In addition to detailed history taking and the more common components of the neurologic examination (motor and sensory function, gait, balance, etc.), careful and thoughtful observation of the patients' appearance, behavior and demeanor can provide insight into the nature of the cognitive status. Observation of patient's level of conscious, general appearance, affect, movement and speech provide important initial evaluation of patient mental status, followed by asking probing questions to sample mood, thought, perception and insight.

Cognitive Assessment

Following observation, the clinician should begin a formal assessment of cognitive abilities. The assessment of cognitive function should be conducted methodically and should assess comprehensively the major domains of neuropsychological function (attention, memory, language, visuospatial skills, executive ability). The patient's age, handedness, educational level, and sociocultural background may all influence cognitive function and should be determined prior to initiating or

Table 4 Useful dementia screening tests for office setting

Screening test	Numbers of items	Scoring system	Cut-off scores	Validity	Limitations
Mini mental state examination (MMSE)	30 items Score range 0–30	Add total number of correct answers Alternate forms for attention tasks – Spell WORLD backwards – Serial subtraction by 7 Lower scores = more impairment	27–30 Normal 24–26 MCI 18–23 Mild dementia 10–17 Moderate dementia 0–9 Severe dementia	Sensitivity 85–100 Specificity 66–100	Scores influenced by age, education, race and ethnicity, language Not ideal to identify mild impairment. Copyright protected, requiring a license fee
Mini-cog	3-word recall combined with clock drawing Score range 0–5	Recall each word = 1 point Correct clock = 2 points Lower scores = more impairment	3–5 Normal 0–2 Impaired	Sensitivity and specificity comparable to MMSE	Test focuses on recall, visuospatial ability and construction. No other domains captured
Short blessed test (SBT)	6 items of orientation-memory and concentration Score range 0–28	Weighted scoring system for total score of 28 Count errors Higher scores = more impairment	0–5 Normal 6–9 Questionable dementia 10–28 Dementia	High correlation (r=0.52) between score and autopsy findings of AD	Test focus on orientation, memory and concentration. May not detect non-amnestic dementias
Saint Louis university mental status (SLUMS)	11 items Score range 0–30	Add total number of correct answers Adjust scores for education less than 12 years Lower scores = more impairment	Cut off of 21–26: mild cognitive impairment 20 and below: dementia for high school education	Sensitivity 96–98 Specificity 61–100	Limited validation on different groups of patients from original study. Tests are complicated and take time to use in an office setting. Not as extensively studied as MMSE
Montreal cognitive assessment (MoCA)	12 items, multiple cognitive domains Score range 0–30	Add total number of correct answers Add 1 point for education less than 12 years Alternate forms available Lower scores = more impairment	26–30 Normal 0–26 Impaired	Sensitivity of 90 for MCI and 100 for dementia	Takes 10 min or more for patient with more severe impairment. Not as extensively studied as MMSE
AD8	8 items, Yes/No Score range 0–8	Add total number of "Yes" responses Higher scores = more impairment	0–1 Normal 2–8 Impaired	Sensitivity 90 Specificity 68	Depends on observant informant. In the absence of informant, the AD8 can be administered to patient
IQCODE	16-items, 5-point Likert scale Score range 0–30	Total score is derived by calculating the average of completed items Higher scores = more impairment	More than 3.44	Sensitivity 76–100 Specificity 65–86	Depends on observant informant.

interpreting the evaluation. In general there are two ways to assess the patient—informant assessments and performance testing.

Using performance testing, the clinician may gain a sense of the objective performance of the patient in relation to published normative values, usually corrected for age and education. If the patient was previously assessed, comparison to previous tests offers the potential to measure change. Brief performance tests while providing a "snap shot" of abilities at the time of examination, are themselves unable to provide information regarding change from previous abilities or how the scores on the tests interfere with the patients social and occupational functioning (i.e., their activities of daily living) (Table 4). The following are examples of general cognitive test commonly used for dementia detection in the clinical setting.

Mini Mental State Exam

The 30-item Mini-Mental State Exam (MMSE) test, which takes around 10 min to complete, has been frequently used for initial assessment of memory problem, and its sensitivity increases if a decline of the score over time is taken into account [9]. The MMSE covers six areas: (1) orientation, (2) registration, (3) attention and calculation, (4) recall, (5) language, and (6) ability to copy a figure. However, although the MMSE is quick and easy to administer, and can track the overall progression of cognitive decline, it may not pick up milder cases of impairment [53], particularly because of its greater emphasis on orientation (10 of 30 points), which is typically not impaired at the earliest stages of dementia. In addition, there are several issues associated with the MMSE, including bias according to age, race, education and socioeconomic status [5]. There are also copyright issues that may limit its use. Several diagnostic tests are now available for use in primary care as alternatives to the MMSE; these are continually being updated and simplified in order to provide brief, easy to administer, and effective diagnostic tools.

Mini-Cog

The Mini Cognitive Assessment Instrument (Mini-Cog) combines an un-cued 3-item recall test with a clock-drawing test that serves as a recall distractor; it can be administered in about 3 min and requires no special equipment [54]. The Mini-Cog, and the MMSE have similar sensitivity (76 % vs. 79 %) and specificity (89 % vs. 88 %) for dementia, correlating with finding achieved using a conventional neuropsychological battery. The Mini-Cog's brevity is a distinct advantage when the goal is to improve recognition of cognitive impairment in primary care [54]. The Mini-Cog is also associated with declines in activities of daily living. In addition, the Mini-Cog also has proven good performance in ethnically diverse populations of the US in which widely used cognitive screens often fail, and is easy to administer to non-English populations. Limitations may include unfamiliarity with how to tell time in illiterate populations and the absence of testing other cognitive domains.

Short Blessed Test

Short Blessed Test (SBT), consisting of the items in the Blessed orientation-memory-concentration test, includes three orientation questions (month, year and time of day), counting from 20 to 1, saying the months backward, and recalling a 5-item name and address memory phase [55]. There was a positive correlation between scores on the 6-item test and plaque counts obtained from the cerebral cortex of 38 subjects at autopsy [56]. This test, which is easily administered by a non-physician, has been shown to discriminate among mild, moderate, and severe cognitive deficits [55]. The SBT is quite sensitive to early cognitive changes due to AD with cut-off scores of 0–4 normal cognition, 5–9 questionable impairment, and 10 or more impairment consistent with dementia [56]. Given its focus of memory and orientation, the SBT may not pick up non-AD forms of dementia.

The Saint Louis University Mental Status

The Saint Louis University Mental Status (SLUMS) is a 30-point, 11-item, clinician-administered screening questionnaire that tests for orientation, memory, attention, and executive functions [57]. The SLUMS is similar in the format of MMSE, but includes additional tasks corresponding to attention, calculations, immediate and delayed recall, animal naming, digit span, clock drawing, figure recognition/size differentiation, and immediate recall of facts from a paragraph. At cuts off score of 27–30 normal, 21–26 mild neurocognitive disorder, and 1–20 dementia for high school education have 0.98 sensitivity and 0.61 specificity for MCI and 0.96 sensitivity and 1.0 specificity for dementia [57]. To date the SLUMS has not been validated outside of the original research sample although it is commonly used in Veterans Administration settings.

The Montreal Cognitive Assessment

The Montreal Cognitive Assessment (MoCA) is a 10-min cognitive screening tool developed to assist physicians in the detection of MCI [58]. MoCA improves sensitivity of detecting early impairments particularly frontal executive functioning. It has high sensitivity and specificity for detecting MCI in those patients who perform within the normal range of the MMSE. Compared with the MMSE, which had a sensitivity of 18 % to detect MCI, the MoCA detected 90 % of MCI subjects and, in patients with mild AD, the MMSE had a sensitivity of 78 %, whereas the MoCA detected 100 % [58]. MoCA is also well-suited as screening test for cognitive impairment in Parkinson disease [59], which memory impairment may be involved later in the stage of disease compared to executive function. The limitation of the MoCA may be in its more complex interpretation of scoring and possible susceptibility to cultural and educational biases.

Neuropsychological Testing

Formal neuropsychological testing provides a more comprehensive assessment of cognitive abilities with estimates of pre-morbid intelligence and provides profiles of performance that assist with differential diagnosis (Table 5). These assessments generally take several hours and are best interpreted by a neuropsychologist. Alternatively, many memory care centers perform their own testing to provide immediate results regarding the cognitive abilities of the patient. While creating a unique, brief psychometric battery might seem appealing, administration of even a brief battery can take 20–30 min. A common strategy is to combine individual cognitive domains to create a brief 20–30 min (depending on level of dementia severity and language ability) battery of tests that could be done in the office setting (Table 6). If this approach is taken, one must be mindful to purchase appropriate license fees and utilize published normative values adjusted for age and education for interpretation.

Informant-Based Tools for Cognitive Evaluation

The diagnosis of dementia is a clinical one, based on the principles of intra-individual decline in cognitive function that interferes with social and occupational functioning. The limitations to all brief performance measures is that they (1) fail to capture "change" and "interference" when used as a dementia screen and (2) may be biased by age, gender, race, education and culture. Informant-based instruments on the other rely on an observant collateral source to assess whether there have been changes in cognition and if said change interferes with function. A particular strength compared to other cognitive screening tests is that informant assessments are relatively unaffected by education and pre-morbid ability or by proficiency in the culture's dominant language. Because each person serves as their own control, there much less bias due to age,

Table 5 Cognitive profiles of common causes of dementia

Cognitive domain	Definition	AD	LBD	FTD	VaD
Episodic memory	Recall of newly learned information after a brief delay				
Free recall	Recall of information without prompts	+++	++	+/−	+
Recognition	Recognition of previously presented information	+++	−	−	−
Prompting	Using cues to prompt recall of information	×	√	√	√
Intrusions	False recall of information not presented in the task.	+++	+++	+++	+
Semantic memory	Knowledge of meaning of words, objects, actions, or ideas	++	+	+	+
Procedural memory	Knowing *how* to perform a task	−	+	−	+
Working memory	Mental manipulation of information	++	+++	+++	++
Insight	Awareness of personal cognitive, mood, and behavioral state	+++	+	+++	−
Attention	Focusing and concentration on a task	++	+++	++	++
Executive functions	Problem-solving tasks that require making choices or switching between different tasks	++	+++	+++	+++
Visuospatial skills	Hand-eye coordination, copying patterns or shapes	++	+++	−	+

Key: ×, no benefit; √, benefit; −, low likelihood of impairment; +, mild impairments; ++, moderate impairments; +++, significant impairments

Table 6 Example of a brief neurobehavioral status examination

Verbal memory	Animal naming Boston naming test Multilingual naming test
Working memory	Digit span forward Digit span backward Word fluency for letters F, A, and S
Episodic memory	Word list recall (Rey Hopkins, California, CERAD) Paragraph recall
Visual-construction	Clock drawing
Psychomotor speed	Trailmaking A
Executive function	Trailmaking B Digit symbol substitution
Abstraction	Similarities and differences Proverb Interpretation
Concentration	Months in reverse order Counting backward from 20
Global measurement (choose one)	Mini-mental status examination Short blessed test Montreal cognitive assessment
Mood (choose one)	Geriatric depression scale PHQ-9 Hospital anxiety and depression scale
Function (choose one)	Functional assessment questionnaire Adcs-activities of daily living scale Barthel index

education, gender or race [60]. The disadvantages of informant assessments are the reliability of the informant and the quality of the relationship between the informant and the patient. Because the informant assessments provide information complementary to cognitive tests, harnessing them together may improve screening accuracy.

A gold standard informant assessment is the Clinical Dementia Rating (CDR) [61] used in many clinical trials and research projects. However the length of the interview makes it impractical for use in the busy office setting. The value of including a reliable informant (spouse, adult child, paid caregiver) in the evaluation of cognitive and affective disorders in older adults has been incorporated into the following questionnaires.

AD-8

The AD8 is a brief screening interview comprises eight Yes/No questions asked of an informant to rate change, and takes approximately 2–3 min for the informant to complete. In the absence of an informant, the AD8 can be directly administered to the patient as a self-rating tool [19–22] with similar large effect sizes (Cohen d for informant = 1.66; for patient = 0.98). The AD8 reliably differentiates between individuals with and without dementia by querying memory, orientation, judgment, and function [19]. The AD8 is highly correlated with the CDR and neuropsychological testing as well amyloid PET imaging and cerebrospinal fluid biomarkers of AD [62]. Use of the AD8 in conjunction with a brief assessment of the participant, such as a word list, could improve detection of dementia in the primary setting to 97 % for dementia and 91 % for MCI [20]. The AD8 has a sensitivity of 84 %, and specificity of 80 % with excellent ability to discriminate between non-demented older adults and those with mild dementia (92 %) regardless of the cause of impairment [20]. The AD8 has been translated into Spanish [63], Portuguese [64], Korean [65] and Chinese [66] with similar psychometric properties.

The Informant Questionnaire on Cognitive Decline in the Elderly

The Informant Questionnaire on Cognitive Decline in the Elderly (IQCODE) measures cognitive decline from a pre-morbid level using informant reports [67]. A more commonly used 16-item short-version has largely replaced the original version. Informants rate the target's cognitive change compared to 10 years prior.

The IQCODE items represent everyday situations in which the patient uses his/her memory or knowledge. Respondents use a 5-point Likert scale to indicate the degree of change (1 = Much Improved to 5 = Much Worse) compared to 10 years prior with a score of 3 representing no change in the ability to complete the item. A total score is derived by calculating the average of completed items. The cut-off for dementia suggested in the literature ranges from 3.4 to 3.9 [68–70]. In clinical situations, a screening cut-off of 3.44+ on the Short IQCODE is a reasonable compromise for balancing sensitivity and specificity. The rating scale was designed to reflect cognitive improvement as well as cognitive decline, to allow for the questionnaire to be used in treatment trials and following acute illnesses [70].

In a comparison of the AD8 and the IQCODE, both were able to detect the presence of cognitive impairment in community settings and were highly correlated with brief assessments of cognitive ability (MMSE, Mini-Cog, Clock Drawing, and Animal Naming) that are commonly used in community settings [71]. Both the AD8 and IQCODE differentiated cognitively normal from individuals with dementia, however, the AD8 was better than the IQCODE in detecting MCI [71]. While the IQCODE covers two aspects of memory (acquisition of new information and retrieval of existing knowledge) and two aspects of intelligence (verbal and performance), the AD8 contains items that relate to memory, problem-solving abilities, orientation, and daily activities.

Concluding Comments

Alzheimer's disease, MCI and related disorders will become a public health crisis and a severe burden on Medicare in the next two decades unless actions are taken to (1) develop disease modifying medications, (2) provide clinicians with valid and reliable measures to detect disease at the earliest possible stage, and (3) reimburse clinicians for their time to evaluate patients [17]. Dementia screening requires a consideration of the population-at-risk and the sensitivity and specificity of the instruments used [11–13]. A large number of false positive individuals might expend limited health care dollars; a large number of individuals receiving false negatives would be denied treatment and miss opportunities to participate in clinical research. Thus, a staged dementia screening approach would make the most sense clinically and economically.

While cognitive disorders are common in older adults, memory complaints may not be readily offered by patients due to denial, lack of insight, fear of stigma and/or a general lack of knowledge about what is "normal" for age. The elements of a comprehensive mental status examination include observational, cognitive and neuropsychiatric assessments. In the absence of a comprehensive approach to evaluating cognitive abilities, it is unlikely a clinician will detect impairment at the mildest stages when intervention may offer the greatest potential for benefit. In addition, the presence of cognitive impairment leads to poorer adherence, higher costs and worse outcomes for other medical conditions compared with age-matched older adults without cognitive impairment. Whether the clinician designs their own unique assessments or utilizes one of the many standardized instruments available, failure to include a mental status examination in the assessment of older adults represents a missed opportunity.

In the environment of healthcare reform, it will be important for clinicians to use brief, sensitive and reliable methods to detect cognitive impairment in their patients across outpatient and inpatient settings. If simple screening for early cognitive impairment in the busy office setting is the goal then a brief interview tool (i.e., AD8) plus a brief performance measure (i.e., Mini-Cog) could be recommended, particularly because they meet the basic requirements of the Personalized Prevention Plan for Medicare beneficiaries.

Acknowledgements This work was supported by grants from the National Institutes of Health (R01 AG040211 and P30 AG008051), the New York State Department of Health (DOH-2011-1004010353 and DOH-2014-1306060830), and the Morris and Alma Schapiro Fund.

References

1. Alzheimer Disease Facts & Figures 2013. www.alz.org. Accessed 25 Jun 2014.
2. U.S. Surgeon General Office. www.surgeongeneral.gov/library/mentalhealth/chapter5/sec1.html. Accessed 25 Jun 2014.
3. Center for Medicare and Medicaid Services—Geographic Variation Public Use File. http://www.cms.gov/Research-Statistics-Data-and-Systems/Statistics-Trends-and-Reports/Medicare-Geographic-Variation/index.html. Accessed 25 Jun 2014.
4. United States Census Bureau. Annual projections of the resident population by age, sex, race and hispanic origin: lowest, middle, highest series and zero international migration series, 1999 to 2100. Accessed 25 Jun 2014.
5. Federal Interagency Forum on Aging-Related Statistics. Older Americans 2010: key indicators of well-being. Federal interagency forum on aging-related statistics. Washington, DC: US Government Printing Office; 2010, July. Accessed 25 Jun 2014.
6. Public Law 111-148. Patient protection and affordable care act. Accessed 25 Jun 2014.
7. U.S. Department of Health and Human Services. National plan to address Alzheimer's disease. Available at: http://aspe.hhs.gov/daltcp/napa/natlplan.shtml. Accessed 25 Jun 2014.
8. Lin JS, O'Connor E, Rossom RC, Perdue LA, Burda BU, Thompson M, Eckstrom E. Screening for cognitive impairment in older adults: an evidence update for the U.S. preventive services task force. Rockville, MD: Agency for Healthcare Research and Quality; 2013 Nov. [Internet].
9. Folstein MF, Folstein SE, McHugh PR. "Mini-mental state". A practical method for grading the cognitive state of patients for the clinician. J Psychiatr Res. 1975;12:189–98.
10. Espino DV, Lichtenstein MJ, Palmer RF, Hazuda HP. Evaluation of the mini-mental state examination's internal consistency in a community-based sample of Mexican-American and European-American elders: results from the San Antonio longitudinal study of aging. J Am Geriatr Soc. 2004;52:822–7.
11. Holsinger T, Deveau J, Boustani M, Williams Jr JW. Does this patient have dementia? JAMA. 2007;297:2391–404.
12. Galvin JE. Dementia screening, biomarkers and protein misfolding: implications for public health and diagnosis. Prion. 2011;5:16–21.
13. Cordell CB, Borson S, Boustani M, Chodosh J, Reuben D, Verghese J, et al. Medicare Detection of Cognitive Impairment Workgroup. Alzheimer's association recommendations for operationalizing the detection of cognitive impairment during the medicare annual wellness visit in a primary care setting. Alzheimers Dement. 2013;9:141–50.
14. Barnett JH, Lewis L, Blackwell AD, Taylor M. Early intervention in Alzheimer's disease: a health economic

study of the effects of diagnostic timing. BMC Neurol. 2014;14:101.

15. Borson S, Frank L, Bayley PJ, Boustani M, Dean M, Lin PJ, et al. Improving dementia care: the role of screening and detection of cognitive impairment. Alzheimers Dement. 2013;9:151–9.

16. Connolly A, Gaehl E, Martin H, Morris J, Purandare N. Underdiagnosis of dementia in primary care: variations in the observed prevalence and comparisons to the expected prevalence. Aging Ment Health. 2011;5:978–84.

17. Galvin JE, Meuser TM, Morris JC. Improving physician awareness of Alzheimer disease and enhancing recruitment: the clinician partners program. Alzheimer Dis Assoc Disord. 2012;26:61–7.

18. Doody RS, Ferris SH, Salloway S, Meusser TM, Murthy AK, Li C, et al. Identifying amnestic mild cognitive impairment in primary care: a feasibility study. Clin Drug Investig. 2011;31:483–91.

19. Galvin JE, Roe C, Coats M, Powlishta KK, Muich SJ, Grant E, et al. The AD8: a brief informant interview to detect dementia. Neurology. 2005;65:559–64.

20. Galvin JE, Roe CM, Xiong C, Morris JC. The validity and reliability of the AD8 informant interview for dementia. Neurology. 2006;67:1942–8.

21. Galvin JE, Roe CM, Coats MA, Morris JC. Patients rating of cognitive ability: using the AD8, a brief informant interview as a self-rating tool to detect dementia. Arch Neurol. 2007;64:725–30.

22. Galvin JE, Roe CM, Morris JC. Evaluation of cognitive impairment in the older adult: combining brief informant and performance measures. Arch Neurol. 2007;64:718–24.

23. National Guideline Clearinghouse (NGC). Guideline synthesis: diagnosis and assessment of Alzheimer's disease and related dementias. Agency for Healthcare Research and Quality 2006. Available at: http://www.guideline.gov. Accessed 14 Aug 2014.

24. Boustani MA, Justiss MD, Frame A, Austrom MG, Perkins AJ, Cai X, et al. Caregiver and noncaregiver attitudes toward dementia screening. J Am Geriatr Soc. 2011;59:681–6.

25. Galvin JE, Fu Q, Nguyen JT, Glasheen C, Scharff DP. Psychosocial determinants of intention to screen for Alzheimer Disease. Alzheimers Dement. 2008;4:353–60.

26. Biagioni M, Galvin JE. Using biomarkers to improve detection of Alzheimer's disease. Neurodegener Dis Manag. 2011;1:127–39.

27. Jack Jr CR, Knopman DS, Jagust WJ, Shaw LM, Aisen PS, Weiner MW, Petersen RC, Trojanowski JQ. Hypothetical model of dynamic biomarkers of the Alzheimer's pathological cascade. Lancet Neurol. 2010;9:119–28.

28. Consensus report of the Working Group on: "Molecular and Biochemical Markers of Alzheimer's Disease". The Ronald and Nancy Reagan Research Institute of the Alzheimer's Association and the National Institute on Aging Working Group. Neurobiol Aging. 1998;19:109–16.

29. Frank RA, Galasko D, Hampel H, Hardy J, de Leon MJ, Mehta PD, et al. Biological markers for therapeutic trials in Alzheimer's disease. Proceedings of the biological markers working group; NIA initiative on neuroimaging in Alzheimer's disease. Neurobiol Aging. 2003;24:521–36.

30. Braak H, Braak E. Neuropathological stageing of Alzheimer-related changes. Acta Neuropathol. 1991;82:239–59.

31. Terry RD, Masliah E, Salmon DP, Butters N, DeTeresa R, Hill R, et al. Physical basis of cognitive alterations in Alzheimer's disease: synapse loss is the major correlate of cognitive impairment. Ann Neurol. 1991;30:572–80.

32. Gomez-Isla T, Hollister R, West H, Mui S, Growdon JH, Petersen RC, et al. Neuronal loss correlates with but exceeds neurofibrillary tangles in Alzheimer's disease. Ann Neurol. 1997;41:17–24.

33. Weinstein G, Seshadri S. Circulating biomarkers that predict incident dementia. Alzheimers Res Ther. 2014;6:6.

34. Kim DH, Yeo SH, Park JM, Choi JY, Lee TH, Park SY, et al. Genetic markers for diagnosis and pathogenesis of Alzheimer's disease. Gene. 2014;545:185–93.

35. Cohen AD, Klunk WE. Early detection of Alzheimer's disease using PiB and FDG PET. Neurobiol Dis. 2014;72(Pt A):117–22.

36. Blennow K, Dubois B, Fagan AM, Lewczuk P, de Leon MJ, Hampel H. Clinical utility of cerebrospinal fluid biomarkers in the diagnosis of early Alzheimer's disease. Alzheimers Dement. 2015;11(1):58–69.

37. Ferreira D, Perestelo-Pérez L, Westman E, Wahlund LO, Sarría A, Serrano-Aguilar P. Meta-review of CSF core biomarkers in Alzheimer's disease: the state-of-the-art after the new revised diagnostic criteria. Front Aging Neurosci. 2014;6:47.

38. Landau SM, Harvey D, Madison CM, Reiman EM, Foster NL, Aisen PS, et al. Comparing predictors of conversion and decline in mild cognitive impairment. Neurology. 2010;75:230–8.

39. Wang L, Miller JP, Gado MH, McKeel DW, Rothermich M, Miller MI, et al. Abnormalities of hippocampal surface structure in very mild dementia of the Alzheimer type. Neuroimage. 2006;30:52–60.

40. Langbaum JB, Chen K, Caselli RJ, Lee W, Reschke C, Bandy D, et al. Hypometabolism in Alzheimer-affected brain regions in cognitively healthy Latino individuals carrying the apolipoprotein E epsilon4 allele. Arch Neurol. 2010;67:462–8.

41. Glodzik L, de Santi S, Tsui WH, Mosconi L, Zinkowski R, Pirraglia E, et al. Phosphorylated tau 231, memory decline and medial temporal atrophy in normal elders. Neurobiol Aging. 2011;32:2131–41.

42. Fagan AM, Roe CM, Xiong C, Mintun MA, Morris JC, Holtzman DM. Cerebrospinal fluid tau/beta-amyloid(42) ratio as a prediction of cognitive decline in nondemented older adults. Arch Neurol. 2007;64:343–9.

43. Shaw LM, Vanderstichele H, Knapik-Czajka M, Clark CM, Aisen PS, Petersen RC, et al. Cerebrospinal

fluid biomarker signature in Alzheimer's disease neuroimaging initiative subjects. Ann Neurol. 2009; 65:403–13.

44. Jack CR, Barrio JR, Kepe V. Cerebral amyloid PET imaging in Alzheimer's disease. Acta Neuropathol. 2013;126:643–57.

45. Sevush S. Relationship between denial of memory deficit and dementia severity in Alzheimer disease. Neuropsychiatry Neuropsychol Behav Neurol. 1999;12:88–94.

46. Derousen C, Thibault S, Lagha-Pierucci S, Baudouin-Madec V, Aneri D, Lacomblez L. Decreased awareness of cognitive deficits in patients with mild dementia of the Alzheimer type. Int J Geriatr Psychiatry. 1999;14:1019–30.

47. Barrett AM, Eslinger PJ, Ballentine NH, Heilman KM. Unawareness of cognitive deficit (cognitive anosognosia) in probable AD and control subjects. Neurology. 2005;64:693–9.

48. Hardy RM, Oyebode JR, Clare L. Measuring awareness in people with mild to moderate Alzheimer's disease: development of the memory awareness rating scale—adjusted. Neuropsychol Rehabil. 2006;16:178–93.

49. Sevush S, Leve N. Denial of memory deficit in Alzheimer's disease. Am J Psychiatry. 1993;150:748–51.

50. Bureau-Chalot F, Novella JL, Jolly D, Ankri J, Guillemin F, Blanchard F. Feasibility, acceptability and internal consistency reliability of the Nottingham health profile in dementia patients. Gerontology. 2002;48:220–5.

51. Yesavage JA. Geriatric depression scale. Psychopharmacol Bull. 1988;24:709–11.

52. James BD, Xie SX, Karlawish JH. How do patients with Alzheimer disease rate their overall quality of life? Am J Geriatr Psychiatry. 2005;13:484–90.

53. deSouza L, Sarazin M, Goetz C, Dubois B. Clinical investigations in primary care. Front Neurol Neurosci. 2009;24:1–11.

54. Borson S, Scanlan JM, Watanabe J, Tu SP, Lessig M. Simplifying detection of cognitive impairment: comparison of the mini-cog and mini-mental state examination in a multiethnic sample. J Am Geriatr Soc. 2005;53:871–4.

55. Katzman R, Brown T, Fuld P, Peck A, Schechter R, Schimmel H. Validation of a short orientation-memory concentration test of cognitive impairment. Am J Psychiatry. 1983;140:734–9.

56. Morris JC, Heyman A, Mohs RC, Hughes JP, van Belle G, Fillenbaum G, Mellits ED, Clark C. The consortium to establish a registry for Alzheimer's disease (CERAD). Part I. Clinical and neuropsychological assessment of Alzheimer's disease. Neurology. 1989;39:1159–65.

57. Tariq SH, Tumosa N, Chibnall JT, Perry III MH, Morley JE. Comparison of the Saint Louis university mental status examination and the mini-mental state examination for detecting dementia and mild neuro-cognitive disorder—a pilot study. Am J Geriatr Psychiatry. 2006;14:900–10.

58. Nasreddine ZS, Phillips NA, Bedirian V, Charbonneau W, Whitehead V, Collin I, et al. The montreal cognitive assessment, MoCA: a brief screening tool for mild cognitive impairment. J Am Geriatr Soc. 2005;53:695–9.

59. Dalrymple-Alford JC, MacAskill MR, Nakas CT, Livingston L, Graham C, Crucian GP, et al. The MoCA: well-suited screen for cognitive impairment in Parkinson disease. Neurology. 2010;75:1717–25.

60. Morales JM, Bermejo F, Romero M, Del-Ser T. Screening of dementia in community dwelling elderly through informant report. Int J Geriatr Psychiatry. 1997;12:808–16.

61. Morris JC. The clinical dementia rating (CDR): current version and scoring rules. Neurology. 1993;43:2412–4.

62. Galvin JE, Fagan AM, Holtzman DM, Mintun MA, Morris JC. Relationship of dementia screening tests with biomarkers of Alzheimer's disease. Brain. 2010;133:3290–300.

63. Carnero Pardo C, de la Vega Cotarelo R, Lopez Alcalde D, Martos Aparicio C, Vilchez Carillo R, Mora Gavilan E, et al. Assessing the diagnostic accuracy (DA) of the Spanish version of the informant-based AD8. Neurologia. 2013;28:88–94.

64. Correia CC, Lima F, Junqueira F, Campos MS, Batos O, Petribu K, et al. AD8-Brazil: cross-cultural validation of the ascertaining dementia interview in Portuguese. J Alzheimers Dis. 2011;27:177–85.

65. Ryu HJ, Kim HJ, Han SH. Validity and reliability of the Korean version of the AD8 informant interview (K-AD8) in dementia. Alzheimer Dis Assoc Disord. 2009;23:371–6.

66. Yang YH, Galvin JE, Morris JC, Lai CL, Chou MC, Lie CK. Application of AD8 questionnaire to screen very mild dementia in Taiwanese. Am J Alzheimers Dis Other Demen. 2011;26:134–8.

67. Jorm AF, Christensen H, Henderson AS, et al. Informant ratings of cognitive decline of elderly people: relationship to longitudinal change on cognitive tests. Age Ageing. 1996;25:125–9.

68. Jorm AF, Jacomb PA. The informant questionnaire on cognitive decline in the elderly (IQCODE): sociodemographic correlates, reliability, validity and some norms. Psychol Med. 1989;19:1015–22.

69. Jorm AF, Scott R, Cullen JS, et al. Performance of the informant questionnaire on cognitive decline in the elderly (IQCODE) as a screening test for dementia. Psychol Med. 1991;21:785–90.

70. Jorm AF. The informant questionnaire on cognitive decline in the elderly (IQCODE): a review. Int Psychogeriatr. 2004;16:275–93.

71. Razavi M, Tolea MI, Margrett J, Martin P, Oakland A, Tscholl DW, Ghods S, Mina M, Galvin JE. Comparison of 2 informant questionnaire screening tools for dementia and mild cognitive impairment: AD8 and IQCODE. Alzheimer Dis Assoc Disord. 2014;28:156–61.

Memory Clinics and Care Management Programs

Yael R. Zweig

Memory Clinics and Care Management Programs

Memory clinics provide a specialized, evidence-based, and multidisciplinary approach to the comprehensive diagnosis, assessment, management and treatment of persons with memory impairments, and provide support to those who care for them. Memory clinics are not universally defined; thus they vary a great deal depending on affiliation, location, and population. Most commonly, memory clinics combine research and clinical care for persons across the continuum of symptomatology with a special focus on early diagnosis and diagnosis of unusual or atypical presentations. Support, counseling, and resources for caregivers are also an integral part of memory clinics.

Memory care in the United States (US) is often provided in the primary care setting, where the majority of older adults receive medical care. Known limitations to memory care in primary care include lack of provider knowledge, time concerns, and ineffective or inappropriate symptom management [1]. Worldwide, most people with dementia do not receive a diagnosis and only 20–50 % of diagnoses are made in primary care. Early diagnosis helps patients and families plan for the future and receive appropriate treatment and intervention earlier in the disease state [2]. Early diagnosis of dementia also allows for opportunities for research participation and may improve care outcomes [3]. Diagnostic disclosure of dementia is accepted by patients and families particularly if they are well prepared and supported during the diagnostic process. The World Alzheimer's Report has recommended countries establish a network of specialized diagnostic centers for this purpose of confirming early dementia diagnoses and providing care management [2].

This chapter will discuss the history and description of memory clinics in the US and abroad, the population served, collaborative care and staffing, patient and caregiver outcomes and care management models. While memory clinics are now present worldwide, this chapter will focus on the US and Europe where they were initially introduced and described.

History

Memory clinics were first established in the US in the 1970s and later in the United Kingdom (UK), with the first UK memory clinic established in 1983 [4]. The first report of memory clinics in the UK and Ireland described 20 clinics which were primarily hospital based specialized services focused on clinical drug trials [5]. Similarly, in the US memory clinics were designed around academic institutions interested

Y.R. Zweig, MSN, ANP-BC, GNP-BC (✉)
Department of Geriatrics, New York University
Langone Medical Center, 550 First Avenue,
New York, NY 10016, USA
e-mail: yael.zweig@nyumc.org

© Springer International Publishing Switzerland 2016
M. Boltz, J.E. Galvin (eds.), *Dementia Care*, DOI 10.1007/978-3-319-18377-0_4

in Alzheimer's disease research. Early services and goals included early diagnosis and treatment, identification and treatment of concomitant disorders outside of dementia, evaluation of new therapeutic agents for treatment, and to provide reassurance to the worried well [6].

Initially memory clinics were more academic in scope but have expanded to provide care post diagnosis as well, particularly after the 1990s with the introduction of cholinesterase inhibitors [7, 8]. A UK survey comparing memory clinics from an initial survey in 1993 and then a repeat survey in 1999–2000 found over time less clinics actively involved in research, more clinics initiating and monitoring treatments, and a higher percentage of early onset dementia services [9]. A more recent continuation survey over the past 10 years has not been reported.

Memory clinics in the US are often part of geriatric, neurology, or psychiatry practices and are not always affiliated with academic medical centers. There are no formal guidelines for what constitutes a "memory clinic" so the range of services is broad. The National Institute on Aging funds Alzheimer's Disease Centers (ADC) at academic institutions across the US. ADCs provide comprehensive research diagnostic evaluations, patient and caregiver information and resources, and volunteer opportunities to participate in clinical trials or other research projects. ADCs may also include satellite programs for underserved populations including minority or rural communities. There are 29 ADCs funded in the US in 19 states as of 2014 [10]. ADCs are research centers and participants who are followed longitudinally and found to have any cognitive decline, would need to be referred for clinical evaluation and treatment. Therefore ADCs often have affiliated clinical memory clinics for referrals from research projects either incorporated in the ADC research center, or affiliated but distinct clinical memory clinics.

In the US, The National Alzheimer's Project Act (NAPA) was signed into law in 2011. The major goals of NAPA are the prevention and treatment of Alzheimer's disease by 2025, optimize care quality and efficiency, expand support for people with AD and their families, finance public awareness and engagement, and track progress to drive improvement [11]. While there is no explicit focus on memory clinics, they do address the NAPA goals and may receive financing through development of innovative models of care, such as one described at University of California, Los Angeles [12].

Memory clinics have been mandated by the England National Dementia Strategy (NDS) in all specialist mental health service for older adults [13]. The NDS is a government initiative launched in 2009 to help achieve goals including raising awareness of dementia, early diagnosis and intervention, and increasing quality of care. The NDS stipulates that the aim of memory clinics is to provide good-quality diagnoses early in the disease course with good quality interventions and to provide the service to those who need it in a given population [4]. After the launch of the NDS in England, the number of memory clinics in the UK increased from 20 in 1995 to at least 58 in 2002 [9]. As of 1999–2000, 44 clinics were in England, five in Scotland, four in Wales, and five in Northern Ireland [9]. A more recent national survey of memory clinics in the Republic of Ireland in 2011 reports the presence of 14 clinics. Of those, the majority are hospital based, located in Dublin, and led by psychiatrists or geriatricians. Less than half of the clinics employ allied health professionals and are active in research [13].

Funding

Individual US states may provide their own funding source for memory services. For example in New York State there are nine Alzheimer's Disease Assistance Centers (ADACs) affiliated with universities and hospitals. ADACs provide diagnosis and assessment of patients, particularly those with atypical or unusual presentations, care management strategies, continuing education to patients, families, and health care professionals, and serve as regional information resource centers [14]. Similarly California funds 10 California

Alzheimer's Disease Centers (CADC) at academic medical centers. Services include diagnosis and treatment of memory disorders, community events for patients and families, and professional training for those in medical specialties. There is additional funding to support Alzheimer's disease research [15]. Florida has an Alzheimer's Disease Initiative that provides funding for caregiver respite and support, memory disorder clinics, adult day programs, and a research database [16]. Memory clinics in the US may receive funding in the same way as other specialty practices by insurance billings or receive monies from participating in clinical trials, grants from state or federal programs as described, or through a fee for service structure.

In England the NDS provided 150 million pounds to Primary Care Trusts (PCTs) to promote early diagnosis and to improve dementia quality of care. One of the mechanisms by which PCTs could achieve these goals is through the provision of memory clinics [17]. Most memory clinics in the UK are funded by the National Health Service (NHS). Other funding sources come from pharmaceutical companies, universities, and medical charities, or some combination of sources [9]. Memory clinic quality standards in the UK are monitored by the Memory Services National Accreditation Programme (MSNAP), and other standards have been adopted in Denmark and the Netherlands [13].

Description

Memory clinics are variable in their overall practice, but the structure of a core staff with a set schedule and location to evaluation patients and families is a shared phenomenon [18]. Jolley [13] describes essential components of a memory clinic including the appropriate place and team with 24 h availability. The "place" should understandably be easily accessible, and examination and conference rooms should be sizeable enough to incorporate the interdisciplinary care team. The memory clinic setting should also include private and quiet accommodations for psychometric testing. The waiting area should be handicap accessible and take into account behavioral triggers for patients with more severe cognitive impairments who can be more easily overstimulated.

An interdisciplinary team is important to provide ongoing consistent care to patients and families outside of the medical scope alone. Staffing and collaborative care will be described later in this chapter. The medical, neurologic, and psychiatric assessments are not standardized but generally includes a comprehensive history of physical and mental health, psychosocial evaluation, medication review, psychometric testing, and assessment of mood, behavior, and function. The patient should undergo standardized psychometric testing and a physical and neurologic exam should be completed. Clinics usually complete or refer for laboratory testing and imaging to evaluate for reversible causes of dementia, or to provide diagnostic clarity. Some clinics complete the entirety of the evaluation in one visit while others complete it over several visits. A collateral source (CS), defined as anyone who can attest to the patient's change in memory, language, or function over time, should be interviewed to provide a history of intra-individual change. Equally the caregiver, if there is one, should be evaluated for stress, burden, and indices of mood [6]. An example of the patient and CS components of a memory clinic assessment and management are described in Table 1.

A survey of memory clinics in the UK reported providing the following functions in order of highest percentage: specialist assessments and/or second opinions, caregiver and patient advice and information, initiating and monitoring treatment, management recommendations, education and training, research and drug trials, and medicolegal assessments [9]. Most clinics reported operating on a weekly to monthly schedule with only 14 % operating more than once per week. There was a trend in the later survey to suggest that newer NHS funded clinics were smaller and evaluate less patients with shorter assessments with a concentration on services rather than research and education [19].

Table 1 Memory clinic assessment and management components

Overview: Comprehensive history from patient and collateral source (CS) including medical, psychiatric, social, and family history; review of prescription and non-prescription medications; evaluation of literacy, culture, and language

Patient evaluation	CS evaluation
– Psychometric testing assessing multiple cognitive domains or formal neuropsychological testing – Mood screening – Comprehensive physical and neurologic exam – Laboratory evaluation CBC, CMP, B12, folate, thyroid function (Urinalysis, syphilis, HIV only if risk factors present) – Structural brain imaging (MRI or CT)	– Functional evaluation and behavior assessment (i.e., Neuropsychiatric Inventory) of patient – Consider additional tools such as Mayo Fluctuation Questionnaire and/or Mayo Sleep Questionnaire based on history – Psychosocial interview to determine resources and supports – Caregiver burden assessment

Development of the plan of care
- Conference with care team, patient, and family to review findings and develop plan
- Provide both verbal and written feedback on specific diagnosis and recommendations including follow-up
- Communicate results with primary care providers and referring providers
- Start cholinesterase inhibitors and memantine where indicated
- Discontinue any medications that may be adversely affecting cognition
- Treat behavioral and psychological symptoms if present
- Use nonpharmacologic interventions before medication to treat behavior unless severity is sufficient to interfere with care or safety
- Address safety needs (wandering, home safety and fall prevention, driving, medication management)
- Assess for risk of abuse
- Discuss advance directives
- Discuss plan to promote mental and physical activity and social engagement
- Utilize referrals to providers who may not be a part of the in-office memory clinic team such as physical and occupational therapists, pharmacists, psychologists, geriatric care managers
- Monitor and continually re-assess caregiver needs (disease information, referrals, financial and legal planning, support groups, home care, respite, day care, meal services)
- Refer for opportunities to participate in research

One of the primary goals of memory clinics is to make or confirm diagnoses in the early stage of disease, or in younger onset, less common, or atypical presentations. Once a diagnosis is established, families often look to memory clinics to help address social or ethical issues such as driving safety, financial planning, decision making ability, jury duty exclusions, and retirement or employment concerns. Memory clinics should have means to help caregivers if and when assessment findings are concerning. This may include management or prevention of current or future burden through education and provision of proactive strategies to prevent crises, community services and resources, support groups, and concrete services such as adult day programs, meal delivery, home care, and respite care. Close relationships with community service and support agencies are crucial. The type of relationship and

follow-up with community services varies depending on patient and caregiver needs and service availability. In the US, the Alzheimer's Association has a 24 h/7 day per week helpline which is free and provides phone based support.

Memory clinics also play an important role in education and training of health care professionals and the public at large. Funding for memory clinics often incorporates the need for community outreach and educational programs for multidisciplinary professionals across the spectrum from prevention and screening through end stage memory care and symptom management. Memory clinics act often as models of best practice standards in the provision of information, teaching, and research [18]. Memory clinics are important rotations for all health professionals in training, as the aging population makes geriatric and dementia education particularly prescient.

Patient and caregiver education should occur at every visit, and memory clinics, particularly those affiliated with academic institutions and research centers, host public seminars on dementia topics of interest. Memory clinics may also partner with community organizations that play a large role in education such as the Alzheimer's Association and Alzheimer's Society [20].

A variety of research projects can be a component of memory clinics, but not required and present in all clinics. Early memory clinics were more research based and the overlap between research and clinical practice has persisted. New interventions can be translated more smoothly into clinical practice in the memory clinic setting [6]. Additionally memory centers can promote research recruitment through its clinical activity and role in community education and outreach.

Population Served

Memory clinics are primarily geared towards the neurodegenerative diagnoses most common in the aging population including Alzheimer's disease, Lewy body dementia, vascular cognitive impairment, and frontotemporal degeneration. Due to the multiple factors associated with memory complaints, memory clinics may also treat concomitant psychiatric illness such as depression and anxiety. However, persons with more prominent psychiatric disorders are less appropriate for memory clinic evaluations [7]. While memory can be affected in many different disorders such as traumatic brain injury, memory clinics are more commonly designed to address mild cognitive impairment or dementia due to neurodegenerative diseases. Memory clinics at academic medical centers are more likely to evaluate patients with unusual or atypical presentations.

Referrals may come from the "worried well", self-referrals from patients, families or caregivers, primary care providers, or other providers such as those in emergency care who have picked up on symptomatology associated with undiagnosed dementia. Self-referrals may be more common in the US depending on insurance reimbursement. Most older adults have Medicare, which traditionally doesn't require a referral to see a specialist. In the UK general practitioners (GP) provide referrals to specialist care. Patients sometimes approach their GP with concern about their memory but more commonly reported was a joint approach with concern from both the patient and their carer. GPs typically support collaboration with the specialist memory team [21]. Self-referrals to memory clinics may help to reduce barriers to early diagnosis. However one concern with self-referrals is the risk of using resources to evaluate the worried well [6].

The socio-demographic profile of patients attending memory clinics is not well-defined, and varies by country and type of memory clinic. Patients from nine memory clinics in Australia were evaluated at baseline and again at 6 months. Patients who were attending memory clinics in this sample were more likely to be men living with a spouse, and had mild dementia, most commonly AD [22]. The sample may have been skewed more male due to female caregivers being proactive about pursuing care. A memory service in the UK similarly collected demographic information at baseline and again at 6 months reported more females, with the most common diagnoses of Alzheimer's disease or mixed dementia, and also more likely in the mild stage [23].

In the US there is no standardized reporting of memory clinics and program descriptions often come from models described in the literature. The University of California, Los Angeles Alzheimer's and Dementia Care program, has described their patient characteristics with a mean age of 81 years, mostly female, and with moderate to severe Alzheimer's disease [12]. The New York University Center for Cognitive Neurology collected patient characteristics for a brief period of time and described a mean age of 78, close to half female, and milder impairments with a wider range of diagnoses describing 38 % carrying an AD diagnosis with and without co-morbid vascular disease [24]. The Healthy Aging Brain Center (HABC) from Indiana described a mean age of 73.8 years, 40 % African American, and 46 % diagnosed with dementia [25].

Telemedicine in Memory Care

Challenges in rural dementia care have been described internationally and include the limited availability of memory care services, long travel distances, and transportation challenges [26]. Additionally there may be waiting lists for care, especially in areas where services are less robust [27]. Telemedicine is an innovative approach to provide care in underserved and rural areas. Telemedicine involves the exchange of medical care from one site to another through the use of telecommunication technology to improve patient's health status [28].

Memory clinics have been described where follow-up care is provided remotely after a comprehensive initial in-office visit has been completed. One example from rural Canada provides an interdisciplinary assessment of dementia through a weekly clinic including a neurologist, neuropsychology team, geriatrician, neuroradiologist, and physical therapist. Patients and their families are evaluated by all team members over the course of one clinic day. Their rural primary care physician is invited to participate in a diagnostic conference call with the team and then telehealth appointments were offered to patients in rural areas for follow-up visits. Patients and caregivers have reported high satisfaction with the in-person assessment and telehealth option for follow-up [26]. Similarly, another Canadian study evaluated patients in rural areas initially for an in-person geriatrician consultation and then in follow-up using a telemedicine system. The majority of participants reported interest in using the videoconferencing system again and felt confident in the physician diagnostic assessment, although expressed more anxiety compared to the in-person session. Overall high satisfaction was reported from patients and physicians in this study with a small sample size [27].

Other studies have reported on memory clinics that do not involve an initial in-office consultation. Rural veterans were evaluated by a memory disorders clinic (MDC) physician using a video-telemedicine system coordinated by their community clinic. A rural clinician remained present with the patient and caregiver, while the MDC physician completed a comprehensive evaluation including history, caregiver interview, neurologic exam, and a consensus diagnosis. The diagnosis was communicated to the patient and caregiver and the primary care provider was invited to a post clinic conference to review treatment and follow-up. In most cases the primary providers followed recommendations and patients and providers expressed positive feedback with the process. This study demonstrated reliability of the procedure, but more evidence is needed to confirm diagnostic consistency [29].

Telemedicine has been hypothesized to reduce costs but has not been comprehensively evaluated in memory care. An Australian study evaluated memory clinics where a specialist travels to a rural area to evaluate patients versus a videoconferencing clinic where the specialist completed similar assessments via videoconference. The videoconference dementia evaluation of patients in rural areas was found to be cost effective if the specialist has to travel two or more hours to provide a face to face consultation [30].

Collaborative Care in the Memory Clinic Setting

The evaluation of patients with memory disorders and their families is inherently collaborative due to the unique nature of managing a progressive chronic disease that affects the person and those caring for them. Additional care challenges include patient lack of insight and behavioral manifestations that are often best managed using nonpharmacologic approaches which require time intensive caregiver education and continued clinician reinforcement. A multidisciplinary approach to care involves professionals performing their own independent assessments and sharing communication without direct interaction [24, 31]. The preferable approaches are interdisciplinary, where professionals exchange information through collaborative communication and work together to deliver quality care, or transdisciplinary, involving frequent and effective communication and crossing of traditional disciplinary boundaries [31]. Patients and families often require care outside of the medical model of diagnosis and medical management alone. The inclusion of social supports, therapeutic interventions, counseling, and nursing services comes from collaborative care among multiple disciplines.

Collaborative care models may include care managers who oversee and coordinate care, as has been described in other chronic diseases such as depression and anxiety [32]. Collaborative care models have also been described as team-based multicomponent interventions that improve patient centered care and help to deliver integrated health and medical care to patients and families [24]. The nature of the diagnostic process in memory clinics is time and labor intensive and not reimbursed as well as other medical specialties. This lends itself well to collaborative care approaches for each member of the care team to provide their own clinical, management, and/or administrative strengths to improve care outcomes.

Collaborative is defined differently among disciplines and the model of care, be it physician led or otherwise, can be malleable depending on the memory care team. Most of the available evidence evaluating collaborative care approaches involves either a physician (MD) or nurse practitioner (NP) collaboration with the NP serving in a care management role [12, 33, 34] or social work care management [35, 36]. Models have been described in which a collaborative memory care clinic has been set up within a primary care practice [34, 37] or as a stand-alone clinic [24, 25]. A home based collaborative care assessment has been described in the Croydon Memory Service Model (CMSM) where any team member, regardless of their clinical background, can complete the initial patient assessment. Once the diagnosis is made, the management of the patient is guided by the multidisciplinary team [23].

Another example of a unique collaborative care model is the Alzheimer's Education Center (ACE) in Spain, which started as a day center and evolved into a memory clinic. It includes a Memory Disorders Unit, with staff such as neurologists, geriatricians, neuropsychologists, social workers, nurses, and technical staff, as well as a comprehensive research team. An outreach team manages publications, education, and seminars and a continuity of care team provides services to patients at the affiliated therapeutic day center [38].

Staffing

A survey of memory clinics from the UK suggests a wide range of staffing with one to nine individuals regularly present at memory clinics. Most commonly reported professionals were psychiatrists as the lead clinician, nurses, psychologists, geriatricians, and neurologists. A smaller percentage included occupational and speech therapists and almost a quarter received input from the Alzheimer's society. Nurses were more likely to be involved compared to an earlier survey of memory clinics in the 1990s [9]. In Ireland most memory clinics are staffed by old age psychiatrists or geriatricians, nurses, and some provide referrals to social work, occupational therapy, or neuropsychology [13]. A comprehensive interdisciplinary memory clinic in Canada described a model utilizing family physicians, consultative geriatricians, nurses, social work, optometry, and pharmacy [39].

Professionals who are more commonly part of interdisciplinary collaborative care memory clinics will be described in more detail.

Physician

Physicians most likely to practice in memory clinics have completed medical school, residency, and a fellowship in either neurology or geriatric psychiatry. Geriatricians are primary care providers with expertise in the care of older adults and may also be part of memory clinic teams. Geriatric psychiatrists are particularly helpful in managing complex behavioral manifestations and memory complaints either as a result of or co-existent with depression, anxiety, or other psychiatric disorders. Behavioral neurologists are subspecialists with training to manage behavior and cognition on the neurological basis of disease. Neurologists, especially those with a subspecialty in movement disorders, can evaluate for Parkinsonism or other movement abnormalities seen in neurodegenerative diseases.

Nurse Practitioner/Physician Assistant

Nurse practitioners (NPs) are registered nurses with Master's degrees, post-Master's degree certificates, and/or doctor of nursing practice degree (DNP). NPs undergo training in specialty areas and obtain national certification and state licensure. Individual states regulate whether NPs can evaluate, manage, and treat patients independently of a physician or in a collaborative or supervisory model [40]. They have prescriptive authority throughout the US [40].

Physician Assistant (PA) programs are generally 2 year post-baccalaureate, and require some level of medical exposure. Training programs provide clinical rotations across the lifespan. PAs must also have national certification and state licensure to practice. State laws dictate scope of practice and physician oversight. They may provide follow-up visits and have prescriptive authority in all the US [40].

The MD-NP/PA collaborative relationship in memory care specifically can be individualized depending on the practice and billing structure. The MD should provide guidance on complex or uncommon diagnoses, review of imaging, and management when the clinical course is complicated or not progressing in an expected fashion. In a primary care practice, the MD may also help to determine when a specialist referral is needed. The memory clinic practice may choose to have the MD make the initial cognitive diagnosis and initiate the medical work-up, and then have the NP/PA focus on evaluating the patient and caregiver in follow-up for medication and symptom management, and re-assessment of behavior, mood, and function. NP/PAs help to prevent complications and emergencies through enhanced in-office availability for appointments or by phone consultation. They also help with care coordination among other health care professionals and support nurses and social workers in referrals or patient and family education that requires more medical expertise.

Registered Nurse

Registered nurses must pass a national exam and undergo training via different pathways. Nurses may complete a 2 year Associate degree in nursing with a more focused scope of practice, a 4 year Bachelor of Science in Nursing, or less common diploma programs. Nurses are able to perform physical exams and take health histories, administer medication, provide patient care services, and educate patients and caregivers. They are trained to care for patients and families across the lifespan in multiple settings [41].

Just as the registered nurse performs routine vital signs on patients in the office, they can also perform the equivalent in a memory context by completing screenings or monitoring tools that allow for objective re-evaluation of change in performance and/or function over time. The nurse may also be the most intimately involved in patient and caregiver phone follow-up and ascertain their own assessment of cognitive decline in the form of missed appointments, confusion about instructions and follow-ups, and medication errors. The registered nurse can help assist with outpatient referrals to disease specific organizations, provide caregiver support, and provide education on medication compliance, safety, behavior management and other dementia related topics.

Medical Assistant

CMAs (certified medical assistants) are eligible for certification with completion of an accredited postsecondary medical assistant training program and a certification exam. CMAs can assist with tasks including monitoring patient vital signs, tracking weight, electrocardiograms, phlebotomy, and assisting with patient needs (i.e., toileting) that arise in the office [42]. CMAs can assist with challenging patient scenarios such as monitoring a patient who wanders while the provider meets with a caregiver. CMAs are also helpful in their crossover potential to alleviate the office staff of more clinically complex administrative duties including electronic medical records, responding to prescription requests, appointment scheduling, referrals, and patient and caregiver education of expectations for the memory clinic appointment.

Psychology and Neuropsychology

Clinical psychologists and Neuropsychologists hold either a PhD or PsyD (doctor of psychology) and a license to practice. Neuropsychologists are specialized clinical psychologists and have advanced knowledge of brain anatomy and neurologic disease [43]. They are important additions to a memory clinic to provide a comprehensive assessment of a person's cognitive ability on psychometric testing. Neuropsychological testing is particularly helpful in diagnostically uncertain cases due to concomitant mood or other diagnoses, milder disease that might not be obvious on simpler testing, and to provide structured interventions using cognitive remediation approaches based on a person's cognitive strengths and weaknesses.

Clinical psychologists can provide caregiver assessment and training, counseling for patients, patient-caregiver dyads, and/or families on caregiver burden, coping strategies, and individualized interventions for management. They can also help run support groups.

Social Work

Clinical social workers hold a Master's degree from an accredited program and are also regulated by states in the US. They may have a LMSW (Licensed Master Social Worker) or LCSW (Licensed Clinical Social worker) with additional supervised training and completion of an exam. The terminology and requirements vary by state [44]. Clinical social workers are an integral part of memory clinics in their knowledge of community services including care agencies and other concrete services. They may collaborate with representatives from Alzheimer's Association chapters or related dementia specific organizations. Often patients and families are most concerned about concrete services and have questions about resources, finances, and strategies for obtaining care. Social workers can help navigate the complex medical and social system of care and make recommendations that are individualized to care needs and stage of cognitive impairment. Social workers can also lead support groups and see patients and families for counseling services.

Physical and Occupational Therapists

Physical therapists must complete a graduate degree program, by 2015 a Doctor of Physical Therapy (DPT), and then pass a national licensure exam. PTs can help with maintenance of physical function in the context of a neurodegenerative disease. They provide individualized exercise interventions for therapeutic exercise, gait training, balance, and fall prevention. PTs can also assess for assistive ambulation devices [45].

Occupational therapists (OT) also must complete a graduate degree, either Master's or doctoral level, and complete a certification exam. OTs help patients function better in their environment and can assess activities of daily living, promote cognitive skills, and evaluate for assistive devices to maximize independence. OTs can also complete on the road assessments of driving ability. Both PTs and OTs can perform home safety assessments and provide caregiver education [46].

Patient and Caregiver Experience and Outcomes

The body of evidence addressing memory clinic outcomes is more robust out of European countries than from the US. This may be because of the difference in funding sources where investigation into memory clinic outcomes is important to allocate money accordingly. Memory clinics have been demonstrated to provide early detection of dementia and related disorders [18], but the diagnostic disclosure process can be complex. Patients with a lack of insight may not have expectations about receiving a diagnosis, however caregivers report specific and concrete expectations about the need for a diagnosis, as well as real life advice and resources. Post encounter interviews with patients and companions from memory clinics in Israel were completed to better define their experience and perception of the process and outcomes [47].

Post encounter interviews with patients and family companions from memory clinics in Israel were completed to better define their experience and perception of the process and outcomes [47]. Patients expressed disappointment with the visit in terms of lack of a perceived benefit and disempowerment with some physician communication styles, such as when the physician spoke directly to their companion. Some patients expressed fear about the diagnosis, particularly Alzheimer's disease. Patients who were satisfied with the process were more likely to have some insight into their memory deficits and were open to their companion's presence. Companions appreciated receiving validation that their suspicions were correct, but also maintained a hope that the diagnosis would not be Alzheimer's disease. Companions expected concrete recommendations on support, long term care planning, and ongoing management and were disappointed if no specific solutions were provided, or if they perceived the diagnostic information was not thoroughly explained. They appreciated the opportunity to vent their feelings of burden and some felt receiving a diagnosis helped to improve their competency [47].

A UK based study performed qualitative interviews of patient-carer dyads from four memory clinics to better ascertain the lived experience of patients with cognitive decline and their carers. Patients initially reported cognitive complaints to their GP who responded appropriately, however in specialty care they reported feeling overwhelmed by neuropsychological testing and imaging. Interpretation of the results was unclear and of particular concern was anxiety around waiting for results complicated by poor communication. Diagnostic disclosure was also anxiety provoking with reports of confusion and uncertainty. Not all patients wanted a diagnosis. The authors recommended memory clinic providers should develop a diagnostic disclosure process that is individualized and person centered and should include clear and relevant information to patients and their caregivers [21]. Best practice recommendations for disclosing a diagnosis of dementia have suggested preparation and pre-diagnostic counseling, involvement of family members, exploring the patient's perspective, disclosing the diagnosis, responding to patient reactions, focusing on quality of life, future planning, and effective communication [48].

A memory clinic in the Netherlands comprised of physicians and a psychologist conducted standardized assessments over three patient visits with a final visit to disclose the diagnosis and treatment plan. Patients and caregivers were interviewed in person and general practitioners (GP) were surveyed by mail to evaluate aspects of care. Patients and caregivers reported the diagnosis was communicated appropriately but was vague; in contrast the GPs expressed satisfaction with diagnostic information provided to them. Patients reported that it did not make a difference whether dementia was diagnosed. Clinician attitudes were rated positively and the memory evaluation as a whole was deemed to be useful. Patients, families, and GPs were not satisfied with information on care support, behavior management, and caregiving.

Quality of care in memory clinics can be graded on communication of the results, diagnostic information provided, clinician attitudes, medical assessment usefulness, and information and advice provided to family members [49]. GPs have reported satisfaction with memory clinics in the comprehensive diagnostic assessment and information provided about the diagnosis, although they were are less satisfied with information about addressing caregiver concerns and community support services [50]. In contrast, a memory clinic utilizing a collaborative care management model with a focus on improving gaps in dementia care, surveyed referring physicians and reported the program provided valuable behavioral and social recommendations [12].

A more recent Netherlands based RCT evaluated the effectiveness of dementia care provided by memory clinics the first year after diagnosis. Patients and caregiver dyads were assigned to either usual care by a GP or a memory clinic. Memory clinics provided pharmacologic and non-pharmacologic management, as did the usual care group. Dutch general practice guidelines did not recommend cholinesterase inhibitors, although several of the usual care providers still prescribed these medications. Overall there was no benefit provided by the memory clinic to patient or caregiver quality of life at 6 and 12 months, or in function, cognition, or behavior [8].

The content of the dementia care was described more comprehensively in the same group of patients. More patients with dementia at memory clinics received cholinesterase inhibitors and Namenda after a cholinesterase inhibitor trial. There was no difference between the groups in referrals for community resources such as home and day care, meal services, or nursing home admissions. The memory clinic group provided more caregiver information on dementia and referred more often to regional meetings for patients and caregivers. The overall difference between the groups was less than anticipated, perhaps explaining the lack of benefit in outcomes in the memory clinic group [51].

A collaborative care based memory clinic described collection of pre- and post-visit evaluations from patients and families. The collaborative care approach provided an impact on three patient domains including patients feeling less stressed about their memory problems, more confident in their knowledge of AD and related disorders, and less depressive symptoms. Caregiver outcomes that improved include less frustration when dealing with the patient, less uncertainty, better sense of control, and more confidence about finding sources of support [24]. A similar type memory clinic utilizing a coordinated care management model found caregivers felt their concerns were listed to, decisions made during the visit were important, referrals were helpful and felt supported in their role and would recommend the program to others after an initial visit [12]. The previously described CMSM service was able to demonstrate appropriate referrals, particularly for those with mild dementia, and an increase in the amount of dementia diagnoses in their community. Six months later, the patients with dementia who participated in the CMSM had improvements in quality of life and in behavioral disturbance, with a small improvement in depression. The caregiver also exhibited an improvement in quality of life [23].

Cost Effectiveness

The theoretical cost effectiveness of memory clinics is that by promoting early recognition and diagnosis of AD and related disorders, patients receive symptomatic treatment earlier with better outcomes. Additionally, caregivers are supported and educated thereby delaying burden, strain, and early institutionalization. The economic evaluations of memory clinics are focused on whether models of care provide an economic advantage. For example, an RCT out of the Netherlands evaluated an integrated approach to dementia care accompanied by an economic evaluation. The intervention provided a multidisciplinary assessment including a home visit by a community mental health team and two outpatient medical visits with an interdisciplinary diagnostic process with care recommendations communicated to the primary care provider [52].

Patients in the intervention gained in a quality of life metric (Quality-adjusted life years (QALY)) by a mean of 0.05 QALY when compared to the usual care group. The probability that the intervention is cost effective was estimated to be between 63 and 80 %. A comprehensive cognitive diagnostic assessment would also evaluate for reversible causes of dementia, provide individual and family targeted interventions based on symptoms or comorbid conditions, and manage unmet needs. These factors should hypothetically contribute to cost savings but were not demonstrated in this study. Patients in the intervention group however did have lower rates of admission to nursing homes and utilized more professional care in the home. One of the challenges in economic analysis is evaluating the economic cost of informal care. Overall, the intervention group did not demonstrate cost effectiveness in reducing cognitive decline or associated behavioral manifestations, but more in the targeted allocation of needed services [52].

A previously described study by Meeuwsen and colleagues evaluating dementia follow-up care in memory clinics compared to GPs also performed an economic evaluation to assess if memory clinics provide any cost saving. Cost effectiveness was again measured using QALY and costs were calculated from multiple information sources. The average cost per patient in the memory clinic group over 12 months was 22,035 euros compared to 23,059 euros in the usual care group. There was no significant different in the

QALY scores between the two groups. Ultimately no evidence was found to suggest memory clinics are more cost effective than GPs in coordinating care and managing post-diagnosis dementia treatment [53]. Compared to study described by Wolfs et al. [52], which did demonstrate cost effectiveness, the patient population in the this study had better cognition and higher mean QALY scores which was hypothesized to explain why the costs were not comparable.

Care Management in Dementia

It is clear that dementia is an ongoing fiscal and societal concern worldwide with the aging population and no curative treatment. Because dementia affects the patient and those who care for them, there is a push towards creating and implementing interventions that provide better patient and caregiver outcomes and cost savings through avoidance of hospitalization and institutionalization. One intervention that has gained traction in the literature is the idea of care management, case management, or care coordination, all of which imply similar services. The term "case management" seems to be appear more often in publications from Europe and Canada, whereas "care management" or "care coordination" are more popular terms in the US. The concept of case management in dementia care has been studied internationally in the US, UK, Netherlands, India, China, Belgium, and Australia [54].

Case management is defined as a collaborative process to meet a persons' health needs through assessment, planning, facilitation, and advocacy [55]. Dementia case management has been defined as any intervention linking a case manager to patients and caregivers and providing advocacy, support, community services information, financial and legal advice, education, and to reduce fragmentation among services [56, 57]. One of the challenges in defining case management is the variability in the services provided and population served, even in a specific example such as dementia care. Case management is also considered to be a professional field. An example

from the US are geriatric care managers (GCM) who are commonly registered nurses or social workers. They have the capability of evaluating patients, often in their home environment, and performing a comprehensive assessment of their medical and social condition. Their assessment often includes housing, home care services, social and personal activities, referral for legal and/or financial services, entitlements, and home safety recommendations [58]. GCMs provide care coordination between providers and help effectively communicate between families. They are often most effective in challenging cases either medically or socially, or with caregivers who are not nearby. One of the major limitations is cost as they are not reimbursed by traditional medical insurance plans in the US.

Case management remains a broad concept with research interventions in a variety of purviews including linking persons to community resources, interventions such as health assessment, needs evaluation, and care coordination, or case management that is guideline based [56]. There have been several systematic reviews of case management programs for people with dementia which will be summarized rather than discussing the merits of each individual trial. Pimouguet and colleagues reviewed all case management randomized controlled trial (RCT) interventions for patients with dementia and their caregivers in the community that evaluated outcomes of informal costs, rate of hospitalization, emergencies, or institutionalization, or another metric of cost effectiveness.

Twelve trials met selection criteria with half of good quality. An overarching theme in all of the trials was assessment and prioritization of patient and caregiver needs by the case manager, caregiver education, and referrals to community resources. Case management was sometimes included in combination with respite care or management of behavioral manifestations. Case managers tended to be nurses or social workers, and worked in a multidisciplinary team most often. Three out of the twelve studies provided economic analysis. There was no evidence that case management interventions reduced costs, or provided savings in health care expenditures or reduction of hospitalization. There was evidence from 4 out of 6 good quality studies that suggested a delay in institutionalization and nursing home admission. This review highlighted that for case management to be effective, there needs to be integration with health care systems, and target populations that would benefit the most such as more cognitively impaired patients and/or caregivers with unmet needs. One of the unmet needs was in fact this question of what population would benefit the most from case management [56].

A later systematic review by Somme and colleagues also examined RCTs of case management programs that reported on longitudinal follow-up for patients with dementia in the community. The authors reviewed six RCTs and reported on patient outcomes, resource utilization, case management integration into the health care system, and the intensity of case management by the reported caseload. Wide variability was noted in the definition of case management in terms of location, staffing, and scope. The studies overall were more likely to report a clinical impact than an impact on resource utilization. The review was not able to determine whether the case manager's professional background, team approach versus case management by an individual, or patient eligibility for case management were related to efficacy. More intensive programs and those that are integrated between health and social service organizations provided more of a benefit [59].

Koch and colleagues replicated the search completed by Pimouguet et al. and also included studies that were not RCTs with a goal of better defining case managers and their role in dementia care, what patients and caregivers want from case management, cost-effectiveness, and opportunities for future research. This review again highlighted the challenges in defining case managers in terms of their clinical background, skill sets, and services. The benefits reported from case management in dementia are broad and specific conclusions were not defined due to the differences in care manager roles, study design and measurement, and outcomes. Case management can improve caregiver outcomes and therefore reduce institutionalization but this is on the assumption that a patient does in fact have a caregiver. Studies with longer follow-up [35] demonstrated a delay in institutionalization so this review theorized that certain outcome measures may have been unrealistic in the short term. Positive findings were seen in reducing caregiver stress and burden. While case management makes sense as an approach that is beneficial in coordinating care, again noted was more research needed to define the population most likely to benefit, and case management skills, location, type, and intensity of interventions [60].

The US Department of Health and Human Services evaluated care coordination models for patients with dementia including medical and psychosocial outcomes and expenditures. Nine RCTs and four observational studies were included with an expansion from prior reviews as described. The review determined common elements described in care coordination including (1) care coordinator, (2) multidisciplinary care team, (3) structured needs assessment, (4) care plan, (5) referrals or direct arrangement of care, and (6) ongoing monitoring and support. The overall results of care coordination were determined to be equivocal with the most successful programs incorporating a care coordination model between medical care and long term support and services into a pre-existing integrated health care environment. Promising results were found in outcomes of caregiver strain, health status, adherence to dementia guidelines, and activities of daily living. Recommendations for future research included larger sample sizes, and longer time frames to evaluate which populations may derive the most benefit [61].

Khanassov and colleagues completed a mixed studies review of case management interventions for dementia in primary care. Twenty three studies were reviewed to determine positive and negative conditions for implementing case management interventions for patients with dementia and their caregivers. Summation of the available evidence concluded the caseload of patients should be reasonable to provide the case manager with the ability to provide individualized and proactive care. The case manager would also benefit from providing their services only to those who need it such as with behavioral manifestations or other concerns. Clear delineation of responsibilities is vital as are interpersonal skills including communication and collaborative ability [54].

The summation of the evidence evaluating case or care management programs in dementia suggest that as a whole, it is an approach that provides a benefit to patients and caregivers but requires more of an evidence base to determine targeted efficacy. Studies that evaluate care management over the long term have demonstrated benefits such as reduction in admission to nursing homes and greater intensity case management produces more of a clinical effect. Moreover, the most effective programs coordinate medical care as well as long term supports and services (day care, home care, social centers, respite care) in an integrated healthcare environment. In clinical practice, utilizing a professional with skills in concrete services, system navigation, and individualized therapeutic interventions makes sense but it is challenging to define more broadly what may work in different environments and settings.

Conclusion

Memory clinics provide an important service in the comprehensive evaluation, assessment, treatment, and management of persons with memory impairments across the disease spectrum and support their family and caregivers. Memory clinics serve as expert resource centers to provide clinical services backed by up to date research evidence and help to educate healthcare providers and the public on neurodegenerative diseases. Most people with dementia worldwide have not received a diagnosis despite the clear benefit an early diagnosis provides [2]. Memory services help bridge the gap from primary care where is it often difficult to make diagnoses that are clinically complex, involve time and resources for investigation, and are often difficult to disclose.

Memory clinics should ideally provide interdisciplinary or transdisciplinary care to promote holistic outcomes to meet the needs of patients and families. Collaborative memory care models have been described within primary care, as stand-alone clinics, or within the home setting. Memory care models may vary depending on location, patient population, and staffing but generally include at least physician and nursing services with support staff and access to outpatient social work and rehabilitation professionals. Part of collaborative care also includes liaising with community supports and services which play a big role in facilitating care for patients and caregivers. Telemedicine may help to expand care options for memory care by providing evaluations remotely or by some combination of in person assessment and remote follow-up.

Memory clinic outcomes are an area of interest in light of the adoption of national dementia strategies. While there appears to be anecdotal value in memory clinic services, more standardized comparisons to general practitioners has not demonstrated a benefit. Cost effectiveness is also unclear with a suggestion that cost savings can be provided in the targeted allocation of needed services. Patients and caregivers report an interest in receiving a diagnosis which is in line with memory clinic goals. The diagnostic process itself can be overwhelming and there remains disconnect in expectations from patients, caregivers, and sometimes GPs in the discussion of supports and services. Dementia care managers may be one way to fill this gap but more investigation is needed to determine how they may best be utilized.

References

1. Rubinstein L. A view from the USA on the Alzheimer's disease international position paper. J Nutr Health Aging. 2010;14:104.
2. World Alzheimer's Report. Early diagnosis and interventions. http://www.alz.co.uk/research/world-report (2011). Accessed 8 Aug 2014.
3. Goldberg SE, Bradshaw LE, Kearney FC, Russell C, Whittamore KH, Foster PE, Mamza J, Gladman JR, Jones RG, Lewis SA, Porock D, Harwood RH. Care in specialist medical and mental health unit compared with standard care for older people with cognitive impairment admitted to general hospital: randomized controlled trial. BMJ. 2013;347:4132.
4. Banerjee S. Memory assessment services. In: Dening T, Thomas A, editors. Oxford textbook of old age

psychiatry. Oxford: Oxford University Press; 2013. p. 319–25.

5. Wright N, Lindesay I. A survey of memory clinics in the British Isles. Int J Geriatr Psychiatry. 1995;10:379–85.

6. Jolley D, Benbow SM, Grizzell M. Memory clinics. Postgrad Med J. 2006;82:199–206.

7. Simpson S, Beavis B, Dyer J, Ball S. Should old age psychiatry develop memory clinics? A comparison with domiciliary work. Psychiatr Bull. 2004;28:78–82. doi:10.1192/pb.28.3.78.

8. Meeuwsen EJ, Melis RJ, Van Der Aa G, Goluke-Willemse GA, De Leest BJ, et al. Effectiveness of dementia follow-up care by memory clinics or general practitioners: randomized controlled trial. BMJ. 2012;34:1–9.

9. Lindesay J, Marudkar M, Van Diepen E, Wilcock G. The second Leicester survey of memory clinics in the British Isles. Int J Geriatr Psychiatry. 2002;17:41–7.

10. US Department of Health and Human Services. http://www.nia.nih.gov/alzheimers/alzheimers-disease-research-centers. Accessed 12 Aug 2014.

11. US Department of Health and Human Services. Office of the Assistant Secretary for Planning and Education. http://aspe.hhs.gov/daltcp/napa/NatlPlan2014.shtml (2014). Accessed 12 Aug 2014.

12. Tan ZS, Jennings L, Reuben D. Coordinated care management for dementia in a large academic health system. Health Aff. 2014;33:619–25.

13. Cahill S, Pierce M, Moore V. A national survey of memory clinics in the republic of Ireland. Int Psychogeriatr. 2014;26:605–13.

14. New York State Department of Health. Alzheimer's Disease Assistance Centers. https://www.health.ny.gov/diseases/conditions/dementia/alzheimer/about_adac.htm (2011). Accessed 12 Aug 2014.

15. California Department of Public Health. California Alzheimer's Disease Program. http://www.cdph.ca.gov/programs/alzheimers/Pages/default.aspx (2014). Accessed 12 Aug 2014.

16. Department of Elder Affairs, State of Florida. http://elderaffairs.state.fl.us/doea/alz.php (2011). Accessed 12 Aug 2014.

17. Mukadam N, Livingston G, Rantell K, Rickman S. Diagnostic rates and treatment of dementia before and after launch of a national dementia policy: an observation study using English national databases. BMJ. 2014;4:1–7.

18. Jolley D, Muniz EC. Memory clinics in context. Indian J Psychiatry. 2009;51:S70–6.

19. Phipps A, O'Brien J. Memory clinics and clinical governance- a UK perspective. Int J Geriatr Psychiatry. 2002;17:1128–32.

20. Lee L, Miller L, Harvey D. Integrating community services into primary care: improving the quality of dementia care. Neurodegener Dis Manag. 2014;4:1–11.

21. Samsi K, Abley C, Campbell S, Keady J, Manthorpe J, et al. Negotiating a Labyrinth: experiences of assessment and diagnostic journey in cognitive impairment and dementia. Int J Geriatr Psychiatry. 2013;29:58–67.

22. Brodaty H, Woodward M, Boundy K, Ames D, Balshaw R. Patients in Australian memory clinics: baseline characteristics and predictors of decline at six months. Int Psychogeriatr. 2011;23:1086–96.

23. Banerjee S, Willis R, Matthews D, Contell F, Chan J, Murray J. Improving the quality of care for mild to moderate dementia: an evaluation of the Croydon memory service model. Int J Geriatr Psychiatry. 2007;22:782–8.

24. Galvin JE, Valois L, Zweig Y. Collaborative transdisciplinary teams approaches for dementia care. Neunodegener Dis Manag. 2014;4:455–69.

25. Boustani MA, Sachs GA, Alder CA, Munger S, Schubert CC, et al. Implementing innovative models of dementia care: the health aging brain center. Aging Ment Health. 2011;15:13–22.

26. Morgan DG, Crossley M, Kirk A, Arcy CD, Stewart N, et al. Improving access to dementia care: development and evaluation of a rural and remote memory clinic. Aging Ment Health. 2014;13:17–30.

27. Azad N, Amos S, Milne K, Power B. Telemedicine in a rural memory disorder clinic-remote management of patients with dementia. Can Geriatr J. 2012;15:96–100.

28. American Telemedicine Association. http://www.americantelemed.org/about-telemedicine/what-is-telemedicine#.U8r6LLGye-c (2012). Accessed 13 Aug 2014.

29. Barton C, Morris R, Rothlind J, Yaffe K. Video-telemedicine in a memory disorders clinic: evaluation and management of rural elders with cognitive impairment. Telemed J E Health. 2011;17:789–93.

30. Comans TA, Martin-Khan MM, Gray LC, Schuffham PA. A break-even analysis of delivering a memory clinic by videoconferencing. J Telemed Telecare. 2013;19:393–6.

31. Dyer J. Multidisciplinary, interdisciplinary, and transdisciplinary educational models and nursing education. Nurs Educ Perspect. 2003;24:186–8.

32. Archer J, Bower P, Gillbody S, Lovell K, Richards D, et al. Collaborative care for depression and anxiety problems. Cochrane Database Syst Rev. 2012;10.

33. Ganz D, Koretz BK, Bail JK, McCreath HE, Wenger NS, et al. Nurse practitioner co-management for patients in an academic geriatric practice. Am J Manag Care. 2013;16:343–55.

34. Callahan CM, Boustani MA, Unverzagt FW, Austrom MG, Damush TM, et al. Effectiveness of collaborative care for older adults with Alzheimer disease in primary care: a randomized controlled trial. JAMA. 2006;295:2148–57.

35. Mittelman MS, Haley WE, Clay OJ, Roth DL. Improving caregiver well-being delays nursing home placement of patients with Alzheimer's disease. Neurology. 2006;67:1592–9.

36. Vickrey BG, Mittman BS, Connor KI, Pearson ML, Della Penna RD, et al. The effect of a disease management

intervention on quality and outcomes of dementia care: a randomized, controlled trial. Ann Intern Med. 2006;145:713–26.

37. Lee L, Hillier LM, Stolee P, Heckman G, Gagnon M, McAiney CA, Harvey D. Enhancing dementia care: a primary care-based memory clinic. J Am Geriatr Soc. 2010;8:2197–204.

38. Boada M, Tarraga L, Hernandez I, Valero S, Alegret M, et al. Design of a comprehensive Alzheimer's disease center in Spain to meet critical patient and family needs. Alzheimers Dement. 2014;10:409–15.

39. Rojas-Fernandez CH, Patel T, Lee L. An interdisciplinary memory clinic: a novel practice setting for pharmacists in primary care. Ann Pharmacother. 2014;48:785–95.

40. American College of Physicians. Hiring a physician assistant or nurse practitioner. http://www.acponline. org/running_practice/practice_management/human_ resources/panp2.pdf (2010). Accessed 16 Jun 2014.

41. American Nurses Association. http://www.nursing-world.org/EspeciallyForYou/What-is-Nursing/Tools-You-Need/RegisteredNurseLicensing.html (2014). Accessed 16 Jun 2014

42. American Association of Medical Assistants. http:// www.aama-ntl.org/ (2014). Accessed 13 Jun 2014.

43. American Neuropsychiatric Association. http://www. anpaonline.org/what-is-neuropsychology. Accessed 17 Jun 2014.

44. National Association of Social Workers. http://www. socialworkers.org/practice/standards/naswclinicalsw-standards.pdf (2005). Accessed 17 Jun 2014.

45. American Physical Therapy Association. http://www. apta.org/ (2014). Accessed 14 Aug 2014.

46. The American Occupational Therapy Association. http://www.aota.org/ (2014). Accessed 14 Aug 2014.

47. Karnieli-Miller O, Werner P, Aharon-Peretz J, Sinaff G, Eidelman S. Expectations, experiences, and tensions in the memory clinic: the process of diagnostic disclosure of dementia within a triad. Int Psychogeriatr. 2012;24:1756–70.

48. Lecouturier J, Bamford C, Hughes JC, Francis JJ, Foy R, Johnston M, Eccles MP. Appropriate disclosure of a diagnosis of dementia: identifying the key behaviours of 'best practice'. BMC Health Serv Res. 2008;8:95.

49. van Hout HPJ, Vernooij-Dassen MJFJ, Hoefnagels WHL, Grol RPTM. Measuring the opinions of memory clinic users: patients, relatives, and general practitioners. Int J Geriatr Psychiatry. 2001;16:846–51.

50. Gardner IL, Foreman P, Davis S. Cognitive dementia and memory service clinics: opinions of general practitioners. Am J Alzheimers Dis Other Demen. 2004;19:105–10.

51. Meeuwsen EJ, Melis RJ, Meulenbroek O, Olde Rikkert MGM. Comparing content of dementia care after diagnosis: memory clinics versus general practitioners. Int J Geriatr Psychiatry. 2014;29:437–8.

52. Wolfs CA, Dirksen CD, Kessels A, Severens JL, Verhey FRJ. Economic evaluation of an integrated diagnostic approach for psychogeriatric patients. Arch Gen Psychiatry. 2009;66:313–23.

53. Meeuwsen E, Melis R, van der Aa G, Goluke-Willemse G, de Leest B, et al. Cost-effectiveness of one year dementia follow-up care by memory clinics or general practitioners: economic evaluation of a randomized controlled trial. PLoS One. 2013;8:1–7.

54. Khanassov V, Vedel I, Pluye P. Case management for dementia in primary health care: a systematic mixed studies review based on the diffusion of innovation model. Clin Interv Aging. 2014;9:915–28.

55. Case Management Society of America. www.cmsa. org (2014). Accessed 18 Aug 2014.

56. Pimouguet C, Lavaud T, Dartigues JF, Helmer C. Dementia case management effectiveness on health care costs and resource utilization: a systematic review of randomized controlled trials. J Nutr Health Aging. 2010;14:669–76.

57. World Alzheimer's Report. Journey of caring, an analysis of long term care for dementia. http://www.alz. co.uk/research/world-report-2013 (2013). Accessed 8 Aug 2014.

58. National Association of Professional Geriatric Care Managers. http://www.caremanager.org/why-care-management/what-you-should-know/ (2014). Accessed 17 Jun 2014.

59. Somme D, Trouve H, Drame M, Gagnon D, Couturier Y, Saint-Jean O. Analysis of case management programs for patients with dementia: a systematic review. Alzheimers Dement. 2012;8:426–36.

60. Koch T, Iliffe S, Manthorpe J, Stephens B, Fox C, et al. The potential of case management for people with dementia: a commentary. Int J Geriatr Psychiatry. 2012;27:1305–14.

61. US Department of Health and Human Services. Care coordination for people with Alzheimer's disease and related dementias: literature review. http://aspe.hhs. gov/daltcp/reports/2013/alzcc.shtml (2013).

Early Stage Dementia: Maximizing Self-Direction and Health

Valerie T. Cotter and Julie Teixeira

An estimated 5.2 million Americans currently have Alzheimer's disease (AD), the most common type of dementia however the number of newly diagnosed individuals is expected to double by the year 2050 [1]. Early stage AD (mild cognitive decline) refers to people in the beginning stages of the disease who experience the following symptoms: noticeable problems coming up with the right word or name, trouble remembering names when introduced to new people, noticeably greater difficulty performing tasks in social or work settings, forgetting material that one has just read, losing or misplacing a valuable object, and increasing trouble with planning or organizing [2].

Another term, early-onset AD (often confused with early stage AD), is not defined by the stage of the disease, but by how it affects people younger than age 65. The prevalence of early stage AD is unclear. Increasing awareness of the disease and its earliest signs, as well as emerging advancements in technology, through brain imaging and biomarker measures, have led to earlier diagnosis of AD and mild cognitive impairment (MCI), a condition that often precedes AD. As individuals are increasingly diagnosed at earlier stages of dementia, they are able to communicate their needs, concerns, and preferences.

Coping in Early Stage Dementia

A diagnosis of early stage dementia typically results in feelings of loss, social stigma and uncertainty, placing major demands on the coping strategies for the individual [3–7]. Both the person with early stage dementia and the care partner acknowledge loss similar to the process of adjustment in grief [8]. Individuals with early stage dementia attempt to manage the illness and its emotional impact through a series of processes that progress through stages of awareness, coping, and evaluation. Through varying levels of awareness, they acknowledge and actively seek to understand and adjust to current and future loss of memory, independence, previous roles and lifestyle, as well as feelings of depression and frustration [9, 10].

The person with early stage dementia can describe a range of specific ways in which they cope with the diagnosis and demands of everyday life, if given the opportunity to express them self [8]. The expression of awareness of impairment and functioning made by the person with dementia and the care partner are influenced by

V.T. Cotter, DrNP, AGPCNP-BC, FAANP (✉)
University of Pennsylvania School of Nursing,
Claire Fagin Hall, Office 350, 418 Curie Blvd.,
Philadelphia, PA 19104, USA
e-mail: cottervt@nursing.upenn.edu

J. Teixeira, BFA, MA
Alzheimer's Association Delaware Valley Chapter,
399 Market Street, Suite 102, Philadelphia,
PA 19106, USA
e-mail: julietex@gmail.com

© Springer International Publishing Switzerland 2016
M. Boltz, J.E. Galvin (eds.), *Dementia Care*, DOI 10.1007/978-3-319-18377-0_5

psychological and social factors [11]. In Clare's recent study [11], mood, self-concept and personality were relevant for the person with dementia; and for the care partner, the quality of relationship with the care recipient, perceptions of disease severity and socio-economic status were important.

As a person copes with early stage dementia, there is a potential for negative beliefs about the self [8, 9, 12]. Reconstruction of a sense of self develops through self-appraisal and reevaluation of abilities, the continuation of old roles and the creation of new roles within relationships [6, 8]. They experience a continuum of reactions and emotional responses to readjust the self-concept through an adaptation-coping model [9]. A recent study has shown that self-concept remains stable in the early stages of dementia, and underscores the importance of a positive self-concept to quality of life [13].

Identity for the individual with early stage dementia may be threatened when physical, psychological, and social consequences of the disease begin to progressively alter sense of self and challenge the individual's ability to hold onto former selves [14]. The multidimensional construct of identity includes representations of oneself, such as roles, traits, identity strength, personal characteristics and autobiography [15]. As the person experiences cognitive and linguistic deficits, one is most likely trying to invent and use alternative communicative resources in order to sustain factors like sense of self and identity [16]. Therefore, identity construction can be viewed as a continually evolving process of negotiation and renegotiation in the individual with AD. A recent study found that people in the early stages of dementia do not differ in many aspects of identity to healthy older people, and reported fewer signs of identity-related distress and anxiety [17].

The person with early stage dementia recognizes how interpersonal relationships change and how others can disregard or disrespect them [12, 18]. Shame, stigma, frustration, embarrassment and feeling unaccepted by others cause individuals to isolate themselves from others [3]. People with early stage dementia have difficulties

negotiating new and existing social relationships with tensions arising between how the person with dementia wishes to be positioned within society and within their own family and social network [9, 12].

Both the person with early stage dementia and care partner rely on each other and find ways to compensate in social situations, look for opportunities to talk about their difficulties, and derive a sense of support from local community activities [9]. Relationships with family members or friends influence how couples interpret the diagnosis of early stage dementia and adjust to loss within their own social context. Partners experience role changes in the relationship with the loss of independence and increased dependence of the person with dementia [6]. Maintaining social roles and contact with a wider social network positively influence coping strategies to prevent isolation and feelings of hopelessness [6, 9].

Hope is central to the adjustment process in early stage dementia when trying to maintain a sense of normalcy and developing cognitive, social and behavioral strategies to improve confidence [19]. Learning and developing can assist in a level of acceptance to balance hope and despair in a realistic manner [9]. It is self-protective when individuals hope for a cure or medication that would stabilize dementia, and attempts to maintain a sense of self and normality [11]. Religion or spirituality inspires feelings of hope, strength, security, or guidance to help cope with the effects of early stage dementia [20].

Strategies to Maintain a Person's Integrity and Autonomy

Diagnostic Disclosure

Early diagnosis and time spent in discussion with the person with dementia and their care partner(s) is important to support optimal adjustment and planning for the future. While clinicians and care partners may be concerned that disclosure of dementia in the earliest stages will overwhelm the person with dementia and cause depression and anxiety, these catastrophic reactions are rare

[21, 22]. Disclosure is complex and should be an ongoing process to promote better understanding of the diagnosis and finding ways to integrate information about support services and future care planning [23, 24]. The following components are recommended in the process of disclosing a diagnosis of dementia: (1) prepare the person with dementia and family for disclosure, (2) explore the patient's perspective, (3) integrate family member(s) into the process to provide an opportunity for patients and care partners to learn to talk together about the diagnosis, (4) disclose the diagnosis tailoring the process and terminology to the preferences of individual patients and their families, (5) respond to patient reactions and be prepared to manage a range of emotional responses and explore these, (6) focus on quality of life and well-being, (7) plan for the future, and (8) communicate effectively [23].

Driving and Dementia

In the earliest stages of AD, an individual may begin to have difficulty with complex tasks such as driving. As judgment, sense of time and place, and physical abilities become impaired, so does the need for a comprehensive safety plan to prevent injuries and allow an individual with AD to maintain independence longer [25]. The following are warning signs of unsafe driving: (1) forgetting how to locate a familiar place and getting lost, (2) failing to observe traffic signals and signs, (3) difficulty with staying in one's own lane, (4) becoming angry and confused while driving, and/or (5) new dents or scratches on the car or garage [25]. These warning signs demonstrate the need for a proactive strategy and plan for how the individual with dementia will get around when he or she no longer can drive. In addition, for the individual in the early stages of AD, putting a plan in place can be an empowering way for the individual to make their voice heard.

Care partners and individuals with dementia may want to consider developing a driving contract or an agreement together. The driving contract would aim to empower the individual with early stage dementia to share directions on what

they would like to happen when he or she can no longer drive [25]. In addition, this agreement would include practical safety steps, such as periodic driving assessments with a driving evaluation specialist, a GPS monitoring system for the car or other safe return program, and alternate transportation systems. It is greatly important for the individual with dementia to consider other options of independent travel as this relates to a sense of independence and control over ones' own mobility [25]. In considering that loss of independence is tied to driving, it is important for the care partner to validate the individual with dementia's feelings with love and support, and to preserve his or her independence, while ensuring their safety and the safety of others [25].

Some individuals will give up driving easily, while others may get angry and project this upon the care partner due to loss of insight that is a part of AD [25]. Impaired insight and judgment make it difficult for the individual with AD to understand that their driving is no longer safe and can cause their mood and personality changes to reflect more pronounced reactions [25]. The care partner will want to stress the positives, acknowledge the pain of this life change, and appeal to the person's desire to act responsibly while demonstrating patience, empathy, and firmness in alternatives offered. In addition, health care professionals and legal authorities may also reinforce a medical diagnosis of AD and accompanying safety directives by writing a letter stating that the diagnosed individual can no longer drive as a care partner safety aid. As a last resort, care partners may have to take the car keys, disable the car or even remove it completely; however, still leaving the individual with dementia a safe reliable alternative route of transportation. See Chapter "Community Mobility and Dementia: The Role for Health Care Professionals" for an extensive discussion on dementia and driving.

Legal and Financial Planning

Planning for the future is important for everyone, but legal and financial plans are especially vital for an individual with AD. Putting a plan into action in the early stages allows the person with early stage dementia to express their wishes for future care and decisions. It is an important key element to empower the individual in the early stages to be able to talk openly with their care partner(s) about their own preferences regarding treatment and care, including end-of-life wishes [26]. This also eliminates unanswered questions as the person with dementia is designating decision makers on his or her own behalf. Allotting this time also gives the care partner space to work through complex issues that may arise in long-term care planning [26].

Legal planning should include (a) making plans for health care and long-term care, (b) making plans for finances and property, and (c) naming another person to make decisions on behalf of the person with dementia [26]. It is recommended that care partners and individuals in the early stages work with a trusted adviser to document one's preferences as the individual in the early stages of dementia is considering who will act in their best interest as their disease progresses [26]. Once all parties have completed these documents, it is imperative that the members of the care team have a copy, including the care partner, trusted family member, attorney, and doctor, as well as the individual in the early stages of AD.

Sometimes these conversations can be very difficult as a range of emotions may be experienced. There may be fear of hurting the other person from a care partner's perspective while the individual in the early stages may feel frustrated or angry with the changes [26]. Successful conversations occur sooner rather than later to allow the wishes of the person with dementia to be included as much as possible and unexpected situations to be avoided in the future [26].

Continuity of Support

Early planning for the future, with support from healthcare professionals, is essential for both the individual with early stage dementia as well as the care partner. Healthcare professionals ought to utilize some of the strategies associated with recovery focused care that encourages the

Table 1 Recovery-oriented practice tips

Actively listen to help the person make sense of their problems
Help the person identify and prioritize their personal (not professional) goals for recovery
Demonstrate a belief in the person's existing strengths and resources in the pursuit of these goals
Identify examples from other service users that inspire and validate the individual's hopes
Pay particular attention to the importance of goals which take the person out of the 'sick role' and enable them to actively contribute to the lives of others
Identify non-mental health resources (friends, contacts, organizations) relevant to the achievement of their goals
Encourage self-management of mental health problems, such as by providing information, reinforcing existing coping strategies
Discuss what the person wants in terms of therapeutic interventions, such as psychological treatments, alternative therapies, joint crisis planning, while respecting their wishes wherever possible
Behave at all times to convey an attitude of respect for the person and a desire for an equal partnership in working together, indicating a willingness to 'go the extra mile'
While accepting that the future is uncertain and setbacks will happen, continue to express support for the possibility of achieving these self-defined goals, maintaining hope and positive expectations

Adapted from [28]

promotion of citizenship and involvement through interaction with health services to help people to self-advocate to whatever extent they are able to [27] (See Table 1). The level of assistance needed from a care partner may vary in the early stages with a goal of empowering the individual to be as independent as possible. The care partner's role involves encouraging the individual in the early stages to tap into their own personal areas of strength and to aid in establishing and maintaining daily routines. For example, a person may need cues and reminders to help with memory: (a) keeping appointments, (b) remembering words or names, (c) recalling familiar places or people, (d) managing money, (e) keeping track of medications, (f) doing familiar tasks, and (g) planning or organizing. A care partner may assist by developing a shared calendar or medication schedule or another type of reminder system. It is important to note that the relationship between the care partner and the individual with dementia will be nurtured not by the systems developed, but by the shared moments in completing tasks as a team [29].

Care partners will go through many emotions as will the person with early stage dementia. It is imperative that they know that they are not alone and that resources are available [29]. A robust health care team and support system is critical to have in place. Being a part of a support group, for instance, provides a community of peers going through similar experiences with support, hope and valuable shared information. Staying engaged in a group setting is healthy for the care partner as well as for the individual with early stage dementia as it fosters encouraged involvement in a supportive and social engagement environment, which fights to combat isolation [29].

Available Resources

Alzheimer's Association

The Alzheimer's Association formed in 1980 is the world's leading voluntary health organization in Alzheimer's care, support and research.

The Alzheimer's Association's mission statement describes the elimination of AD through the advancement of research, the importance of providing and enhancing quality care and support for both the family and person with dementia, as well as the importance of dementia care education [1]. Nationally, each chapter of the Alzheimer's Association has early stage initiatives as it recognizes that individuals in the early stages of dementia need programs geared to their specific concerns (See Table 2).

The formation of chapter Early-Stage Advisory Councils as well as the national Alzheimer's Association Early-Stage Advisory Group allow individuals in the early stages to give advice about the best ways the association can assist individuals living with AD or related disorders. The Early-Stage Peer-to-Peer Outreach Program is a program designed to connect newly diagnosed individuals in the early stages of AD via telephone with others in the same stage [30]. The telephone calls provide a time to share personal experiences, ask questions, as well as for the volunteer to discuss Alzheimer's Association programs and services, thus also providing another element of meaning for the volunteer.

Table 2 Alzheimer's association early stage resources

Early-Stage Advisory Council	www.alz.org/about_us_early_stage_advisory_group.asp
Early-Stage Peer-to-Peer Outreach Program	www.alz.org/sewi/in_my_community_59796.asp
Living with Alzheimer's: For Persons with Dementia	www.elearning.alz.org
Early Stage Support Groups	www.communityresourcefinder.org
24/7 Helpline	1-800-272-3900
ALZConnected®	www.alzconnected.org
TrialMatch®	www.alz.org/research/clinical_trials/find_clinical_trials_trialmatch.asp
Green-Field Library Virtual Library	www.alz.org/library/index.asp
Alzheimer's Navigator®	www.alzheimersnavigator.org/?_ga=1.28660287.2076691233.1410202757
Living with Alzheimer's: For Younger-Onset	www.elearning.alz.org
Legal and Financial Planning for Alzheimer's Disease	www.elearning.alz.org
Comfort Zone® and Comfort Zone Check-In®	www.alz.org/care/alzheimers-dementia-gps-comfortzone.asp
MedicAlert® and Alzheimer's Association Safe Return®	www.alz.org/care/dementia-medic-alert-safe-return.asp
Care Team Calendar	www.alz.org/care/alzheimers-dementia-care-calendar.asp

The Alzheimer's Association also offers free education programs to the public, which provides knowledge, tools, and strategies on how to cope with a diagnosis of dementia for both the individual with early stage dementia as well as the family. The *Living with Alzheimer's: For Persons with Dementia* is one of these interactive programs; the first part of this three part series discusses topics such as symptomology, resource planning, and the importance of a robust care team in the early stages of the disease [30].

Early stage dual support groups is a program intended for the individual in the early stages of dementia as well as their family or friends; however, care partners do not have to attend. The goal is to learn more about the disease, share their experiences, reduce feelings of isolation, and provide assistance in coping and long term planning. Although the formats of these programs can vary, one 9-week session program demonstrated improved quality of life, family communication and self-efficacy, and decreased depressive symptoms for the person in the early stages [31]. It is imperative that healthcare professionals reach out to their local chapters for more information on their early stage initiatives, as this can vary from chapter to chapter.

Buddy Programs in Medical Education

Some educational institutions have created programs aimed at improving general knowledge of, and attitudes toward the person with cognitive impairment by introducing medical students to individuals in the early stages of dementia. The Northwestern University Feinberg School of Medicine (NUFSM) developed the first buddy program in 1997 to provide an opportunity for first year medical students and individuals with early stage dementia to participate in an experiential learning and mentorship program [32, 33]. The Buddy Program aims to achieve the following goals: (1) provide the individual with dementia the opportunity for social engagement and, (2) provide the medical student with hands-on education pertaining to the early stages of dementia, as well as care partner needs [32].

By imparting and sharing their personal experiences and knowledge to the medical student, the Buddy Program provides a sense of meaning, purpose, and contribution for the person with early stage dementia. The program acknowledges the value of the sharing relationship over the hierarchical relationship as the word 'mentor' was chosen for the person with dementia to recognize that the individual with early stage dementia has the continued capacity to make meaningful contributions to society and others despite cognitive decline [33].

Medical students' journals and personal reflections demonstrated the impact that their mentors had on them during their participation in the Buddy Program. Of the 96 Buddy Programs between the years 1997 and 2005, research results showed that the student's monthly journal entries best reflected the students' growth from participating in the program marked by a growth in basic knowledge regarding dementia as well as growth in compassion and empathy for individuals with dementia and their families [33].

Boston University created the first educational initiative known as the Partnering in Alzheimer's Instruction Research Study (PAIRS) Program to replicate Northwestern University's Buddy Program. Research results between the years 2007 and 2011 again showed that medical students observed and reflected upon the emotional and physical strain of the caregiver as well as it increased their understanding of communication skills and understanding of AD [34]. Overall, the forward movement of the buddy programs provides a vehicle for social engagement for the individual with early stage dementia and respite for the care partner, and provides experiential education for the medical student. The Buddy program model also represents a unique educational initiative response to the increased prevalence of AD and related dementias [34].

Cognitive Support

Strategies designed to promote learning and enhance memory performance or a cognitive rehabilitation (CR) approach promotes positive coping skills and well-being for individuals with early stage dementia [35]. Some components of memory are relatively preserved despite severe episodic memory deficits thus cognitive support may yield memory performance. A cognitive training program with 21 adults with very mild or mild AD was found to make modest changes in improving working memory, processing speed (sustained attention), and learning ability (switching attention tasks) [36]. Individual cognitive training was relatively more effective than group cognitive training; however, it can be offered in both forms [36]. These results further support the evidence that both learning and re-learning is possible in early stage AD [37, 38].

Awareness of one's difficulties in early stage AD may have an important impact on functioning and response to CR [39]. Increased awareness has been associated with depression and reported behavior problems in a study of early stage AD [39]. The results indicate that variations in awareness level in early stage AD are influenced by psychological factors, but not to impairment in executive function [39]. Excess disability or decreased self-confidence due to cognitive difficulties can lead to anxiety, depression, and withdrawal from activities [40].

Creative Art Approaches

Art therapy has been practiced and researched as a therapeutic modality for individuals with dementia. Art therapy uses art expression to facilitate creation of one's own spontaneous images within a trusting therapeutic relationship. The emphasis is on communication instead of aesthetic merit of images [41]. Art therapy uses mediums such as painting, drawing, and sculpture with the goal of furthering one's emotional and mental well-being and taps into the natural and inherent healing qualities integral in the art making process [42]. The process of art therapy facilitates the expression and integration of emotions and ideas to promote emotional growth, communication, and problem solving skills which help to preserve a sense of one's identity [42].

The individual with dementia will often express forgotten memories through engagement with art materials [41] as creativity reinforces essential connections between brain cells [43]. It also theoretically helps exercise the areas of the brain still functioning well, thus increasing quality of life by providing opportunities for sensory stimulation and self-expression [44]. Art therapy approaches such as individualized reminiscence and life story work help preserve a person's identity [41]. It is important for individuals with dementia to be reminded of the higher levels of health and function they previously achieved through the process of life review and reminiscence [41]. In addition, individualized reminiscence and life story work helps to enhance insight and understanding for an individual with dementia by evoking embedded memories through the engagement of art materials [41].

Memories in the Making® (MIM) is a therapeutic arts program for individuals with dementia in both the early and middle stages [45]. Individuals engaged in this program are guided by trained facilitators to recreate memories, tell stories, and socialize through expression with watercolors and acrylics on various papers [46]. By expressing pleasure verbally and nonverbally, individuals demonstrate increased self-esteem with having created something of value to self and others [46].

Expressive art therapy techniques such as journaling, memory books, self-boxes, life maps, and time capsules create effective meaning-making process which is central to the individual with dementia's autobiographical or narrative identity [47]. Counselors, patients, care partners, and family members can participate in the process of the life review through shared recollection of memory.

Physical Fitness

Engagement in physical exercise programs may provide cognitive and social stimulation for individuals with early stage AD [48]. Benefits of engaging in physical exercise are not limited to, but include improved energy levels and increased mood; creates a calming effect through a familiar activity; and promotes emotional bonding with an exercise partner [48]. Physical fitness is one area where individuals with dementia can achieve significant gains leading to esteem-building experiences for them and their families [48]. More recent research suggests that low levels of regular physical activity may slow cognitive decline and even reduce risk for development of incident dementia [49].

Care partners can also be a source of encouragement and supervision for individuals with early stage dementia with regards to adherence to exercise regimes in home-based settings. Individuals with early stage dementia are more independent and self-directed in their daily activities thus care partners may provide reminders, guidance, support, or even be an exercise buddy for them [49]. A daily walking program with care partner support also results in less perceived stress for the care partner [49].

Conclusion

Both the individual in the early stages of dementia and care partner(s) will go through a range of emotions that progress through stages of awareness, coping and self-evaluation. There are varying factors that can influence ones psychological responses pertaining to a diagnosis of dementia. It is important to focus on autonomy and empowering the individual with early stage dementia to be as independent as possible in areas of strength. This is demonstrated through the importance of early detection and diagnostic disclosure as well as having joint conversations about difficult topics with the individual in the early stages to further empower personal choice and voice. Therefore, it is imperative that the individual in the early stages and care partner(s), with support from healthcare professionals, work together as a team thus enhancing a sense of control over this change of life situation through joint interventions and strategies.

References

1. Alzheimer's Association. 2014 Alzheimer's disease facts and figures. Alzheimers Dement. 2014;10(2): 1–75.
2. Alzheimer's Association. Seven stages of Alzheimer's 2014 [cited 2014 September 2]. Available from: http://www.alz.org/alzheimers_disease_stages_of_alzheimers.asp
3. Alzheimer's Association. Voices of Alzheimer's disease: a summary report on the Nationwide Town Hall Meetings for people with early stage dementia; 2008.
4. Beard RL. In their voices: identity preservation and experiences of Alzheimer's disease. J Aging Stud. 2004;18(4):415–28. PubMed PMID: WOS: 000224598900004.
5. Pratt RW, Wilkinson H. A psychosocial model of understanding the experience of receiving a diagnosis of dementia. Dementia. 2003;2(2):181–99.
6. Robinson L, Clare L, Evans K. Making sense of dementia and adjusting to loss: psychological reactions to a diagnosis of dementia in couples. Aging Ment Health. 2005;9(4):337–47. PubMed PMID: 16019290.
7. Husband HJ. Diagnostic disclosure in dementia: an opportunity for intervention? Int J Geriatr Psychiatry. 2000;15(6):544–7. PubMed PMID: 10861922.
8. Clare L, Roth I, Pratt R. Perceptions of change over time in early-stage Alzheimer's disease: implications for understanding awareness and coping style. Dementia. 2005;4(4):487–520.
9. Clare L. We'll fight it as long as we can: coping with the onset of Alzheimer's disease. Aging Ment Health. 2002;6(2):139–48. PubMed PMID: 12028882.
10. Werezak L, Stewart N. Learning to live with early dementia. Can J Nurs Res. 2002;34(1):67–85. PubMed PMID: 12122774.
11. Clare L, Nelis SM, Martyr A, Roberts J, Whitaker CJ, Markova IS, et al. The influence of psychological, social and contextual factors on the expression and measurement of awareness in early-stage dementia: testing a biopsychosocial model. Int J Geriatr Psychiatry. 2012;27(2):167–77. PubMed PMID: 21425345.
12. Harman G, Clare L. Illness representations and lived experience in early-stage dementia. Qual Health Res. 2006;16(4):484–502. PubMed PMID: 16513992.
13. Clare L, Whitaker CJ, Nelis SM, Martyr A, Markova IS, Roth I, et al. Self-concept in early stage dementia: profile, course, correlates, predictors and implications for quality of life. Int J Geriatr Psychiatry. 2013; 28(5):494–503. PubMed PMID: 22767455.
14. Macrae H. Managing identity while living with Alzheimer's disease. Qual Health Res. 2010; 20(3):293–305. PubMed PMID: 19940091.
15. Morin A. Levels of consciousness and self-awareness: a comparison and integration of various neurocognitive views. Conscious Cogn. 2006;15(2):358–71. PubMed PMID: 16260154.

16. Hyden LC, Orulv L. Narrative and identity in Alzheimer's disease: a case study. J Aging Stud. 2009;23(4):205–14. PubMed PMID: WOS: 000271796300001.

17. Caddell LS, Clare L. A profile of identity in early-stage dementia and a comparison with healthy older people. Aging Ment Health. 2013;17(3):319–27. PubMed PMID: 23171274.

18. Clare L. Managing threats to self: awareness in early stage Alzheimer's disease. Soc Sci Med. 2003; 57(6):1017–29. PubMed PMID: 12878102.

19. Cotter VT. Hope in early-stage dementia: a concept analysis. Holist Nurs Pract. 2009;23(5):297–301. PubMed PMID: 19713788.

20. Snyder L. Satisfactions and challenges in spiritual faith and practice for persons with dementia. Dementia. 2003;2(3):299–313.

21. Carpenter BD, Xiong C, Porensky EK, Lee MM, Brown PJ, Coats M, et al. Reaction to a dementia diagnosis in individuals with Alzheimer's disease and mild cognitive impairment. J Am Geriatr Soc. 2008;56(3):405–12. PubMed PMID: 18194228.

22. Vernooij-Dassen M, Derksen E, Scheltens P, Moniz-Cook E. Receiving a diagnosis of dementia: the experience over time. Dementia. 2006;5(3): 397–410.

23. Lecouturier J, Bamford C, Hughes JC, Francis JJ, Foy R, Johnston M, et al. Appropriate disclosure of a diagnosis of dementia: identifying the key behaviours of 'best practice'. BMC Health Serv Res. 2008;8:95. PubMed PMID: 18452594. Pubmed Central PMCID: 2408568.

24. Zaleta AK, Carpenter BD, Porensky EK, Xiong C, Morris JC. Agreement on diagnosis among patients, companions, and professionals after a dementia evaluation. Alzheimer Dis Assoc Disord. 2012;26(3):232–7. PubMed PMID: 22037598. Pubmed Central PMCID: 3277665.

25. Alzheimer's Association. Dementia & Driving Resource Center 2014 [cited 2014 September 19]. Available from: http://www.alz.org/care/alzheimers-dementia-and-driving.asp

26. Alzheimer's Association. Plan for Your Future, Make Your Wishes Known 2014 [cited 2014 September 19]. Available from: http://www.alz.org/i-have-alz/plan-for-your-future.asp

27. Irving K, Lakeman R. Reconciling mental health recovery with screening and early intervention in dementia care. Int J Ment Health Nurs. 2010; 19(6):402–8. PubMed PMID: 21054726.

28. Shepherd G, Boardman, J., & Slade, M. Making Recovery a Reality London: Sainsbury Centre for Mental Health; 2008 [cited 2014 September 19]. 2008 [Available from: http://www.centreformentalhealth.org.uk/pdfs/Making_recovery_a_reality_policy_paper.pdf.

29. Alzheimer's Association. Building a Care Team 2014 [cited 2014 September 19]. Available from: http://www.alz.org/i-have-alz/building-a-care-team.as

30. Alzheimer's Association. Early Stage 2014 [cited 2014 September 8]. Available from: http://www.alz.org/delval/in_my_Community_15417.asp

31. Logsdon RG, Pike KC, McCurry SM, Hunter P, Maher J, Snyder L, et al. Early-stage memory loss support groups: outcomes from a randomized controlled clinical trial. J Gerontol B Psychol Sci Soc Sci. 2010;65(6):691–7. PubMed PMID: 20693265. Pubmed Central PMCID: 2954328.

32. Morhardt D. Educating medical students on Alzheimer's disease and related disorders: an overview of the Northwestern University Bubby Program. Dementia. 2006;5:448–56.

33. Morhardt DJ. The effects of an experiential learning and mentorship program pairing medical students and persons with cognitive impairment: A qualitative content analysis. Dissertations Paper 727; 2013.

34. Jefferson AL, Cantwell NG, Byerly LK, Morhardt D. Medical student education program in Alzheimer's disease: the PAIRS Program. BMC Med Educ. 2012;12:80. PMID: 22906234. Pubmed Central PMCID: 3500260.

35. Dunn JC, Clare L. Learning face-name associations in early-stage dementia: comparing the effects of errorless learning and effortful processing. Neuropsychol Rehabil. 2007;17(6):735–54.

36. Kanaan SF, McDowd JM, Colgrove Y, Burns JM, Gajewski B, Pohl PS. Feasibility and efficacy of intensive cognitive training in early-stage Alzheimer's disease. Am J Alzheimers Dis Other Demen. 2014;29(2):150–8. PubMed PMID: 24667905.

37. Clare L, Wilson BA, Carter G, Roth I, Hodges JR. Relearning face-name associations in early Alzheimer's disease. Neuropsychology. 2002;16(4):538–47. PubMed PMID: 12382992.

38. Clare L, Woods RT, Moniz Cook ED, Orrell M, Spector A. Cognitive rehabilitation and cognitive training for early-stage Alzheimer's disease and vascular dementia. Cochrane Database Syst Rev. 2003;(4):CD003260. PubMed PMID: 14583963.

39. Clare L. Does awareness of cognitive difficulties influence the outcome of cognitive rehabilitation for people with early-stage Alzheimer disease? Neurobiol Aging. 2004;25:S72-S. PubMed PMID: WOS: 000223058700243.

40. Reifler BV, Larson E. Alzheimer's disease treatment and family stress: excess disability in dementia of the Alzheimer's type. New York: Hemisphere; 1990.

41. Mottram P. Art therapy with clients who have dementia. Dementia. 2003;2:272–7.

42. Harlan JE. The therapeutic value of art for persons with Alzheimer's disease and related disorders. Loss Grief Care. 1993;6(4):99–106.

43. Hannemann BT. Creativity with dementia patients. Can creativity and art stimulate dementia patients positively? Gerontology. 2006;52(1):59–65. PubMed PMID: 16439826.

44. Stewart EG. Art therapy and neuroscience blend: working with patients who have dementia. Art Ther J Am Art Ther Assoc. 2004;21(3):148–55.

45. Alzheimer's Association. Memories in the Making 2014 [cited 2014 September 8]. Available from: http://www.alz.org/delval/in_my_Community_63511.asp

46. Rentz CA. Memories in the making: outcome-based evaluation of an art program for individuals with dementing illnesses. Am J Alzheimers Dis Other Demen. 2002;17(3):175–81. PubMed PMID: 12083348.

47. Caldwell RL. At the confluence of memory and meaning- Life review with older adults and families: using narrative therapy and the expressive arts to re-member and re-author stories of resilience. Fam J. 2005;13(2):172–5.

48. Arkin SM. Student-led exercise sessions yield significant fitness gains for Alzheimer's patients. Am J Alzheimers Dis Other Demen. 2003;18(3):159–70.

49. McCurry SM, Pike KC, Logsdon RG, Vitiello MV, Larson EB, Teri L. Predictors of short- and long-term adherence to a daily walking program in persons with Alzheimer's disease. Am J Alzheimers Dis Other Demen. 2010;25(6):505–12. PubMed PMID: 20660515. Pubmed Central PMCID: 2935497.

Part II

Clinical Management of Dementia

Treatment of Dementia: Pharmacological Approaches

Nicole J. Brandt and Daniel Z. Mansour

Background

Every 68 s someone receives a diagnosis of Alzheimer's disease [1]. An estimated 5.2 million Americans of all ages had Alzheimer's disease (AD) in 2013. This includes an estimated five million people age 65 and older and approximately 200,000 individuals under age 65 who have younger-onset Alzheimer's [2]. For persons with Alzheimer's disease and other dementias the aggregate costs for healthcare, long-term care and hospice are projected to increase from $203 billion in 2013 to $1.2 trillion in 2050. Of note, Medicare and Medicaid cover about 70 % of the costs of care [2]. These statistics are staggering when coupled with the fact that there are no curative medications currently available [3].

N.J. Brandt, PharmD, MBA, CGP, BCPP, FASCP (✉)
School of Pharmacy, Geriatric Pharmacotherapy,
Pharmacy Practice and Science University of
Maryland, 20 North Pine Street N529, Baltimore,
MD 21201, USA

Clinical and Educational Programs of Peter
Lamy Center Drug Therapy and Aging,
20 North Pine Street N529, Baltimore,
MD 21201, USA
e-mail: nbrandt@rx.umaryland.edu

D.Z. Mansour, PharmD
School of Pharmacy, Geriatric Pharmacotherapy,
Pharmacy Practice and Science University of
Maryland, 20 North Pine Street N529, Baltimore,
MD 21201, USA
e-mail: dmansour@rx.umaryland.edu

Unfortunately there has not been an innovative pharmacologic treatment approach in almost 20 years and still to date there is no disease modifying medications. It is not for the lack of trying with existing and new molecules, but because there have been obstacles in neuropsychiatric research to produce data that are clinically actionable and sustainable [4]. A peculiar human trait, cognitive impairment, for instance becomes practically immeasurable in mice, the in-vitro models most often used in trials [4]. One other obstacle we face is that a plethora of negative research data have gone unpublished and are therefore practically useless [4]. There are currently many compounds that evolve around a number of fairly newly discovered hypotheses explaining AD. Many of these molecules have been excluded during phase III of clinical trials due to emergence of severe side effects that rendered the molecules' risk-benefit profile unfavorable [5]. In the IDENTITY double-blind, placebo controlled clinical trial, Semagacestat had a promising inhibitory effect on γ-secretase [6], a key enzyme in the synthesis of amyloid-beta peptide [7].

Worsening of functional abilities as well as development of skin cancers and infections emerged that brought further investigation to a halt sometime before the very first weeks of what would have been a 76 week trial [6]. These examples highlight challenges with respect to treating Alzheimer's disease and associated symptoms. The goal of this chapter is to

© Springer International Publishing Switzerland 2016
M. Boltz, J.E. Galvin (eds.), *Dementia Care*, DOI 10.1007/978-3-319-18377-0_6

review the current and promising pharmacologic approaches to managing various aspects of
Alzheimer's disease, namely the cognitive, functional and behavioral.

Present Pharmacologic Approaches

Currently, there are two classes of medications
that are used in the treatment of Alzheimer's disease, acetylcholinesterase inhibitors (AChEIs)
and N-methyl-D-Aspartate (NMDA) receptor
agonist [8]. They are pharmacologically distinct
and can be prescribed concurrently in patients in
the moderate to severe stages of the illness.
AChEIs act on inhibiting acetylcholinesterase, an
enzyme directly involved in the destruction of
acetylcholine leading to increasing its concentration in the nucleus basalis of Meynert in the brain
and hence ameliorating the cognitive and functional aspects of AD [9]. This pharmacological
category includes tacrine (Cognex)®, donepezil
(Aricept)®, rivastigmine (Exelon)® and galantamine (Razadyne)®. The effect of NMDA-
receptor agonist exerts a glutamate-like effect
said found to improve cognition. The only pharmacological agent currently available in this
class is memantine (Namenda)® [10].

Acetylcholinesterase Inhibitors

According to the cholinergic hypothesis, AD is
thought to develop secondary to lack of acetylcholine in the brain [7]. Hence, research targeting
the inhibition of acetylcholine esterase has been
the focus of neuro-medicine for the last four
decades. However, the theory has brought attention to many other biomarkers that similarly could
affect clinical outcomes in AD such as the dopa-
minergic, amyloid and the tau hyperphosphorylation hypotheses [11]. Consequently, the notion
that AD initiation and progression is hardly a factor of a single mechanism or pathologic pathway
is believed to be true [12]. To this day, however,
acetylcholinesterase inhibitors have been the
mainstay of treatment for all stages of AD.

Tacrine (Cognex)®

Tacrine oral capsule was the first acetylcholinesterase inhibitor that gained approval to treat mild
to moderate AD by the United States Food and
Drug Administration (US FDA) in 1993 [13].
The approval followed an evaluation of the effect
of the drug in one study (n=2,706) with
Alzheimer's disease and in another (n=9,861) in
a treatment investigational new drug (TIND) program. More than 190,000 patients in the US
received tacrine during the first 2 years following
marketing approval that year [14].

Dosing of Tacrine
Patients would be started on 40 mg/day in four
divided doses for 4 weeks then increased to
80 mg/day in four divided doses for the following
4 weeks. Given that patient was tolerating treatment with no elevation of liver transaminases,
doses would be increased to 120 mg/day then
160 mg/day in four divided doses in 4-week
intervals. If elevation of liver transaminases to
occur, a clinical decision then ensues to either to
stop titrating the dose upward, decrease dose by
40 mg/day or discontinue medication depending
on how many times the normal levels of transaminases had been violated. Levels as high as
five times the normal levels of ALT have been
dismissed as collateral to treatment and patients
were allowed to remain on the medicine or to be
rechallenged if discontinued due to suspected
hepatic injury [15].

Adverse Reactions of Tacrine
The most common tacrine-associated adverse
events were elevated liver transaminases levels
particularly Alanine Aminotransferase (ALT)
during the first 3 months. ALT is almost exclusively found in the liver while Aspartate
Aminotransferase (AST), besides found in the
liver, is also found in muscles and other organs.
ALT levels increased as much at three times the
upper limit normal in 25 % of the patients treated
with tacrine, which was deemed clinically significantly risky and required routine monitoring
early in treatment [14, 15].

The elevations were almost always asymptomatic, rarely accompanied by significant increases in bilirubin, and were related to duration on drug rather than to dose (90 % occurred within the first 12 weeks of treatment). And, to a lesser degree, aspartate aminotransferase AST plus peripheral cholinergic events involving (nausea, vomiting, diarrhea, dyspepsia, anorexia, and weight loss) were also recorded. Tacrine fell out of favor and was totally withdrawn from US market in May 2012 [14].

Donepezil (Aricept)®

This medication was approved in 1996 by the US FDA and has been the market lead in treating all stages of AD. A study in ambulatory patients with severe Alzheimer's disease (n = 343) for 24 weeks, randomized, double blind, placebo controlled concluded that donepezil was better than placebo in affecting cognitive improvement and global function [16]. Another US study in patients in the nursing home with Alzheimer's disease that were randomized, double-blinded and placebo controlled (n = 248) for 24 weeks also concluded improvement in cognition, activities of daily living (ADLs) and global function but with no improvement in behavior [17]. Donepezil has also been shown to have benefit in other forms of dementia such as Lewy Body and Parkinson's disease dementia [18, 19].

Dosing of Donepezil

Donepezil is to be started at 5 mg/day for 4–6 weeks then it may be increased to 10 mg/day if tolerated [20]. In July 2010, US FDA approved a higher dose of 23 mg/day for treatment of moderate to severe AD as another dosing option based on a clinical study in patients with mild to severe AD. There were two primary endpoints examined, namely the Severe Impairment Battery (SIB) and the Clinician's Interview-Based Impression of Change Plus Caregiver Input (CIBIC-Plus). The former is to measure cognition while the latter evaluates global function. Although the study did not show improvement in global function, it did however, show a statistically significant improvement in cognition for patients on donepezil 23 mg/day compared to 10 mg/day which was enough to gain FDA approval in 2010 [21–23].

Adverse Reactions of Donepezil

Overall, donepezil like other AChEIs has been known to cause gastrointestinal symptoms such as nausea, vomiting, diarrhea as well as syncope and vivid nighttime dreams [20]. Declines in cognitive and functional impairment as well as the incidence of adverse drug reactions have been associated with the discontinuation of donepezil [24].

Rivastigmine (Exelon)®

A Cochrane review (n = 4,775) that included patients with mild to moderate AD dementia in nine randomized, double-blind, placebo controlled trials concluded that oral rivastigmine slowed decline in cognitive function, improved ADL and decreased the severity of dementia [25]. Rivastigmine gains its uniqueness among other AChEIs in that it inhibits two cholinesterase enzymes namely, acetyl and butyryl cholinesterase (BuChE), both constituents in the production of acetylcholine. In a study in Switzerland (n = 18) where the Computerized Neuropsychological Test Battery (CNTB) test was used to evaluate the relationship between the inhibition of AChE and BuChE activities in the cerebrospinal fluid (CSF) and cognitive change following the administration of rivastigmine. A statistically significant correlation was shown between the change in CNTB summary scores and inhibition of AChE activity ($r = -0.56$, $p < 0.05$) and BuChE activity ($r = -0.65$, $p < 0.01$) in CSF. Improvement in speed-, attention- and memory-related subtests of the CNTB correlated significantly with inhibition of BuChE but not AChE activity in CSF [26]. Weak or absent correlation with change in cognitive performance was noted for inhibition of plasma BuChE. These results indicate that cognitive improvement with rivastigmine in AD is associated with central inhibition of cholinesterase and support a role for central BuChE in addition to AChE inhibition in modulating cholinergic function in AD [26].

Rivastigmine followed donepezil in approval by the US FDA and in April 2000 it was approved to treat mild to moderate AD in oral capsule as well as oral liquid formulations. The liquid formulation eased the administration of rivastigmine to patients who had difficulty swallowing a solid dosage form. In 2006, rivastigmine became the first acetylcholinesterase inhibitor to be approved to treat mild to moderate dementia associated with Parkinson's disease and in 2007, it was the first to be formulated in a transdermal patch (RV-TDP) form resulting in less gastrointestinal adverse drug reaction [27], less concern with QTc interval prolongation [28], less caregiver burden and more treatment adherence by patients [29].

Dosing of Rivastigmine

The oral dose for mild to moderate AD is 1.5 mg every 12 h for 2 weeks for a total of 3 mg/day then increase by 1.5 mg per dose every 2 weeks as tolerated not to exceed 6 mg/dose or 12 mg/day. Of note, the therapeutic dose range is between 6 and 12 mg/day and often a longer titration schedule is needed (e.g. every 4 weeks). The transdermal dose for mild to moderate AD is 4.6 mg/patch to dry skin every 24 h for 4 weeks then increase to 9.5 mg/day for 4 weeks. The maintenance dose is generally 9.5–13.3 mg/day. In patients with moderate to severe AD, the maintenance dose is 13.3 mg/day. If treatment is interrupted for at least 3 days, the lowest dosing should be restarted [25].

Adverse Reactions of Rivastigmine

Overall, the transdermal patch has been associated with fewer adverse events of nausea, vomiting, and dizziness compared to the oral route. A slow titration of the oral route as well as giving the medication with or after food may ameliorate these adverse effects [25].

Galantamine (Razadyne)®

Galantamine is an acetylcholinesterase inhibitor approved by the US FDA in 2003 for treatment of mild to moderate dementia of AD. A multicenter double-blind trial (n=636) patients with mild to moderate disease were randomly given either placebo or galantamine then increased the dose to maintenance at 24–32 mg/day. The study concluded that galantamine significantly improved cognition and global function as well as daily function [30].

Galantamine has also shown α7-nicotinic receptor agonist activity, the clinical relevance of which is yet to be established. It is considered a step forward in studying neurogenesis, as well as reduction of neuroinflammation, oxidative stress and brain injury [31, 32].

Dosing of Galantamine

This medication is available in both an immediate release as well as extended release with the total daily starting dose of 8 mg/day and titrating every 4 weeks up to a target dose of 16–24 mg/day. If patient is moderately renally or hepatically impaired, dose should not exceed 16 mg/day. Like other cholinesterase inhibitors, galantamine should be restarted at the lowest dose if there is an interruption in therapy of 3 days or more.

Adverse Reactions of Galantamine

Similar to other AChEIs, galantamine has shown to cause gastrointestinal symptoms such as diarrhea, nausea and vomiting. Weight losses have been reported; however, it may not be attributed to the use of galantamine and other causes of weight loss should be investigated first according to a recent study [33]. Galantamine has also caused dizziness, bradycardia and syncope, tiredness and somnolence, which could potentially make older adults more prone to falls.

Memantine (Namenda)®

In 2003, oral memantine has been approved for the treatment of moderate to severe stages of AD in the N-methyl-ᴅ-aspartate (NMDA) class, which includes amantadine, ketamine and dextromethorphan (a commonly used cough suppressant). In a 28-week double-blind placebo-controlled trial (n=252), memantine reduced clinical deterioration. In another placebo-controlled trial (n=404), patients with moderate to severe AD, already taking stable doses of donepezil were randomized; some (n=203) were given memantine 20 mg/day and some (n=201) were given placebo. For about 1 year after, the memantine group improved on measures of global, functional, and cognitive scores, compared to placebo and was deemed to be statistically significant [34, 35].

In 2012, an extended release form of memantine was approved by the US FDA and made available as (Namenda XR). The pivotal study that led to its approval was a 24-week, double-blind multinational trial that looked into patients already taking a AChEI (n=667) who were given memantine XR28 mg/day for 24 weeks. Patients who were given memantine significantly outperformed placebo-treated patients on the severe impairment battery (p=0.001), the Clinician's Interview-Based Impression of Change Plus Caregiver Input (CIBIC-Plus) (p=0.008), Neuropsychiatric Inventory (NPI) (p=0.005) and verbal fluency test (p=0.004) [36].

Dosing of Memantine

The non-extended release memantine is to be started consider with 5 mg/day then increased in 5 mg increments every week to a maximum dose of 20 mg/day in two divided doses. The recommended dose for patients with renal impairment should be lowered to 10 mg/day in two divided doses since memantine is excreted renally. The extended-release form, however, should be started at 7 mg redundant once per day then increase by 7 mg weekly to a maximum dose of 28 mg/day but should be limited to 14 mg/day in patients with renal compromise.

Adverse Reactions of Memantine

Although generally well tolerated, memantine may cause adverse gastrointestinal symptoms such as constipation and may also cause dizziness, confusion and headache, Furthermore, in light that this medication is indicated for moderate-severe stages of AD, it is important to monitor change in behaviors. This medication has been shown to improve target symptoms such as agitation but it has been shown to worsen this as well [36].

Summary

Medication therapy can only delay but not reverse the disease process. This medicinal advancement offers the person with dementia as well as the caregiver the opportunity of time to make important life and financial decisions that would otherwise not be feasible. The choice of pharmacologic agents is typically based on stage of illness, tolerability, adverse effect profile, ease of use, and cost of medication. Careful considerations need to be employed when prescribing due to the likelihood of continued use possibly until death or admission to hospice [37].

Future Drug Therapy Approaches to Treating Alzheimer's Disease

There are multiple targets for future pharmacologic approaches that will be highlighted (Table 1). These approaches may include but are not limited to: (1) inhibition of amyloid-beta peptide (Aβ) accumulation, (2) inhibition of the production of tau/phospho-tau, (3) inhibition of insulin receptors, and (4) anti-inflammatory approaches. Ongoing debate ensues about the pathophysiology of AD and the impact of the various approaches discussed below.

Inhibition of Amyloid-Beta Peptide Accumulation

Amyloid-beta peptide (Aβ) is thought to form due to the cleavage of amyloid precursor proteins (APP) to β-secretase and then breaking of the product (sAPPβ) in a pathological manner. Under healthy conditions, APP breaks to sAPPα and form sAPPα and C83 by α-secretatse. sAPPα then breaks to AICD and an intracellular domain with the aid of Υ-secretase and both moieties appear to be mostly benign. In patients

Table 1 Targeted approaches to treating Alzheimer's disease

Approach	Main concept	Examples	Discussion
Inhibition of amyloid-beta peptide accumulation	By increasing clearance of amyloid-beta peptide either by inhibition of γ-secretase or inhibition of β-secretase or decrease of APP production resulting in inhibition of amyloid-beta peptide aggregation	Semagacestat AN-1792 Bapineuzumab	Semagacestat, a γ-secretase inhibitor, would have inhibited amyloid-beta peptide production and accumulation. Instead, it resulted in severe adverse reactions, e.g. cancer, that prompted the clinical trial in its infancy. Both active (e.g. AN-1792) and passive immunization (e.g. Bapineuzumab) resulted in a reduction in functional decline. However, the trials were deemed non-conclusive. A dose–response relationship has not been able to be established as well as the activation of CD4+ T cells response has been a challenge in this pathway of treatment
Inhibition of tau hyperphosphorylation	By inhibition of tau phosphotylating kinases, tau hyperphosphorylation is reduced and hence more microtubule stabilization and less axonal death	Lithium Minocycline	Lithium, a potent glycogen synthase kinase (GSK3β) inhibitor is thought to reduce tau hyperphsphorylation accordingly. Minocycline, an antimicrobial with anti- neuroinflammatory characteristics may have some promising effect via reduction of tau-hyperphosphorylation by virtue of its inhibitory effect of on neuronal cytokines
Targeting insulin receptors	By overcoming brain insulin receptor resistance, glucose levels in the brain are better controlled	Insulin Pioglitazone	Since hyperglycemia and diabetes have been linked increased risk of acquiring AD, insulin is naturally a powerful regimen to curtail increase in blood glucose. Pioglitazone in higher than indicated doses has been associated with improved in cognitive, behavioral and functional levels in a recent case study
HMG CO-A	Decrease cholesterol concentrations/pleiotropic effects (lowers amyloid-beta peptide production)	Atorvastatin Pitavastatin	Long-term use of statins seems to prevent dementia [38]. Atorvastatin has been noted to reduce inflammatory response which in turn decreases the production of amyloid-beta peptide hence improving memory, Zhang et al. [39]. Pitavastatin has the same pleiotropic effect as Atorvastatin but may, in comparison, have a long-term effect, Kurata et al. [40]
Inflammation	NSAIDs	Ibuprofen Indomethacin Rofecoxib	Ibuprofen reduces intraneuronal oligomeric amyloid-beta peptide, reduces cognitive deficits, and prevents hyperphosphorylated tau immunoreactivity [41]. Efficacy of NSAIDs and COX-2 inhibitors is not proven and therefore cannot be recommended for the treatment of AD [42]

with AD, β-secretase, particularly BACE1, acts on APP in lieu of α-secretase forming sAPPβ and C99, which by the aid of Υ-secretase, amyloid-beta peptide forms and accumulates into oligomers to what is known as plaques found in post mortem patients with AD [43].

Active or passive immunization has been thought to may be capable of reducing the level of amyloid-beta peptide. Vaccination of non-human subjects with full-length Aβ42 (e.g. AN-1792) resulted in production of low titers of anti Aβ-antibodies and was associated with a variation of amyloid plaque removal results when compared to unimmunized patients. Safety concerns emerged over activating CD4+ T cells while administering the vaccine. This observation of producing a safe and effective AD vaccine where induction of high titers of anti-Aβ antibodies without activation of harmful autoreactive CD4+ T cells is a challenge in immunology that is yet to be overcome [44]. Determination of dose in conjunction with the degree of plaque removal was also a challenge in vaccination trials. This study was halted due to development of meningoencephalitis in a small subset of patients after a phase II trial of the vaccine and the vaccine was deemed ineffective and unsafe until further studies were conducted. On a positive note, patients who were administered the vaccine reported a reduction in functional decline. New evidence suggests that amyloid-beta peptide accumulation may only be how the brain is adapting to long term chronic stress stimuli and that further studies on the effect of stress may be necessary [45].

An additional example of applying the passive vaccination methodology is the use of Bapineuzumab, which is a humanized anti Aβ — monoclonal antibodies. It has been observed to reduce the burden of amyloid-beta peptide in the brains in two phase II trials but did not improve clinical outcomes in patients with AD [46].

Inhibition of Tau/Phospho-tau

Tau is a protein that holds microtubules intact, and microtubules, as part of the axon, are essential for transmitting nerve signals to other axons.

When tau is hyperphosphorylated, it dissociates and causes microtubules to break; hence, the axon dies and a neurofibrillary tangle is formed. This category of treatment has targeted the enzymes that were thought to promote the abnormal hyperphosphorylation of tau in an effort to save axonal structure and function e.g. GSK3, CDK5 and MARK.

Lithium, which is indicated in bipolar disorder, was suspected to inhibit tau-hyperphosphorylation via potent glycogen synthase kinase (GSK3β) inhibition, resulting in stabilization of neuronal microtubules, improvement in axonal transport and decrease in neuronal death [47]. However, Lithium failed to show change in global performance as measured by the ADAS-Cog subscale in a randomized, placebo-controlled study [48]. Another example, Minocycline, a common antimicrobial with anti-inflammatory properties usually used to treat acne, has been also tested in treating AD. Its significance is derived from its anti-neuro-inflammatory effect particularly on interleukin-1β and tumor necrosis factor-α in neurons which in turn reduces tau-hyperphosphorylation and consequently, minimizing axonal death [49]. Certainly, the findings, although significant, still warrant further investigation [50].

Of interest, *Helicobacter pylori* filtrate, a bacterium linked to causing gastroeosophageal reflux disorder, has been linked to increase in tau-hyperphosphorylation. In one study, application of GSK3 inhibitors efficiently attenuated *Helicobacter pylori*-induced tau-hyperphosphorylation [51].

Inhibition of Insulin Receptors

Insulin has a key role in learning and memory as well as directly regulating ERK, a kinase required for the type of learning and memory compromised in early Alzheimer's disease (AD). Insulin resistance, on the other hand, has been identified as a major risk factor for the onset of AD [52]. Hence, hyperglycemia and diabetes have been linked to increased risk of AD. A recent study has linked insulin resistance to accumulation of amyloid-beta peptide plaques [53] where insulin and pharmaceutically structured insulin have been a material for research against AD. Increase in the administration of insulin in type 1 diabetes may have been linked to protection against AD and one possible mechanism was via tau-hypophosphorylationreduction [54].

Peroxisome proliferator-activated receptor-gamma (PPAR-γ) agonists, e.g., rosiglitazone and pioglitazone, have also been known to regulate insulin function especially insulin resistant subjects. Hence, they have been marketed as a treatment for diabetes. However, in studying their effect on treating AD, a 6- and 12-month phase III trials of rosiglitazone, failed to show significant benefit at therapeutic doses [55] and no evidence of efficacy at 2 or 8 mg against AD [56]. However, in a recent case study, a 73 year-old male with mild cognitive impairment and with family history of questionable maternal AD and MMSE score of 24, has shown significant improvement in cognition as well as functionality but only at doses beyond US FDA approved (i.e., up to 60 mg/day of pioglitazone) [57].

Anti-inflammatory Approaches

There is ongoing research and debate with respect to various anti-inflammatory approaches to potentially modifying the disease course. An overview is highlighted below.

HMG-CoA Reductase Inhibitors ("Statins")

This class of medications has been shown to reduce atherosclerotic deposits in brain blood vessels. (e.g., atorvastatin and pitavastatin). An interest in HMG-CoA was perhaps sparked due to post-mortem atherosclerotic findings in patients with AD. Answering the question of a possible link between dyslipidemia and amyloid-beta peptide aggregation has been studied and has been inconclusive [58].

In one study, long-term use of statins seems to prevent dementia [38]. Furthermore, atorvastatin has been noted to reduce inflammatory response which in turn decreases the production of amyloid-beta peptide hence improving memory [39].

Pitavastatin has the same pleiotropic effect as atorvastatin but may, in comparison, have a long-term effect [40]. Another study demonstrated the weakness of the cholesterol-AD hypothesis continuing the debate of the benefit versus risk of this medication class [59].

Aspirin-Generated Lipoxin A$_4$

Aspirin-generated Lipoxin A$_4$ (LXA$_4$), an endogenous lipid mediator with potent anti-inflammatory characteristics, in a dose of 15 μ/kg s.c. twice a day has resulted in return to homeostasis by reducing NF-kB activation, decreasing the levels of inflammation-producing cytokines and chemokines and increasing the levels of IL-10 and transforming growth factor-β. Such changes resulted in the microglia showing phagocytic characteristics to amyloid-beta peptide deposits and eventually resulting in reduction in synaptotoxicity and enhanced cognition [60, 61].

Anti-neuroinflammatory (e.g. SCM-198)

The compound SCM-198 may have an anti-neuroinflammatory effect on microglia. Microglia are non-neuronal cells that are thought to keep neurons physically in place, provide nutrients and oxygen to neurons, act as an insulator between one neuron and another as well as act as a barrier against potential infections to the nervous system. As such they are recently believed to have a physiological role as well. SCM-198 led to less neuron loss and decreased the loss of tau and extracellular signal-regulated kinase in neurons. It also directly protected against amyloid-beta peptide 1-40-induced neuronal death and enhanced cognitive performance in rats [62].

Summary

Ongoing pursuit of disease modifying agents ensues to combat the public health concerns of this devastating illness. As practitioners, it is imperative that we continue to review new approaches to treating this disease. Patients and caregivers continue to look for treatment approaches not only from traditional medicine but also through alternative approaches.

Role of Nutraceuticals in Treating Dementia

Nutraceuticals are defined as, "food or part of a food that provides medical or health benefits including the prevention and/or treatment of a disease [63]." Sales of nutraceuticals in the U.S. have been growing annually over the last 9 years with 5.5 % growth from 2011 to 2012. In one U.S. study cohort of patients aged 80 and above, 59.4 % reported multivitamin use, 66.6 % used at least one vitamin or mineral supplement, and 27.4 % used some type of other dietary supplement (e.g. Ginkgo) [64, 65].

Many of these supplements may seem innocuous but the possibility of adverse effects or drug interactions, especially in combination with prescription medications, is of paramount concern. For example, vitamin E and gingko biloba may both increase a patient's risk of bleeding and should be discontinued if a patient is on anticoagulation therapy [66, 67]. Due to such risks, it is imperative that health care providers ask their patients about OTC and herbal use and consider co-morbid conditions/medications when initiating nutraceutical therapy. The subsequent sections will review literature surrounding the use of commonly used nutraceuticals for cognitive health.

B Vitamins

Elevated serum homocysteine (Hcy) has been associated with an increased incidence of dementia and AD [68]. Folic acid (B9), cyanacobalamin (B12), and pyridoxine (B6) aid in the metabolism of Hcy and have been shown to decrease Hcy levels by 25–33 % [69]. That is why Hcy can be used as a surrogate marker for vitamin B12, B6, and folate levels [70]. The combination of these vitamins has also been shown to decrease plasma levels of amyloid-beta peptide protein 1–40 (Aβ 40), a beta amyloid protein thought to contribute to the pathophysiology of AD [71]. Thus, it has been hypothesized that B vitamins can help prevent or treat dementias, namely Alzheimer's disease.

A systematic review of 19 randomized, controlled trials (RCTs) concluded that vitamin B12, B6, and folic acid supplementation alone or in combination does not improve cognitive function in individuals with or without existing cognitive impairment [72]. A prior systematic review derived the same conclusion [73]. One RCT not included in the systematic analyses used brain atrophy as measured by MRI as a surrogate marker for cognitive function. This study found that a 2-year course of B12, B6, and folate slowed the rate of brain atrophy in elderly patients with mild cognitive impairment [74].

It is important to note that neither this study nor any of the RCTs included in the systematic reviews listed B12 deficiency as an eligibility criterion. This is relevant because there is evidence that B12 deficiency may be correlated with increased risk of cognitive decline [75]. B12 therapy should be initiated in deficient patients for this reason and because of other health concerns including anemia, neuropathy, and neurologic disorders [76]. However, evidence that vitamin B12 supplementation can improve the cognitive function in B12 deficient patients with coexisting dementia is insufficient [77]. Moreover, fully reversible dementias are exceedingly rare [78]. However, acute states of confusion secondary to B12 deficiency that are fully reversible with B12 therapy are possible [79]. If B12 supplementation is indicated, oral B12 has been shown to be equally efficacious compared to traditional intramuscular dosing and is more cost effective as well [80, 81].

With respect to the other B vitamins, folic acid by itself or in combination with B12 has no beneficial impact on measures of cognition or mood in older patients with normal cognition, or mild to moderate cognitive decline, including different forms of dementia [82]. Furthermore, recent evidence suggests that folic acid supplementation may actually be detrimental to cognition in older people with low or normal vitamin B12 levels [83]. Folic acid supplementation in a patient that is B12 deficient can mask this deficiency and lead to irreversible neurologic damage [82]; however the mechanism underlying cognitive impairment from excess folic acid in those with normal B12 is unclear [83]. Vitamin B6 alone has not been shown to positively impact cognition either, although it is less studied than folate and B12 [84].

Vitamin D

Vitamin D deficiency is prevalent and it is estimated that approximately 70–90 % of older adults with AD are affected. Low serum concentrations of vitamin D are cross-sectionally associated with global cognitive impairment and an increased risk of AD [85]. Vitamin D binds to the Vitamin D Receptor (VDR) which triggers neuronal protection against AD through several possible mechanisms, namely: anti-inflammatory action; antioxidant effect; control of calcium homeostasis by regulating the concentration of intracellular calcium in hippocampal neurons; anti-trophic effect by regulating neurotrophic agents; and prevention of acetylcholine defect by increasing the activity of choline acetyltransferase in the brain [85, 86].

As noted, vitamin D not only has an impact on bone health but also brain health. A pre- post study of older patients seen in a memory clinic over a 2-year period showed that the vitamin D3 group had higher 25OHD concentrations than at baseline. This translated into higher final scores and greater score changes on the MMSE, CAB, and FAB than the control group [87]. A recent small 6 month pilot study looked at the effectiveness of the combination of memantine plus vitamin D on cognition in patients with Alzheimer's disease. Overall, patients with AD who took memantine plus vitamin D for 6 months had a four point gain in MMSE Score while vitamin D alone and memantine alone had no change [88].

Overall, vitamin D appears to be a viable option for older adults who are vitamin D deficient. The clinical conundrum surrounds, which is the optimal formulation to use for supplementation. Emerging evidence supports the use of cholecalciferol (D3) vs. ergocalciferol (D2) due to the sustained therapeutic levels [89]. Regardless of the formulation it is imperative to avoid supratherapeutic levels of vitamin D. Excess vitamin D carries the risk of causing hypercalcemia, which may manifest as anorexia, diarrhea, constipation, nausea, bone, muscle and joint pain, continuous headaches, irregular heartbeat, and even acute renal failure [90, 91].

Vitamin E

Alpha tocopherol, Vitamin E is another fat soluble vitamin that functions as an antioxidant scavenging toxic free radicals. Free radicals may contribute to the pathology of cognitive impairment including AD. In patients with plasma levels of total tocopherols, total tocotrienols, or total vitamin E in the highest tertile, there was a reduced risk of developing AD vs. the lowest tertile [92].

A recent Cochrane review evaluating vitamin E for Alzheimer's dementia and mild cognitive impairment (MCI) included three RCTs, 2 in AD, 1 in MCI. Endpoints in the three studies included death, institutionalism, Clinical Dementia Rating, ADLs, MMSE, and progression to MCI/AD. The overall conclusion of the authors noted: "No convincing evidence that vitamin E is of benefit in the treatment of AD or MCI. Future trials assessing vitamin E treatment in AD should not be restricted to Alpha-tocopherol [93]."

The TEAM-AD VA Cooperative Randomized Trial, looked at the effect of Vitamin E and memantine on functional decline. They enrolled mild-moderate AD patients who were then randomized to receive either 2,000 IU/day of α-tocopherol (n = 152), 20 mg/day of memantine (n = 155), the combination (n = 154), or placebo (n = 152). Despite not reaching adequate study numbers, the authors were able to show the ADCS-ADL Inventory scores declined by 3.15 units less in the α-tocopherol group versus the placebo group. Furthermore, there was a reduction in caregiver time in the α-tocopherol group as well. The results of the TEAM-AD study suggest that high-dose vitamin E use is not associated with a significant increase in adverse effects or increased mortality [94].

Historically, vitamin E at doses of ≥400 IU/day has been associated with an increase in the incidences of heart failure, coagulation disturbances, and all-cause mortality [95, 96]. Caution should be used in patients on anticoagulants and antiplatelet medications due to the increased risk of bleeding. Therefore, at this time, high dose vitamin E should be used cautiously due to potential for adverse consequences coupled with limited efficacy.

Omega-3 Fatty Acids

Omega-3 fatty acids (FAs) have become increasingly popular in the U.S. in recent years with fish oil supplement sales alone rising from $425 million in 2007 to over $1 billion in 2012 [97]. Omega-3 fatty acids (FAs) refer to an array of molecules among which docosahexaenoic acid (DHA) and eicosapentanoic acid (EPA) are thought to be the most biologically relevant. Interest in their effect on cognition arose when epidemiologic studies observed a consistent association of higher fish consumption and a decreased risk for AD [98].

In regards to AD, studies of the transgenic mouse model of AD have illustrated that DHA enriched diets significantly reduced total amyloid-beta peptide by 70 % compared to regular diets [99]. It has been postulated that this decrease is due to DHA's modulation of certain neuronal proteins that regulate amyloid-beta peptide production [100]. AD pathophysiology has been linked to oxidative stress, inflammation, and elevated cholesterol levels as well [101]. EPA replaces arachidonic acid (AA) and leads to the synthesis of less potent inflammatory mediators (prostanoids). Moreover, several omega-3 FAs have been shown to decrease cholesterol [102].

However, these mechanisms of neuroprotection by omega-3 FAs may be of little clinical significance. This is because RCTs have failed to consistently show benefits of supplementation on slowing cognitive decline in healthy patients or those with mild-moderate AD. One meta-analysis of three RCTs examining omega-3 FA supplementation on memory in cognitively healthy adults over age 60 concluded that omega-3 FAs did not improve cognition or slow cognitive decline compared to placebo over 6–40 months follow up [103]. A RCT evaluated the efficacy of omega-3 FA therapy in patients with mild-moderate AD. Two experimental groups were included in the study: omega-3 FA (675 mg DHA and 975 mg EPA) alone and omega-3 FA (same dose) plus 600 mg of alpha-lipoic acid (LA) per day. Compared to placebo, omega-3 FA and alpha-lipoic acid (LA) dual therapy significantly slowed decline in MMSE and instrumental activities of daily living (IADLs) over 12 months. The omega-3 FA only group showed less decline in IADLs as well. Neither treatment improved ADAS-cog scores or ADLs though, and the sample size was only 39 patients [101].

In conclusion, there is a paucity of evidence supporting use of omega-3 FAs in older patients for the purpose of cognitive enhancement or slowing cognitive decline. More evidence exists supporting supplementation in patients with AD, especially mild AD, but this evidence is variable and inconsistent. Most of the studies with omega-3 FAs make a point to mention that the supplements are well tolerated and at most cause occasional GI upset, typically in the form of belching. Overall, given the minimal downside to treatment and possible benefits, omega-3 FA therapy may be considered in patients with mild-moderate AD.

Ginkgo Biloba

Ginkgo biloba sales ranked fifth among all herbals in 2012 exceeding $25 million in sales [65]. The use of Ginkgo for purported memory benefits is even higher in Europe with 15 % of patients in one German study reporting use [104]. The mechanism of action of Ginkgo seems to be related to antioxidative properties provided by flavonoids, terpenoids, and organic acids [105]. In animal models, EGb 761 Ginkgo extract has been shown to normalize cognitive deficits in models of AD [106] and improve spatial memory and protect hippocampal neurons in models of vascular dementia [107]. Research concerning Ginkgo use in preventing and treating cognitive impairment (CI) and dementias is vast but often contradictory.

A meta-analysis of RCTs examining Ginkgo use in cognitive impairment and dementia patients found that all doses of Ginkgo improved measures of cognition at 12 weeks, but not at 24 weeks. Furthermore, benefits in ADL measures were seen in 4/5 studies at 12–24 weeks follow up and clinical global improvement (CGI) was significantly superior to placebo at 24 weeks. Though the results seem promising, the authors concluded, "overall many of the trials used unsatisfactory methods, were small, and we cannot exclude publication bias [108]." Another systematic review combined the results of four RCTs including older patients with Alzheimer or vascular dementia with neuropsychiatric features (n = 1,294). Patients treated with EGb761 Ginkgo extract showed improvements in cognitive performance and behavioral symptoms that were associated with advances in ADLs and a reduced caregiver burden [109]. One RCT included in the review used donepezil as an active control to EGb761 and revealed no statistical difference between the two in the aforementioned endpoints [109]. But does Ginkgo slow cognitive decline in AD as well as cholinesterase inhibitors? Authors of one meta-analysis concluded that, "delay in symptom progression, rates of clinically significant treatment response and numbers needed to treat (NNT) found for EGb 761 are in the same range as those reported for acetylcholinesterase inhibitors (AChEIs) [110]." A more recent RCT found MMSE and Seven Minute Test (SMT) scores at 24 weeks to be significantly higher in patients receiving rivastigmine 4.5 mg/day compared to those receiving G. biloba 120 mg/day [111].

The efficacy of Ginkgo in treating dementia remains unclear. Studies examining the use of Ginkgo to prevent the onset of AD and other dementias seem to unanimously conclude that Ginkgo is not superior to placebo [112, 113]. Conflicting evidence exists and is further complicated by an array of formulations, dosing, and treatment durations in individual study designs. Supplements in the U.S. likely have inconsistent levels of active ingredient compared to the EGb 761 Ginkgo extract used in European studies [114]. Overall, it appears Ginkgo supplementa-

tion is unlikely to benefit dementia patients, at least not as much as existing pharmacologic therapies (i.e. AChEIs), and is even less likely to benefit healthy patients.

Pharmacologic Management of Behaviors Associated with Dementia

Managing behavioral health in persons with dementia is a growing public health concern. Challenging neuropsychiatric symptoms such as agitation are often overwhelming for caregivers and result in institutionalization and increased healthcare utilization [115]. Various psychopharmacological medications are used to treat these symptoms such as antidepressants, antipsychotics, anticonvulsants, anxiolytics and cholinesterase inhibitors. There are limited studies of these medications in persons with dementia and most of their use is off-label and not FDA approved [116, 117].

Despite these limitations, there is widespread use of psychopharmacological medications in persons with dementia. For instance, antipsychotics, had an increase in use over the past decade: 27.6 % of all Medicare beneficiaries in nursing homes as of 2001 had a prescription for at least one antipsychotic agent [118]. Antidepressants have a high prevalence of use as well, with 49.1 % of nursing home residents having a prescription for an antidepressant in 2009 [119]. Anxiolytics and sedative-hypnotics also have a high prevalence in some populations [120] and anticonvulsants are used in nursing home populations, albeit to a lesser degree than the other psychopharmacological drug classes [121].

On March 29, 2012, the Centers for Medicare and Medicaid Service (CMS) launched a national initiative aimed to improve behavioral health and minimize the use of medications such as antipsychotics, to manage persons with dementia. Behavioral health refers to an overall state in which a person's behavior is relatively stable and not markedly disruptive or damaging to self and others. There are many factors that influence behavior such as the brain, body as

Table 2 Resources for caring for older adults with dementia

Resource	Description	Website
Advancing excellence	Provides facilities and providers resources and tools to help them reduce the use of antipsychotics	http://www.nhqualitycampaign.org/star_index.aspx?controls=medicationsexploregoal
Alzheimer's association dementia care practice recommendations for assisted living residences and nursing homes	Covers fundamentals of dementia care for areas such as preventing falls, family support, pain management, food and fluid consumption, and resident wandering	http://www.alz.org/national/documents/brochure_dcprphases1n2.pdf
Assessments and best practices in care of older adults	Contains numerous assessment tools to assess dementia, pain, fall risk, nutrition, etc. in older adults	http://www.nursingcenter.com/lnc/static?pageid=730390
Iowa Geriatric Education Center—improving antipsychotic appropriateness in dementia patients	Contains lectures, reference guides, and other information on appropriateness, risks, and benefits of antipsychotic medications in dementia patients	https://www.healthcare.uiowa.edu/igec/iaadapt/
Qualidigm, in collaboration with the University of Massachusetts Medical School "Caring for residents with dementia: a guide for behavior management and evidence-based medication use"	Educational materials about caring for residents with dementia, specifically relating to behavior management and atypical antipsychotic medication use in the nursing home	https://www.nursing-home-antipsychotic.org/

well as personal experience and learning, inborn traits, the environment, and the actions and reactions of other people. That is why it is imperative to perform a comprehensive biopsychosocial assessment to have a better understanding of the person's possible origins of the behaviors and unmet needs. Concerns exist that nursing homes and other settings (i.e. hospitals, ambulatory care) may use medications as a "quick fix" for behavioral symptoms or as a substitute for a comprehensive care approach that involves a thorough assessment of underlying physical, functional, and psychosocial causes and individualized, person-centered interventions. Table 2 provides resources and tools that may assist with the assessments as well as interventions.

Generally, any medication may be effective and safe when they are used appropriately to address significant, specific underlying medical and psychiatric causes of new or worsening behavioral symptoms. Unfortunately, this may not be the case especially when given *without* an appropriate indication for use or comprehensive assessment being performed. Furthermore, medications may also be harmful when used without adequate monitoring for therapeutic effectiveness or adverse effects. Review of the role of the various commonly used psychopharamacological medications will be discussed.

Antipsychotics

Antipsychotics are commonly prescribed despite FDA black box warnings in persons with dementia over the age of 65 to treat neuropsychiatric symptoms such as psychosis, hallucinations and agitation [122]. A 2012 Cochrane review evaluated each of the atypical (second generation) antipsychotics with respect to effectiveness and adverse effects in persons with dementia. Risperidone 1–2 mg/day and 2 mg/day showed benefit in aggression and psychosis yet the 2 mg/day had a greater drop out rate. Compared to placebo there was a greater incidence of adverse effects such as extrapyramidal symptoms, somnolence as well as infections (upper respiratory and urinary tract) in the treatment group. Among those treated with Olanzapine, 1–15 mg/day, there was benefit in aggressiveness, anxiety, euphoria compared to placebo. However there was an increase in adverse effects such as hostility, abnormal gait, somnolence, and urinary incontinence. There are fewer trials on the use of Aripiprazole 2–15 mg/day yet there may be some benefit on psychosis compared to placebo yet an overall increase in adverse effects. Furthermore, Quetiapine 50–100 mg/day, which is commonly used has poor efficacy data and has been noted to worsen cognition compared to placebo [123].

Limited efficacy coupled with increased risk of complications such as movement disorders, falls, hip fractures, cerebrovascular accidents, and death has been why antipsychotics have undergone increasing scrutiny [124–127]. Furthermore, antipsychotic medications may be being used without an adequate rationale, or for the purpose of limiting or controlling behavior of an unidentified cause which leave them or any other psychopharmacological medication for that matter any ability to be effective. Alternatives to antipsychotics will be discussed below in light that their use should be evaluated critically as well.

Antidepressants

Depression is commonly seen in dementia patients, and has a prevalence of approximately 17 % in Alzheimer's patients and an even higher prevalence in patients with subcortical dementias [128]. Therefore, it is imperative that healthcare professionals not only screen for depression but also suicide risk [129]. The severity of dementia is predictive of depression, with prevalence of depression increasing along with the severity of the dementia [130]. Furthermore, it is possible that underlying depression can exacerbate dementia symptoms [129] as depression has been linked to both aggression and agitation in dementia patients [130].

This theory as well as presence of apathy, sleep issues, agitation and depression has lead to an increased use of various antidepressants to address these behaviors in attempts to avoid the use of antipsychotics. There is mixed efficacy of various antidepressants but generally speaking selective serotonin reuptake inhibitors (SSRIs) appear to be used more often due to tolerability as well as clinical evidence in persons with dementia [129].

Citalopram has been compared in randomized double blind clinical trials to perphenazine, or placebo for the treatment of moderate-severe target symptoms such as aggression, agitation, hostility, suspiciousness, hallucinations, or delusions in 85 hospitalized patients for a 17-day period. The citalopram treatment group showed statistically significant improvement in agitation/aggression and lability/tension factors, compared to other treatment arms, as well as statistically significant improvement in cognition, agitation, retardation, psychosis, lability from baseline. There were no differences in adverse effects between the three treatments noted [131].

Citalopram has also been compared to risperidone in the treatment of behavioral symptoms of non-depressed, hospitalized dementia patients (n = 103) for 12 weeks. In-patients were recruited if they presented with one or more moderate-severe neuropsychiatric symptoms of aggression, agitation, hostility, suspiciousness, hallucinations, or delusions. There was a 44 % completion rate and both treatment groups showed statistically significant improvements in agitation symptoms (aggression, hostility or agitation) as well as psychotic symptoms (e.g. suspiciousness, hallucinations, or delusions) however the side effect burden was significantly higher in the risperidone group compared to the citalopram group. Caution was noted by the authors about the interpretation of these efficacy findings on psychotic symptoms with serotonergic antidepressants [132].

Trazodone, was compared to haloperidol, and behavior management therapy (BMT) versus placebo for treatment of agitation in 149 AD outpatients for 16 weeks. There was no significant difference between the different treatment modalities in terms of improving agitation. The overall dropout rates were similar between each arm, but reasons for dropout differed. Trazodone arm dropout was largely due to increased agitation (50 %), and caregiver difficulties and increased agitation (35 %) resulted in drop out of the BMT arm. BMT had significantly fewer adverse events (bradykinesia and parkinsonian gait) as compared to the other treatment arms [133].

Caution should be taken when using antidepressant such as those noted above due to the increased risk of adverse effects such as falls that is dose dependent in older persons with dementia [134]. Furthermore, their chronic use has increased use not only for depression but also in more than 33 % of the time for off-label indications such as sleep and appetite [135]. This is important to note because there are limited safety studies looking at the prolonged use of antidepressants such as SSRIs in older persons with dementia.

Anticonvulsants

Anticonvulsants have been an alternative medication class utilized in patients with agitation and mood lability with varying degrees of success in persons with dementia. Carbamazepine has shown to improve agitation compared to placebo yet there were more adverse events noted such as ataxia and somnolence. Furthermore, carbamazepine is a narrow therapeutic agent with multiple drug interactions which can be concerning especially in older adults [136]. Porsteinson's review of four clinical trials noted there was no clinically significant benefit to using Divalproex sodium and furthermore it increased the risk of adverse effects. For instance, Tariot et al. [137], showed that divalproex did not improve agitation and furthermore the study was discontinued early due

to significantly higher adverse event rate in the divalproex group, predominantly somnolence.

Anxiolytics

There is limited data on the efficacy of anxiolytic medications like benzodiazepines in persons with dementia [129]. Nonetheless, there may be an acceptable role for these medications in anxious patients, or in patients who occasionally need sedation due to agitation or medical procedures [129]. Caution is advised, however, because despite short-term indications for anxiolytics, many patients are prescribed these drugs on a chronic basis [138, 139].

Furthermore, it is estimated that 42 % of benzodiazepine use in nursing homes is without appropriate indication [140]. This is particularly problematic in older adults, because they can cause dependence, worsen cognition and memory, cause delirium, and interfere with breathing. Furthermore, they increase the risk of falls, which is associated with higher mortality rates in older adults [138]. Benzodiazepines have also been shown to paradoxically increase agitation in older adults with dementia [141]. Not only do they cause a constellation of potential adverse effects on their own, benzodiazepines are frequently prescribed in conjunction with antipsychotic medications, potentially leading to increased side effects as well as deleterious effects on cognition [142]. When and if needed, lorazepam and oxazepam are the preferred benzodiazepines due to their pharmacokinetic preferred profile [129]. Regardless of the chosen agent, anxiolytics used to control behavioral symptoms should be regularly evaluated and tapering attempted after 6 months [143].

Cognitive Enhancers (Cholinesterase Inhibitors and Memantine)

Medications such as cholinesterase inhibitors and memantine are indicated to treat the cognitive issues seen with different types of dementia and discussed above. Limited studies have suggested that they may have a secondary benefit on various neuropsychiatric symptoms. Rivastigmine (mean dose, 9.4 mg/day) did not show any difference in mean change in delusions, hallucinations, apathy, depression or overall neuropsychiatric scores. There was also no difference in the dropout rate yet nausea, vomiting, anorexia, andsomnolence were significantly more common in rivastigmine [144]. Donepezil (mean dose, 9.5 mg/day) did show a difference at 24 weeks in patients with moderate to severe Alzheimer's disease compared to placebo (63 vs. 42 %) on neuropsychiatric scores. Only 8 % of donepezil and 6 % placebo dropped out due to adverse events such as diarrhea, headache, and arthralgias [145]. Galantamine (24 mg/day) did show an improvement at 6 months in 74 % of galantamine vs. 59 % placebo patients. Of note, 20 % of galantamine vs. 8 % placebo group dropped out due to adverse events such as nausea and vomiting [146]. There is also some limited data that memantine (20 mg/day) improves NPI compared to placebo (55 vs. 45 %) and was well tolerated [35].

Medication Management and Safety

Throughout this chapter, discussion has focused on specific treatment approaches available over-the-counter as well as via prescriptions for managing dementia and behavioral symptoms. One of the major safety concerns for people with dementia is the taking of medications. The person with dementia might not remember to take his or her medications regularly, or might take too many by mistake. The following tips may be helpful in making sure that the person with dementia takes his or her medications as prescribed.

- Use a pillbox or other type of reminder system.

– If necessary, get the help of family or friends to fill the pillbox.
- Keep a routine for both filling the pillbox (for example, every Saturday night) and for taking the medications (for example, keeping the pillbox in the same place, and taking the medications at the same time each day) to make this a habit.
- Remind the person to take medications, by leaving notes or calling the person each day. There are a number of reminder systems (telephone or mobile alerts, watch or clock alarms, "smart" bottle caps) that are available.

Table 3 provides more information about medication management and safety for people with dementia. In addition to medication management, it is instrumental to have a comprehensive medication review conducted to ensure that medications may not be worsening the behaviors or cognitive health. The American Geriatrics Society publishes the Beers Criteria which provides a list of potentially inappropriate medications in older adults. One domain of that list focuses on medications that can worsen cognitive impairment/dementia [147]. For example, diphenhydramine, a commonly used over the counter medication, due to its anticholinergic properties has been implicated as an agent that should be avoided in older adults.

Conclusion

Medication management for patients with dementia and their caregivers is a daunting challenge. This is due to the fact that there are no treatments that alter the disease trajectory and furthermore as the disease progresses behavior management becomes a challenge. It is critical that all members of the healthcare team play an active role in monitoring medications, both for their continued need as well as for the emergence of adverse effects.

Table 3 Medication management and safety resources

Topic	Website description	Website
Medication safety and Alzheimer's disease:	This website describes how to work with your doctor and pharmacist regarding medicines	http://www.alz.org/care/dementia-medication-drug-safety.asp
Staying safe	This brochure addresses safety concerns with medicines that you need to consider when caring for someone with Alzheimer's disease	http://www.alz.org/national/documents/brochure_stayingsafe.pdf
Alzheimer's disease and medications fact sheet	Several prescription drugs are currently approved by the U.S. Food and Drug Administration (FDA) to treat people who have been diagnosed with Alzheimer's disease. These treatments might improve the person's symptoms and keep them more independent for a longer period of time; they also might reduce the burden on the caregiver. However, it is important to understand that none of these medications stops the disease itself. Being familiar with all of the person's medications is critical to improving the quality of his or her life	http://www.nia.nih.gov/alzheimers/publication/alzheimers-disease-medications-fact-sheet
Drugs, herbs and supplements information site	This site provides information about prescription and over-the-counter medication information. Some over-the-counter medications, herbs and supplements have possible serious side effects and can interact with prescription medications to make them less effective. Therefore, it is very important to tell the doctor about all of the medications, including over-the-counter, herbs, vitamins, home remedies and nutritional supplements that the person is taking	http://www.nlm.nih.gov/medlineplus/druginformation.html
Anticholinergic Pocket Card (AKA as medications to avoid in persons with dementia)	This reference card lists commonly used anticholinergic drugs (drugs that interfere with chemicals in the brain associated with memory functioning) that can worsen the symptoms of Alzheimer's disease. It also includes some background information and describes common adverse effects. This is from the University of Iowa Health Effectiveness Research Center, and was supported by the Agency for Healthcare Research and Quality	http://medmanagement.umaryland.edu/anticholinergic

References

1. U.S. Food and Drug and Administration (US). Science guides Alzheimer's disease drug development [Internet]. Bethesda, MD: U.S. Department of Health and Human Services, Food and Drug Administration; [updated 2014 Dec 5; cited 2015 Feb 8]. Available from: http://www.fda.gov/Drugs/ResourcesForYou/SpecialFeatures/ucm361513.htm

2. Alzheimer's Association, Gaugler J, James B, Johnson T, Scholz K, Weuve J. Facts and figures includes a special report on women and Alzheimer's Disease [Internet]. Chicago, IL: Alzheimer's Association, Main Office; 2014 [cited 2015 February 8]. Available from: http://www.alz.org/downloads/Facts_Figures_2014.pdf?utm_content=bufferb49b5&utm_medium=social&utm_source=twitter.com&utm_campaign=buffer

3. Petrella JR. Neuroimaging and the search for a cure for Alzheimer disease. Radiology. 2013;269(3):671–91.

4. Becker RE, Greig NH. Lost in translation: neuropsychiatric drug development. Sci Transl Med. 2010; 2(61):61rv6.

5. Caraci F, Bosco P, Leggio GM, Malaguarnera M, Drago F, Bucolo C, Salomone S. Clinical pharmacology of novel anti-Alzheimer disease modifying

medications. Curr Top Med Chem. 2013;13(15): 1853–63.

6. Henley DB, Sundell KL, Sethuraman G, Dowsett SA, May PC. Safety profile of semagacestat, a gamma-secretase inhibitor: IDENTITY trial findings. Curr Med Res Opin. 2014;30(10):2021–32.

7. Wagner SL, Zhang C, Cheng S, Nguyen P, Zhang X, Rynearson KD, Wang R, Li Y, Sisodia SS, Mobley WC, Tanzi RE. Soluble γ-secretase modulators selectively inhibit the production of the 42-amino acid amyloid β peptide variant and augment the production of multiple carboxy-truncated amyloid β species. Biochemistry. 2014;53(4):702–13.

8. Riordan KC, Hoffman Snyder CR, Wellik KE, Caselli RJ, Wingerchuk DM, Demaerschalk BM. Effectiveness of adding memantine to an Alzheimer dementia treatment regimen which already includes stable donepezil therapy: a critically appraised topic. Neurologist. 2011;17(2):121–3.

9. Liu AK, Chang RC, Pearce RK, Gentleman SM. Nucleus basalis of Meynert revisited: anatomy, history and differential involvement in Alzheimer's and Parkinson's disease. Acta Neuropathol. 2015;129(4): 527–40.

10. Olivares D, Deshpande VK, Shi Y, Lahiri DK, Greig NH, Rogers JT, Huang X. N-methyl D-aspartate (NMDA) receptor antagonists and memantine treatment for Alzheimer's disease, vascular dementia and Parkinson's disease. Curr Alzheimer Res. 2012;9(6): 746–58.

11. Doraiswamy PM. The role of the N-methyl-D-aspartate receptor in Alzheimer's disease: therapeutic potential. Curr Neurol Neurosci Rep. 2003;3(5): 373–8.

12. Martorana A, Koch G. Is dopamine involved in Alzheimer's disease? Front Aging Neurosci. 2014; 6:252.

13. Crismon ML. Tacrine: first drug approved for Alzheimer's disease. Ann Pharmacother. 1994;28(6): 744–51.

14. Gracon SI, Knapp MJ, Berghoff WG, et al. Safety of tacrine: clinical trials, treatment IND, and postmarketing experience. Alzheimer Dis Assoc Disord. 1998;12(2):93–101.

15. Tacrine Drug Monograph. In: Micromedex [database on the Internet]. Ann Arbor, MI: Truven Health Analytics; 2015 [cited 8 February 2015]. Available from: www.micromedexsolutions.com. Subscription required to view.

16. Black SE, Doody R, Li H. Donepezil preserves cognition and global function in patients with severe Alzheimer disease. Neurology. 2007;69:459.

17. Winblad B, Kilander L, Eriksson S, Minthon L, Båtsman S, Wetterholm AL, Jansson-Blixt C, Haglund A. Severe Alzheimer's Disease Study Group. Donepezil in patients with severe Alzheimer's disease: double-blind, parallel-group, placebo-controlled study. Lancet. 2006;367(9516):1057–65.

18. Rolinski M, Fox C, Maidment I, McShane R. Cholinesterase inhibitors for dementia with Lewy

bodies, Parkinson's disease dementia and cognitive impairment in Parkinson's disease. Cochrane Database Syst Rev. 2012;(3):CD006504.

19. Ikeda M, Mori E, Kosaka K, Iseki E, Hashimoto M, Matsukawa N, Matsuo K, Nakagawa M. Donepezil-DLB Study Investigators. Long –term safety and efficacy of donepezil in patients with dementia with Lewy bodies: results from 52-week, open-label, multicenter extension study. Dement Geriatr Cogn Disord. 2013;36(3–4):229–41.

20. Donepezil Drug Monograph. In: Micromedex [database on the Internet]. Ann Arbor, MI: Truven Health Analytics; 2015 [cited 8 February 2015]. Available from: www.micromedexsolutions.com. Subscription required to view.

21. Farlow MR, Salloway S, Tariot PN, Yardley J, Moline ML, Wang Q, Brand-Schieber E, Zou H, Hsu T, Satlin A. Effectiveness and tolerability of high-dose (23 mg/d) versus standard-dose (10 mg/d) donepezil in moderate to severe Alzheimer's disease: a 24-week, randomized, double-blind study. Clin Ther. 2010;32(7):1234–51.

22. Sabbagh M, Cummings J, Christensen D, Doody R, Farlow M, Liu L, Mackell J, Fain R. Evaluating the cognitive effects of donepezil 23 mg/d in moderate and severe Alzheimer's disease: analysis of effects of baseline features on treatment response. BMC Geriatr. 2013;13:56.

23. Nguyen MD, Salbu RL. Donepezil 23 mg: a brief insight on efficacy and safety concerns. Consult Pharm. 2013;28(12):800–3.

24. Geldmacher D. Long-term cholinesterase inhibitor therapy for Alzheimer's disease: practical considerations for the primary care physician. Prim Care Companion J Clin Psychiatry. 2003;5(6):251–9.

25. Birks J, Grimley Evans J, Iakovidou V, Tsolaki M, Holt FE. Rivastigmine for Alzheimer's disease. Cochrane Database Syst Rev. 2009;(2):CD001191.

26. Giacobini E, Spiegel R, Enz A, Veroff AE, Cutler NR. Inhibition of acetyl- and butyryl-cholinesterase in the cerebrospinal fluid of patients with Alzheimer's disease by rivastigmine: correlation with cognitive benefit. J Neural Transm. 2002; 109(7–8):1053–65.

27. Moretti DV, Frisoni GB, Binetti G, Zanetti O. Comparison of the effects of transdermal and oral rivastigmine on cognitive function and EEG markers in patients with Alzheimer's disease. Front Aging Neuroscience. 2014;6:179.

28. Riepe MW. High-dose cholinergic therapy with rivastigmine patch does not prolong QTc time in patients with Alzheimer's disease. J Clin Psychiatry. 2014;75(3):288.

29. Adler G, Mueller B, Articus K. The transdermal formulation of rivastigmine improves caregiver burden and treatment adherence of patients with Alzheimer's disease under daily practice conditions. Int J Clin Pract. 2014;68(4):465–70.

30. Raskind MA, Peskind ER, Wessel T, Yuan W. Galantamine in AD: a 6-month randomized, placebo-

controlled trial with a 6-month extension. Neurology. 2000;54(12):2261–8.

31. Kita Y, Ago Y, Higashino K, Asada K, Takano E, Takuma K, Matsuda T. Galantamine promotes adult hippocampal neurogenesis via M1 muscarinic and α7 nicotinic receptors in mice. Int J Neuropsychopharmacol. 2014;12:1–12.

32. Han Z, Li L, Wang L, Degos V, Maze M, Su H. Alpha-7 nicotinic acetylcholine receptor agonist treatment reduces neuroinflammation oxidative stress, and brain injury in mice with ischemic stroke and bone fracture. J Neurochem. 2014;131(4):498–508.

33. Droogsma E, van Asselt DZ, van Steijn JH, Schuur T, Huinink EJ. Effect of long-term treatment with galantamine on weight of patients with Alzheimer's dementia. J Nutr Health Aging. 2013;17(5):461–5.

34. Reisberg B, Doody R, Stöffler A, Schmitt F, Ferris S, Möbius HJ, Memantine Study Group, et al. Memantine in moderate-to-severe Alzheimer's disease. N Engl J Med. 2003;348:1333.

35. Tariot PN, Farlow MR, Grossberg GT, Graham SM, McDonald S, Gergel I. Memantine treatment in patients with moderate to severe Alzheimer disease already receiving donepezil: a randomized controlled trial. JAMA. 2004;291:317–24.

36. Grossberg GT, Manes F, Allegri RF, Gutiérrez-Robledo LM, Gloger S, Xie L, Jia XD, Pejović V, Miller ML, Perhach JL, Graham SM, et al. The safety, tolerability and efficacy of once-daily memantine (28 mg): a multinational, randomized, double-blind, placebo-controlled trial in patients with moderate-to-severe Alzheimer's disease taking cholinesterase inhibitors. CNS Drugs. 2013;27:469.

37. Mansour D, Wong R, Kuskowski M, Dysken M. Discontinuation of acetylcholinesterase inhibitor treatment in the nursing home. Am J Geriatr Pharmacother. 2011;9(5):345–50.

38. Corrao G, Ibrahim B, Nicotra F, Zambon A, et al. Long-term use of statins reduces the risk of hospitalization for dementia. Atherosclerosis. 2013;230(2):171–6.

39. Zhang Y, Fan Y, Wang M, Wang D, Li X. Atorvastatin attenuates the production of IL-1β, IL-6, and TNF-α in the hippocampus of an amyloid β1-42-induced rat model of Alzheimer's disease. J Clin Interv Aging. 2013;8:103–10.

40. Kurata T, Miyazaki K, Kozuki M, Morimoto N, Ohta Y, Ikeda Y, Abe K. Atorvastatin and pitavastatin reduce senile plaques and inflammatory responses in a mouse model of Alzheimer's disease. Neurol Res. 2012;34(6):601–10.

41. McKee A, Carreras I, Hossain L, Ryu H, Klein W, Oddo S, LaFerla F, Jenkins B, Kowall N, Dedeoglu A. Ibuprofen reduces Abeta, hyperphosphorylated tau and memory deficits in Alzheimer mice. Brain Res. 2008;1207:225–36.

42. Jaturapatporn D, Isaac M, McCleery J, Tabet N. Aspirin, steroidal and non-steroidal antiinflammatory drugs for the treatment of Alzheimer's disease. Cochrane Database Syst Rev. 2012;2:CD006378.

43. Hardy J, Selkoe D. The amyloid hypothesis of Alzheimer's disease: progress and problems on the road to therapeutics. Science. 2002;297(5580):353–6.

44. Davtyan H, Petrushina I, Ghochikyan A. Immunotherapy for Alzheimer's disease: DNA- and protein-based epitope vaccines. Methods Mol Biol. 2014;1143:259–81.

45. Castello MA, Jeppson JD, Soriano S. Moving beyond anti-amyloid therapy for the prevention and treatment of Alzheimer's disease. BMC Neurol. 2014;14(1):169.

46. Counts SE, Lahiri DK. Editorial: overview of immunotherapy in Alzheimer's Disease (AD) and mechanisms of IVIG neuroprotection in preclinical models of AD. Curr Alzheimer Res. 2014;11(7):623–5.

47. Jing P, Zhang JY, Ouyang Q, Wu J, Zhang XJ. Lithium treatment induces proteasomal degradation of over-expressed acetylcholinesterase (AChE-S) and inhibit GSK3β. Chem Biol Interact. 2013;203(1):309–13.

48. Hampel H, Ewers M, Bürger K, Annas P, Mörtberg A, Bogstedt A, Frölich L, Schröder J, Schönknecht P, Riepe MW, Kraft I, Gasser T, Leyhe T, Möller HJ, Kurz A, Basun H. Lithium trial in Alzheimer's disease: a randomized, single-blind, placebo-controlled, multicenter 10-week study. J Clin Psychiatry. 2009;70(6):922–31.

49. Cai Z, Yan Y, Wang Y. Minocycline alleviates beta-amyloid protein and tau pathology via restraining neuroinflammation induced by diabetic metabolic disorder. J Clin Interv Aging. 2013;8:1089–95.

50. Hashimoto K. Can minocycline prevent the onset of Alzheimer's disease? Ann Neurol. 2011;69(4):739–40.

51. Xiu-Lian W, Ji Z, Yang Y, Yan X, Zhi-Hua Z, Mei Q, Xiong Y, Xu-Ying S, Qing-Zhang T, Rong L, Jian-Zhi W. Helicobacter pylori filtrate induces Alzheimer-like tau hyperphosphorylation by activating glycogen synthase kinase-3β. J Alzheimers Dis. 2014(Jul 30).

52. Dineley K, Jahrling J, Denner L. Insulin resistance in Alzheimer's disease. Neurobiol Dis. 2014;72 Pt A:92–103.

53. Willette AA, Johnson SC, Birdsill AC, Sager MA, Christian B, Baker LD, Craft S, Oh J, Statz E, Hermann BP, Jonaitis EM, Koscik RL, La Rue A, Asthana S, Bendlin BB (2014). Insulin resistance predicts brain amyloid deposition in late middle-aged adults. Alzheimers Dement. 2014;pii: S1552-5260(14)02420-0.

54. Rdzak GM, Abdelghany O. Does insulin therapy for type 1 diabetes mellitus protect against Alzheimer's disease? Pharmacotherapy. 2014;34(12):1317–23.

55. Harrington C, Sawchak S, Chiang C, Davies J, Donovan C, Saunders AM, Irizarry M, Jeter B, Zvartau-Hind M, van Dyck CH, Gold M. Rosiglitazone does not improve cognition or global function when used as adjunctive therapy to AChE inhibitors in mild-to-moderate Alzheimer's disease: two phase 3 studies. Curr Alzheimer Res. 2011;8(5):592–606.

56. Gold M, Alderton C, Zvartau-Hind M, Egginton S, Saunders AM, Irizarry M, Craft S, Landreth G, Linnamägi U, Sawchak S. Rosiglitazone monotherapy in mild-to-moderate Alzheimer's disease: results from a randomized, double-blind, placebo-controlled phase III study. Dement Geriatr Cogn Disord. 2010;30(2):131–46.

57. Read S, Wu P, Biscow M. Sustained 4-year cognitive and functional response in early Alzheimer's disease with pioglitazone. J Am Geriatric Soc. 2014;62(3):584–6.

58. Reed B, Villeneuve S, Mack W, DeCarli C, Chui HC, Jagust W. Associations between serum cholesterol levels and cerebral amyloidosis. JAMA Neurol. 2014;71(2):195–200.

59. Wood WG, Li L, Müller WE, Eckert GP. Cholesterol as a causative factor in Alzheimer's disease: a debatable hypothesis. J Neurochem. 2014;129(4):559–72.

60. Medeiros R, Kitazawa M, Passos GF, Baglietto-Vargas D, Cheng D, Cribbs DH, LaFerla FM. Aspirin-triggered lipoxin A4 stimulates alternative activation of microglia and reduces Alzheimer disease-like pathology in mice. Am J Pathol. 2013;182(5):1780–9.

61. Rochette L, Ghibu S, Richard C, Zeller M, Cottin Y, Vergely C. Direct and indirect antioxidant properties of α-lipoic acid and therapeutic potential. Mol Nutr Food Res. 2013;57(1):114–25.

62. Hong ZY, Shi XR, Zhu K, Wu TT, Zhu YZ. SCM-198 inhibits microglial over activation and attenuates Aß. J Neuroinflammation. 2014;11(1):147.

63. Chauhan B, Kumar G, Kalam N, Ansari S. Current concepts and prospects of herbal nutraceutical: a review. J Adv Pharm Technol Res. 2013;4(1):4–8.

64. Nahin R, Fitzpatrick A, Williamson J, Burke G, Dekosky S, Furberg C. Use of herbal medicine and other dietary supplements in community-dwelling older people: baseline data from the ginkgo evaluation of memory study. J Am Geriatr Soc. 2006;54(11):1725–35.

65. Lindstrom A, Ooyen C, Lynch M, Blumenthal M. Herb supplement sales increase 5.5% in 2012: Herbal supplement sales rise for 9th consecutive year. HerbalGram. 2013;99:60–5.

66. Szuwart T, Brzoska T, Luger TA, Filler T, Peuker E, Dierichs R. Vitamin E reduces platelet adhesion to human endothelial cells in vitro. Am J Hematol. 2000;65(1):1–4.

67. Roland P, Nergård C. Ginkgo biloba–effect, adverse events and drug interaction. Tidsskrift For Den Norske Lægeforening: Tidsskrift For PraktiskMedicin, NyRække. 2012;132(8):956–9.

68. Selhub J. The many facets of hyperhomocysteinemia: studies from the Framingham cohorts. J Nutr. 2006;136(6 suppl):1726S–30.

69. Homocysteine Lowering Trialists' Collaboration. Lowering blood homocysteine with folic acid based supplements: meta-analysis of randomised trials. BMJ. 1998;316(7135):894–8.

70. Klee G. Cobalamin and folate evaluation: measurements of methylmalonic acid and homocystein vs vitamin B12 and folate. Clin Chem. 2000;46:1277–83.

71. Flicker L, Martins RN, Thomas J, et al. B-vitamins reduce plasma levels of beta amyloid. Neurobiol Aging. 2008;29(2):303–5.

72. Ford AH, Almeida OP. Effect of homocysteine lowering treatment on cognitive function: a systematic review and meta-analysis of randomized controlled trials. J Alzheimers Dis. 2012;29(1):133–49.

73. Balk EM, Raman G, Tatsioni A, Chung M, Lau J, Rosenberg IH. Vitamin B6, B12, and folic acid supplementation and cognitive function: a systematic review of randomized trials. Arch Intern Med. 2007;167(1):21–30.

74. Smith AD, Smith SM, de Jager CA, Whitbread P, Johnston C, Agacinski G, et al. Homocysteine-lowering by B vitamins slows the rate of accelerated brain atrophy in mild cognitive impairment: a randomized controlled trial. PLoS One. 2010;5(9), e12244.

75. O'Leary F, Allman-Farinelli M, Samman S. Vitamin B12 status, cognitive decline and dementia: a systematic review of prospective cohort studies. Br J Nutr. 2012;108(11):1948–61.

76. Gröber U, Kisters K, Schmidt J. Neuroenhancement with vitamin B12—underestimated neurological significance. Nutrients. 2013;5(12):5031–45.

77. Malouf R, AreosaSastre A. Vitamin B12 for cognition. Cochrane Database Syst Rev. 2003;(3):CD004326.

78. Clarfield AM. The decreasing prevalence of reversible dementias: an updated meta-analysis. Arch Intern Med. 2003;163:2219–29.

79. Kibirige D, Wekesa C, Kaddu-Mukasa M, Waiswa M. Vitamin B12 deficiency presenting as an acute confusional state: a case report and review of literature. Afr Health Sci. 2013;13(3):850–2.

80. Castelli MC, Friedman K, Sherry J, Brazzillo K, Genoble L, Bhargava P, Riley M. Comparing the efficacy and tolerability of a new daily oral vitamin B12 formulation and intermittent intramuscular vitamin B12 in normalizing low cobalamin levels: a randomized, open-label, parallel-group study. Clin Ther. 2011;33(3):358–71.

81. Masucci L, Goeree R. Vitamin B12 intramuscular injections versus oral supplements: a budget impact analysis. Ont Health Technol Assess Ser. 2013;13(24):1–24.

82. Malouf M, Grimley EJ, Areosa SA. Folic acid with or without vitamin B12 for cognition and dementia. Cochrane Database Syst Rev. 2003;(4):CD004514.

83. Moore E, Ames D, Watters D, et al. Among vitamin B12 deficient older people, high folate levels are associated with worse cognitive function: combined data from three cohorts. J Alzheimers Dis. 2014;39(3):661–8.

84. Malouf R, Grimley Evans J. The effect of vitamin B6 on cognition. Cochrane Database Syst Rev [serial online]. 2003;(4):CD004393.

85. Annweiler C, Rolland Y, Schott AM, Blain H, Vellas B, Herrmann FR, et al. Higher vitamin D dietary intake is associated with lower risk of Alzheimer's disease: a 7-year follow-up. J Gerontol A Biol Sci Med Sci. 2012;67:1205–11.

86. Annweiler C, Karras SN, Anagnostis P, Beauchet O. Vitamin D supplements: a novel therapeutic approach for Alzheimer patients. Front Pharmacol. 2014;5:1–4.

87. Annweiler C, Fantino B, Gauiter J, Beaudenon M, Thiery S, Beauchet O. Cognitive effects of vitamin D supplementation in older outpatients visiting a memory clinic: a pre-post study. J Am Geriatr Soc. 2012;60(4):793–5.

88. Annweiler C, Herrmann FR, Fantino B, Brugg B, Beauchet O. Effectiveness of the combination of memantine plus vitamin D on cognition in patients with Alzheimer disease: a pre-post pilot study. Cogn Behav Neurol. 2012;25:121–7.

89. Lehmann U, Hirche F, Stangl GI, Hinz K, Westphal S, Dierkes J. Bioavailability of vitamin D(2) and D(3) in healthy volunteers, a randomized placebo-controlled trial. J Clin Endocrinol Metab. 2013;98(11):4339–45.

90. Alshahrani F, Aljohani N. Vitamin D deficiency sufficiency and toxicity. Nutrients. 2013;5(9):3605–16.

91. Granado-Lorencio F, Rubio E, Blanco-Navarro I, Pérez-Sacristán B, Rodríguez-Pena R, GarcíaLópez F. Hypercalcemia, hypervitaminosis A and 3-epi-25-OH-D3 levels after consumption of an "over the counter" vitamin D remedy. A case report. Food Chem Toxicol. 2012;50(6):2106–8.

92. Mangialasche F, Kivipelto M, Fratiglioni L, et al. High plasma levels of vitamin E forms and reduced Alzheimer's disease risk in advanced age. J Alzheimers Dis. 2010;20(4):1029–37.

93. Farina N, Isaac M, Clark A, Rusted J, Tabet N. Vitamin E for Alzheimer's dementia and mild cognitive impairment. Cochrane Database Syst Rev [serial online]. 2012;11:CD002854.

94. Dysken M, Sano M, Asthana S, et al. Effect of vitamin E and memantine on functional decline in Alzheimer Disease: The TEAM-AD VA cooperative randomized trial. JAMA. 2014;311(1):33–44.

95. Miller III E, Pastor-Barriuso R, Dalal D, et al. Meta-analysis: high-dosage vitamin E supplementation may increase all-cause mortality. Ann Intern Med. 2005;142(1):37–46.

96. Lonn E, Bosch J, Yusuf S, et al. Effects of long-term vitamin E supplementation on cardiovascular events and cancer: a randomized controlled trial. JAMA. 2005;293:1338–47.

97. Doyle K. Fish oil sales don't reflect evidence. Reuters. 2013. Available at: http://www.reuters.com/article/2013/12/16/us-fish-oil-sales-dont-reflect-evidence-idUSBRE9BF1DH20131216

98. Barberger-Gateau P, Raffaitin C, Letenneur L, Berr C, Tzourio C, Dartigues JF, Alpérovitch A. Dietary patterns and risk of dementia: The Three-City cohort study. Neurology. 2007;69:1921–30.

99. Lim GP, Calon F, Morihara T, et al. A diet enriched with the omega-3 fatty acid docosahexaenoic acid reduces amyloid burden in an aged Alzheimer mouse model. J Neurosci. 2005;25:3032–40.

100. Ma QL, Teter B, Ubeda OJ, Morihara T, Dhoot D, Nyby MD, Tuck ML, Frautschy SA, Cole GM. Omega-3 fatty acid docosahexaenoic acid increases SorLA/LR11, a sorting protein with reduced expression in sporadic Alzheimer's disease (AD): relevance to AD prevention. J Neurosci. 2007;27:14299–307.

101. Shinto L, Quinn J, Montine T, Dodge H, Woodward W, Baldauf-Wagner S, Waichunas D, Bumgarner L, Bourdette D, Silbert L, Kaye J. A randomized placebo-controlled pilot trial of omega-3 fatty acids and alpha lipoic acid in Alzheimer's disease. J Alzheimers Dis. 2014;38(1):111–20.

102. Anderson BM, Ma DW. Are all n-3 polyunsaturated fatty acids created equal? Lipids Health Dis. 2009;8:33.

103. Sydenham E, Dangour A, Lim W. Omega 3 fatty acid for the prevention of cognitive decline and dementia. Cochrane Database Syst Rev [serial online]. 2012;(6):CD005379.

104. Franke A, Heinrich I, Lieb K, Fellgiebel A. The use of Ginkgo biloba in healthy elderly. Age (Dordr) [serial online]. 2014;36(1):435–444.

105. Maidment I. The use of ginkgo biloba in the treatment of dementia. Psychiatrist. 2001;25:353–6.

106. Stackman R, Eckenstein F, Frei B, Kulhanek D, Nowlin J, Quinn J. Prevention of age-related spatial memory deficits in a transgenic mouse model of Alzheimer's disease by chronic Ginkgo biloba treatment. Exp Neurol. 2003;184:510–20.

107. Rocher MN, Carré D, Spinnewyn B, Schulz J, Delaflotte S, Pignol B, Chabrier B, Auguet M. Long-term treatment with standardized Ginkgo biloba Extract (EGb 761) attenuates cognitive deficits and hippocampal neuron loss in a gerbil model of vascular dementia. Fitoterapia. 2011;82(7):1075–80.

108. Birks J, Grimley EJ. Ginkgo biloba for cognitive impairment and dementia. Cochrane Database Syst Rev. 2007;18(2), CD003120.

109. Ihl R. Effects of Ginkgo biloba extract EGb 761® in dementia with neuropsychiatric features: review of recently completed randomised, controlled trials. Int J Psychiatry Clin Pract. 2013;17 Suppl 1:8–14.

110. Kasper S, Schubert H. Ginkgo biloba extract EGb 761 in the treatment of dementia: evidence of efficacy and tolerability. Fortschritte Der Neurologie-Psychiatrie [serial online]. 2009;77(9):494–506.

111. Nasab N, Bahrammi M, Nikpour M, Rahim F, Naghibis S. Efficacy of rivastigmine in comparison to ginkgo for treating Alzheimer's dementia. J Pak Med Assoc [serial online]. 2012;62(7):677–80.

112. DeKosky ST, Williamson JD, Fitzpatrick AL, Kronmal RA, Ives DG, Saxton JA, Lopez OL, Burke G, Carlson MC, Fried LP, et al. Ginkgo biloba for prevention of dementia: a randomized controlled trial. JAMA. 2008;300(19):2253–62.

113. Vellas B, Coley N, Ousset P, Berrut G, Dartiques J, Dubois B, et al. Long-term use of standardised ginkgo biloba extract for the prevention of Alzheimer's disease (GuidAge): a randomised placebo-controlled trial. Lancet Neurol. 2012; 11(10):851–9.

114. EGb 761: ginkgo biloba extract, Ginkor. Drugs R D. 2003;4(3):188–93.

115. Alzheimer's Association, Public Policy Office, Robert Egge, Vice President (US). Letter addressed to US Senate Finance Committee and House Committee on Ways and Means [Internet]. Washington, DC: Alzheimer's Association, Public Policy Office; 2013 August 19 [cited 2015 February 8]. Available from: http://www.alz.org/national/documents/Medicare-PAC-Reform-8-19-13.pdf

116. Cummings JL. Alzheimer's disease. N Engl J Med. 2004;351:56–67.

117. Glick ID, Murray SR, Vasudevan P, Marder SR, Hu RJ. Treatment with atypical antipsychotics: new indications and new populations. J Psychiatr Res. 2001;35(3):187–91.

118. Briesacher BA, Limcangco MR, Simoni-Wastila L, Doshi JA, Levens SR, Shea DG, Stuart B. The quality of antipsychotic drug prescribing in nursing homes. Arch Intern Med. 2005;165(11):1280–5.

119. Hanlon JT, Handler SM, Castle NG. Antidepressant prescribing in US nursing homes between 1996 and 2006 and its relationship to staffing patterns and use of other psychotropic medications. J Am Med Dir Assoc. 2010;11(5):320–4.

120. Sørensen L, Foldspang A, Gulmann NC, Munk-Jørgensen P. Determinants for the use of psychotropics among nursing home residents. Int J Geriat Psychiatry. 2001;16(2):147–54.

121. Harms SL, Eberly LE, Garrard JM, Hardie NA, Bland PC, Leppik IE. Prevalence of appropriate and problematic antiepileptic combination therapy in older people in the nursing home. J Am Geriat Soc. 2005;53(6):1023–8.

122. Levinson DR. Medicare atypical antipsychotic drug claims for elderly nursing home residents. Department of Health and Human Services Office of Inspector General Report (OEI-07-08-00150)05-04-2011. http://oig.hhs.gov/oei/reports/oei-07-08-00150.asp. Retrieved 3 Feb 2015

123. Ballard C, Waite J, Birks J. Atypical antipsychotics for aggression and psychosis in Alzheimer's disease. Cochrane Database Syst Rev. 2012;(5):CD003476.

124. Schneider LS, Dagerman K, Insel PS. Efficacy and adverse effects of atypical antipsychotics for dementia: meta-analysis of randomized, placebo-controlled trials. Am J Geriatr Psychiatry. 2006;14:191–210.

125. Schneider LS, Tariot P, Dagerman K. Effectiveness of atypical antipsychotic drugs in residents with Alzheimer's disease. N Engl J Med. 2006;355: 1525–38.

126. Ray WA, Chung CP, Murray KT, Hall K, Stein CM. Atypical antipsychotic drugs and the risk of sudden cardiac death. N Engl J Med. 2009;360:225–35.

127. Rochon PA, Normand SL, Gomes T, Gill SS, Anderson GM, Melo M, et al. Antipsychotic therapy and short-term serious events in older adults with dementia. Arch Intern Med. 2008;168:1090–6.

128. Alexopoulos GS. Depression in the elderly. Lancet. 2005;365:1961–70.

129. Rabins PV, Blacker D, Rovner BW, Rummans T, Schneider LS, Tariot PN, Blass DM. American Psychiatric Association practice guideline for the treatment of patients with Alzheimer's disease and other dementias, 2nd Edition. Am J Psychiatry. 2007;164:1–56.

130. Majić T, Pluta JP, Mell T, Treusch Y, Gutzmann H, Rapp MA. Correlates of agitation and depression in nursing home residents with dementia. Int Psychogeriatr. 2012;24(11):1779–89.

131. Pollock BG. Comparison of citalopram, perphenazine, and placebo for the acute treatment of psychosis and behavior disturbances in hospitalized, demented patients. Am J Psychiatry. 2002; 159:460–5.

132. Pollock BG, Mulsant BH, Rosen J, Mazumdar S, Blakesly LE, Houck PR, et al. A double-blind comparison of citalopram and risperidone for the treatment of behavioral and psychotic symptoms associated with dementia. Am J Geriatr Psychiatry. 2007;15(11):942–52.

133. Teri L, Logsdon RG, Peskind E, Raskind M, Weiner MF, et al. Treatment of agitation in AD: a randomized, placebo-controlled clinical trial. Neurology. 2000;55:1271–8.

134. Sterke CS, van Beeck EF, van der Velde N, Ziere G, Petrovic M, Looman CW, van der Cammen TJ. Newinsights: dose-responserelationship between psychotropic drugs and falls: a study in nursing home residents with dementia. J Clin Pharmacol. 2012;52(6):947–55.

135. Eguale T, Buckeridge DL, Winslade NE, Benedetti A, Hanley JA, Tamblyn R. Drug, patient, and physician characteristics associated with off-label prescribing in primary care. Arch Intern Med. 2012;172(10):781–8.

136. Tariot PN, Erb R, Podgorski CA, Cox C, Patel S, Jakimovich L, Irvine C. Efficacy and tolerability of carbamazepine for agitation and aggression in dementia. Am J Psychiatry. 1998;155:54–61.

137. Tariot PN, Schneider LS, Mintzer J, Cutler AJ, Cunningham MR, Thomas JW, Sommerville KW. Safety and tolerability of divalproex sodium in the treatment of signs and symptoms of mania in elderly patients with dementia: results of a double-blind, placebo controlled trial. Curr Ther Res Clin Exp. 2001;62:51–67.

138. Uchida H, Suzuki T, Mamo DC, Mulsant BH, Kikuchi T, Takeuchi H, et al. Benzodiazepine and antidepressant use in elderly patients with anxiety disorders: a survey of 796 outpatients in Japan. J Anxiety Disord. 2009;23(4):477–81.

139. Wetzels RB, Zuidema SU, de Jonghe JF, Verhey FR, Koopmans RT. Prescribing pattern of psychotropic

drugs in nursing home residents with dementia. Int Psychogeriatr. 2011;23(8):1249–59.

140. Stevenson DG, Decker SL, Dwyer LL, Huskamp HA, Grabowski DC, Metzger ED, Mitchell SL. Antipsychotic and benzodiazepine use among nursing home residents: findings from the 2004 national nursing home survey. Am J Geriatr Psychiatry. 2010;18(12):1078–92.

141. Paton C. Benzodiazepines and disinhibition: a review. Psychiatrist. 2002;26:460–2.

142. Huber M, Kölzsch M, Rapp MA, Wulff I, Kalinowski S, Bolbrinker J, et al. Antipsychotic Drugs predominate in pharmacotherapy of nursing home residents with dementia. Pharmacopsychiatry. 2012;45(5): 182–8.

143. American Geriatrics Society, & American Association for Geriatric Psychiatry. Consensus statement on improving the quality of mental health care in U.S. nursing homes: management of depression and behavioral symptoms associated with dementia. J Am Geriatr Soc. 2003;51(9):1287–98.

144. McKeith I, Del Ser T, Spano P, Emre M, Wesnes K, Anand R, et al. Efficacy of rivastigmine in dementia with Lewy bodies: a randomized, double blind, placebo-controlled international study. Lancet. 2000;356:2031–6.

145. Feldman H, Gauthier S, Hecker J, Vellas B, Subbiah P, Whalen E. A 24-week, randomized, doubleblind study of donepezil in moderate to severe Alzheimer's disease. Neurology. 2001;57:613–20.

146. Erkinjuntti T, Kurz A, Gauthier S, Bullock R, Lilienfeld S, Damaraju CV. Efficacy of galantamine in probable vascular dementia and Alzheimer's disease combined with cerebrovascular disease: a randomized trial. Lancet. 2002;359:1283–90.

147. American Geriatrics Society. Updated Beers Criteria for potentially inappropriate medication use in older adults. J Am Geriatr Soc. 2012;60:616–31.

Treatment of Dementia: Non-pharmacological Approaches

Elizabeth Galik

Behavioral symptoms associated with dementia such as physical and verbal aggression, mood disturbances, psychotic symptoms, agitation, resistance to care, and sleep disorders are common and distressing for both individuals with dementia and their caregivers. Behavioral symptoms are also commonly referred to as behavioral disturbance, behavioral and psychological symptoms of dementia (BPSD), and neuropsychiatric symptoms. While behavioral symptoms are frequently time limited, it is estimated that almost all individuals with dementia will develop them at some point during the course of their illness [1, 2]. Additionally, the majority of individuals with dementia will require non-pharmacological and/or pharmacological interventions in an attempt to decrease or eliminate these behaviors.

Pharmacologic management of behavioral symptoms among individuals with dementia has been minimally effective and is fraught with significant risks, such as, falls, fractures, delirium, parkinsonism, stroke, pneumonia, and death [3–8]. The International Association of Gerontology and Geriatrics, the Center for Medicare and Medicaid (CMS), and the National Alzheimer Project Act (NAPA) advocate for the use of non-pharmacologic interventions as first line treatment in the management of behavioral symptoms, seek to minimize psychotropic medication use among individuals with dementia, and call for high quality research and education on non-pharmacologic strategies for the management of these symptoms [9–11]. Additionally, the American Psychiatric Association (APA) and the American Association for Geriatric Psychiatry (AAGP) strongly support the use of non-pharmacological interventions in all individuals with dementia through published treatment guidelines and position statements [12, 13].

In 2012, the Centers for Medicare and Medicaid Services (CMS) launched the *National Partnership to Improve Dementia Care and Reduce Antipsychotic Use in Nursing Homes*. Through this initiative, there has been a 17 % reduction in antipsychotic medication use among long term nursing home residents [14]. While the decrease in antipsychotic use was encouraging, reduction of antipsychotic drug use is only one part of providing quality dementia care. The ultimate goal of the *National Partnership to Improve Dementia Care and Reduce Antipsychotic Use in Nursing Homes* is to increase the use of non-pharmacological interventions, encourage the use of person-centered care and optimize residents' quality of life. To achieve this goal, it is critical to supplement medication reduction with non-pharmacological interventions to improve dementia care and decrease challenging behavioral symptoms.

While policy initiatives have helped to reduce pharmacological interventions to treat BPSD

E. Galik, PhD, CRNP (✉)
University of Maryland School of Nursing,
655 West Lombard Street, Baltimore,
MD 21201, USA
e-mail: galik@son.umaryland.edu

© Springer International Publishing Switzerland 2016
M. Boltz, J.E. Galvin (eds.), *Dementia Care*, DOI 10.1007/978-3-319-18377-0_7

among nursing home residents, health care providers, professional caregivers, and family caregivers continue to consider pharmacologic interventions as a primary way in which to manage challenging behavioral symptoms [15, 16]. While staff support the use of non-pharmacological interventions, they acknowledge insufficient knowledge about these approaches to manage BPSD and lack confidence in their ability to consistently implement them [16–18].

Additional challenges to the implementation of non-pharmacological interventions for BPSD include environments that exacerbate BPSD, lack of physical activity, boredom, excessive fear of the resident causing harm to self or others, and caregiver burden [19, 20]. Implementation of non-pharmacological interventions to modify or treat behavioral symptoms of dementia will require knowledge about available interventions, appropriate intervention selection strategies, and behavior change on the part of the clinician as well as the family caregiver. Given that the majority of people with dementia live in the community and for approximately 75 % of these individuals, care is provided by family and friends, [21] a partnership between the clinician and family caregiver is critical to support their emotional well-being and behavioral stability. Ongoing education, use of resources (e.g., adult day programs) and engaging the family in plan to monitor the patient's mood, behavior, and function will help prevent distress and the associated behavioral symptoms.

This chapter will review common BPSD that may be responsive to non-pharmacological interventions, describe the impact of behavioral symptoms on the patient, family, and professional caregivers, summarize the origins and risk factors associated with behavioral symptoms among individuals with dementia, and outline a step approach to the assessment of behavior problems in preparation for the implementation of non-pharmacological interventions. Categories of non-pharmacological interventions for the management of BPSD will be discussed and these include: (1) Sensory stimulation; (2) Cognitive stimulation and training; (3) Emotion-oriented interventions; (4) Physical Activity and Exercise; and (5) Behavioral training and educational interventions. Using the latest evidence regarding feasibility of intervention implementation and efficacy, a step approach to the selection and implementation of non-pharmacological interventions will also be summarized.

Categories of Common Behavioral Symptoms

Individuals with dementia frequently experience a variety of non-cognitive neuropsychiatric and behavioral symptoms. The common types of behavioral symptoms seen among individuals with dementia include affective/mood disturbances, psychotic symptoms, agitation/resistance to care, and sleep pattern disturbance. The most prevalent behavioral symptoms include depression, apathy and agitation, while caregivers identify that the most distressing symptoms associated with BPSD include psychotic symptoms, and agitation which includes verbal and physical aggression [22].

Affective/Mood Disturbances

Depression is one of the most common BPSD of dementia, and often presents as an atypical symptom constellation (depression without sadness or masked depression) characterized by anhedonia, irritability, anxiety, psychomotor agitation, worsening of cognitive symptoms, sleep disturbance, weight loss, and mood congruent delusions. Sadness, tearfulness, and self-depreciation are much less common or prominent, and suicidality is rare. The reported rates of depression in Alzheimer's disease, the most common cause of dementia, vary widely. In several studies when patients with dementia have been evaluated thoroughly for symptoms of depression, the prevalence of clinically significant depression ranged from 18 to 32 % [2]. Depression is most common among individuals with vascular dementia, Parkinson's disease dementia, and Lewy body dementia [23–25].

Apathy is the most common behavioral symptom seen among all types of dementia syndromes and is associated with moderate to severe cognitive impairment [26]. Apathy within the context of dementia is characterized by emotional indifference, lack of interest in usual activities and relationships, decreased motivation and initiative, and social withdrawal [27–29] . Clinical apathy has been minimally responsive to pharmacological interventions, but does seem to improve modestly with structured activities and one-on-one personal interactions [30].

Psychotic Symptoms

Delusions and illusions occur in 30–40 % of patients with Alzheimer's disease at some point during the course of the illness [31]. Approximately, 25 % of individuals with Alzheimer's disease experience hallucinations [31]. Hallucinations associated with Alzheimer's disease are typically visual, especially among individuals with underlying eye disease, such as glaucoma or macular degeneration. Auditory hallucinations can also occur in Alzheimer's disease and typically are distressing for the patient and family. Among patients with more severe dementia who have significant expressive aphasia, psychotic symptoms may result in troubling behaviors such as aggressive behaviors, barricading in a room, hiding belongings, or refusing to eat. Psychotic symptoms are even more common among individuals with Lewy body dementia with visual hallucinations experienced by up to 80 % of these individuals [25].

Agitation/Resistance to Care

Agitation is defined as increased motor activity with elevated feelings of internal tension and frustration [32]. Agitation includes a variety of symptoms, such as verbal aggression, verbally non-aggressive behaviors (i.e. repetitive vocalizations), physical aggression, resistance to care, wandering, and impulsive behaviors. Physically aggressive and resistant behaviors are associated with severe cognitive impairment, functional dependency, restraint use, and

male gender [33–36]. Female gender is more commonly associated with verbal aggression and repetitive vocalizations [37].

Additionally, many of these agitated behavioral symptoms are most likely to occur during personal care interactions and frequently challenge and frustrate caregivers [17, 34, 38, 39]. Individuals with moderate to severe cognitive impairment typically experience challenges in communicating and understanding spoken language, and misinterpret touch that occurs during provision of care activities [35, 40]. Physical assistance with care is perceived as a threat that often results in a fear, fight or flight response [41], resistance to care and other behavioral symptoms [42, 43].

Sleep Pattern Disturbance

Sleep pattern disturbances include insomnia, daytime lethargy, and day-night reversal and occur in approximately 25–35 % of individuals with dementia [44, 45]. Sleep disturbances typically coexist with other previously mentioned BPSD and are associated with patient impairments in function, cognition, and caregiver burden [44, 45].

Impact of Behavioral Symptoms

For the individual with dementia, BPSD negatively impacts quality of life, increases risk of injury, exacerbates functional decline, leads to inappropriate use of psychotropic medications, and increases the likelihood of early institutionalization [8, 22, 46–48]. For caregivers, both family and professional, BPSD is known to increase caregiver burden, time spent in caregiving activities, risk of injury, risk of depression, and decrease satisfaction with the caregiving role [17, 38, 49–51]. In a Canadian study, 89 % of nursing assistants experienced at least one incident of combative behavior while providing care to residents with dementia during the previous month [17]. Most of the incidents occurred during assistance with activities of daily living and the most common behaviors were slapping, squeezing, punching, hitting, and shoving [17]. Exposure to persistent behavioral symptoms can also lead to decreased job satisfaction and staff turnover among direct care workers in long term care and home care settings [38, 51, 52].

Origins and Triggers of Behavioral Symptoms in Dementia

Prior to the implementation of an individualized non-pharmacological intervention and/or pharmacologic management of BPSD, it is important to consider potential origins or common triggers for the behavioral symptom. Determine whether the patient is experiencing an underlying medical condition or disease state that can cause or aggravate behavioral symptoms. Common conditions such as constipation, infection, exacerbation of a chronic medical illness, dehydration, pain, delirium, depression, anxiety, or an adverse medication side effect can impact a patient's behavior and should be assessed and treated appropriately. For example, a patient who was has poorly managed diabetes and polyuria may become increasingly resistant to care due to more frequent urinary incontinence and toileting. A patient with dementia and chronic obstructive pulmonary disorder may experience mood lability due to long term anti-inflammatory treatment with prednisone. Simply put, active medical problems should be ruled out or addressed before consideration is given to implementation of non-pharmacological and/or pharmacological interventions.

Environmental factors, such as uncomfortable temperature, inadequate lighting, loud noise, tethering that restrict movement or mobility (i.e. intravenous lines, catheters, restraints), and the patient's lack familiarity with an environmental setting must be considered as potential aggravating factors for behavioral symptoms. The loud and unfamiliar environment of an acute care setting or a crowded public venue can be over-stimulating for an individual with dementia and may result in catastrophic behavioral responses. The use of restraints or other tethering devices among individuals with dementia is to be avoided.

The caregiver's approach may also influence the behavior of the individual with dementia. This is often the challenge faced when patients refuse or resist assistance with activities of daily living. Caregivers who possess an understanding of the cognitive symptoms of dementia (memory loss, aphasia, motor apraxia, agnosia) are more likely to successfully adjust their expectations to the patient's underlying capabilities [51, 53, 54]. Caregivers who talk to rapidly, give multiple step directions, attempt to reason and rationalize with the patient, perform care tasks for the patient rather than actively engaging the patient in the process, and/or utilize too many caregivers to complete care activities are more likely to encounter challenging patient behavioral symptoms.

Assessment of BPSD: A Three Step Process

The assessment of BPSD requires a holistic and systematic approach. The first step involves an accurate description of the target behavior(s). Table 1 summarizes common behavioral symptoms and gives specific examples of clinical presentations. It is not uncommon for an individual with dementia to exhibit behaviors in more than one category. In addition to a description and classification of the target behavior, it is also important to collect data on the onset, frequency, duration, setting, antecedents associated with the behavior, aggravating and relieving factors. Behavior is rarely random or unprovoked, and a thorough description and history associated with the behavior is necessary in order to design an effective non-pharmacological management strategy.

Following a clear description of the target behavioral symptom, the second step involves a thorough assessment of the patient and his/her underlying medical conditions prior to the initiation of any specific non-pharmacological and/or pharmacological treatment. This assessment should include a medical history (with particular attention to medication reconciliation, review of systems), personal and occupational history,

Table 1 Common behavioral and psychological symptoms of dementia with clinical presentation

Behavioral classification	Common clinical presentation in dementia
Depressive symptoms	Loss of appetite, weight loss, anhedonia, irritability, anxiety, psychomotor agitation or retardation, self-deprecating statements, tearfulness, mood congruent delusions (in more severe cases) [29, 55, 56]
Apathy	Social withdrawal, flat or restricted affect, difficult to motivate, psychomotor retardation, lack of interest [27, 28, 57]
Verbally aggressive	Screaming, yelling, cursing, derogatory comments, name calling, threaten [32, 58, 59]
Verbally non-aggressive	Persistent requests for help or attention, repetitive calling out, complaining, rambling speech [32, 58, 59]
Physically aggressive	Hitting, kicking, biting, scratching, grabbing, pinching, spitting, squeezing, pushing, throwing things [32, 58, 59]
Physically non-aggressive	Pacing, wandering, intrusive behaviors (getting into other's personal space or rooms), elopement, searching, gathering/collecting [58–61]
Resistance to care	Pull away, turn away, avoidance of care, refusal of care, grab object, clench mouth [43, 62, 63]
Disinhibition	Disrobing, inappropriate/unwanted verbal or physical sexual advances [2, 36]
Sleep pattern disturbance	Insomnia, day–night reversal, early morning awakening [44, 45]
Delusion	Fixed false belief held despite evidence to the contrary; paranoia, persecutory delusions, delusions of infidelity, delusions of people stealing [64, 65]
Hallucination	A sensory experience without a stimuli; visual and auditory are most common in dementia [64, 65]
Illusion	A misperception/misinterpretation of an actual stimulus; for example a slamming door is perceived as a gunshot [65]

physical examination, mental status and cognitive examination, and any relevant laboratory tests or diagnostic studies that may clarify treatable medical conditions that are consistent with the patient and family goals of care. A sudden change in the patient's level of consciousness, attention, cognition, functional ability, and/or behavior is often the first sign of a delirium or complicating medical problem.

As a third step in the process, rating scales provide a standardized and accurate way to assess not only the behavioral symptoms, but also the patient's underlying cognitive, functional and physical capabilities. This baseline information is critical in the identification of appropriate non-pharmacological interventions that are feasible to implement. For example, before recommending a physical activity intervention to decrease night-time wandering and insomnia, underlying physical and cognitive capability must be known to match appropriate activities with the patient's remaining strengths, preferences, and abilities. Additionally, rating scales can also be used to monitor symptoms and

track non-pharmacological intervention efficacy over time. Ideally, rating scales/instruments should be simple to administer, and have evidence of reliability and validity with individuals with dementia. Table 2 summarizes instruments that are psychometrically sound and commonly used with individuals with dementia.

Non-pharmacological Interventions for Behavioral Symptoms

Given our increasing knowledge of the morbidity and mortality risks associated with pharmacological interventions, particularly antipsychotics, several professional organizations and practice guidelines support the use of non-pharmacological interventions as first line treatment for individuals with BPSD [13, 74–76] and should also be used in concurrently when pharmacological interventions may be needed. Whenever possible, non-pharmacological interventions should be identified and adapted to the patient's preferences, known motivating factors, strengths, and

Table 2 Rating scales to assess cognition, behavior, and functional ability of individuals with dementia

Domain	Instrument	Rating scale description
Cognition	Mini-Mental Status Examination (MMSE)	A 30 point cognitive screening instrument that assesses orientation, registration, recall, calculation, language, and visual spatial skills. Takes 10 min to administer. Widely used; however has significant ceiling and floor effects and underestimates cognitive abilities among individuals with significant aphasia [66]
	Montreal Cognitive Assessment (MOCA)	A 30 point scale that assesses visual spatial skills/ executive function, naming, memory, attention, language, abstraction, recall, and orientation. Can be administered in 10–15 min [67]
	Severe Impairment Rating Scale (SIRS)	An 11 item, 22 point scale that measures the cognitive ability in individuals with severe dementia [68]
Physical/functional	Tinetti Gait and Balance	An observed performance measure of the ability gait and balance that takes 10–15 min to administer [69]
	Barthel Index	A 14 item measure of physical function that assesses an individual's ability for self-care with activities of daily living. Can be used as a performance measure or with verbal report from a reliable source. A total score of 100 on the Barthel Index indicates complete independence, while a score of 0 indicates total dependence [70]
	Basic Physical Capability Scale	A performance based measured designed to assess the underlying physical and cognitive capability of older adults. The scale has established validity and reliability with older adults across care settings and with varying levels of cognitive impairment [71, 72]
Behavioral/psychological	Cornell Scale for Depression in Dementia	A 19 item survey designed to assess depressive symptoms in individuals with dementia [55]
	Apathy Evaluation Inventory	An instrument that provides an assessment of global apathy in addition to cognitive, behavioral, and emotional apathy [57]
	Cohen-Mansfield Agitation Inventory	An instrument that was designed for use in the nursing home and measures the frequency of 29 agitated behaviors [58]
	Neuropsychiatric Inventory (NPI)	Assesses the frequency and severity of 10 behavioral symptoms common among individuals with dementia including delusions, hallucinations, dysphoria, anxiety, agitation/aggression, euphoria, disinhibition, irritability/lability, apathy, and aberrant motor activity. Commonly used in research. Can be lengthy to administer [73]
	Resistiveness to Care Scale	Is a 13 item observation, likert scale designed to assess aggressive and resistive behaviors that occur during care activities [43]

abilities [32]. Non-pharmacological interventions for BPSD are known to have fewer risks associated with their use than pharmacological alternatives [74–77]. There are several hundred research studies that have investigated the efficacy of non-pharmacological interventions particularly for BPSD, and many of them have demonstrated positive findings, such as improvements in mood, quality of life, functional abilities, sleep, and cognition, and behavioral symptoms among individuals with dementia [74–78]. Similarly, caregivers of individuals with dementia have also shown some benefits from non-pharmacological interventions including reduction of caregiver burden, and increased knowledge of dementia and effective caregiving strategies [53, 54].

Unfortunately, many of the studies involving non-pharmacological interventions have significant methodological flaws, such as small sample size, single group studies, lack of blinding in the measurement of outcomes, measurement challenges, multi-component interventions that are poorly described and may lack replicability, and lack of long term efficacy and sustainability data [76, 77]. Multi-component interventions also make it difficult to determine which parts of the intervention constellation were actually effective. Many of the behavioral training studies conducted in the long term care setting are efficacy trials of non-pharmacological interventions that are carried out by research staff that is external to the institution [20]. Future research should focus on testing these intervention in real world settings where trained staff of the facilities function as the behavioral interventionists. Nevertheless, knowledge gained by these studies lays the groundwork for future research with higher quality study designs that are also feasible to disseminate and implement in real world settings.

There is no universally accepted categorization of non-pharmacological interventions designed for individuals with dementia. For the purpose of this chapter, non-pharmacological interventions have been organized into the following categories: sensory stimulation, cognitive stimulation and training, emotion-oriented interventions, physical activity and exercise, and behavioral education and training interventions.

Sensory Stimulation

Sensory stimulation consists of activities designed to engage, refocus, or redirect individuals with dementia to meaningful and/or pleasant activities [79]. Some of the most common forms of sensory stimulation include aromatherapy, music, massage and touch, animal assisted therapy, one-to-one interaction, and the use of Snoezelen rooms, which are also known as multisensory rooms [76]. A recent study among

nursing home residents with dementia demonstrated that direct care workers were most likely to use one-to-one personal interaction and music to address behavioral symptoms; however, the most efficacious of these sensory stimulation techniques included hand massage, activities consistent with past life routines (i.e. folding towels, setting the table), and one-to-one personal interaction and music [80].

While music interventions have been effective in decreasing behavioral symptoms particularly during meals and caregiving activities, the benefits achieved are typically only during the music activity and does not extend beyond the length of the sensory experience [76, 81, 82]. The effectiveness of aromatherapy seemed to be mixed with some studies finding no improvement in behavioral symptoms [76, 83]. The use of animal assisted therapy has increased among older adults with dementia over the past 5 years; however, the efficacy is often mixed and many studies lack rigorous study designs [76, 84–87]. Modest improvements in behavior, mood and physical activity of individuals with dementia have been seen with the implementation of animal assisted therapies [84, 87]. While there has been some evidence that the use of Snoezelen rooms can improve mood symptoms and decrease agitation, caregivers of individuals with dementia frequently do not make use of them, and patients may be resistant to their use [76, 88, 89]. While sensory stimulation interventions generally are considered low risk, not all individuals respond positively to these activities and in some cases, over-stimulation can occur and result in increased agitation and other behavioral symptoms [76].

Cognitive Stimulation and Training

The development of cognitive stimulation and training arose from the theory of neuronal plasticity which suggests that despite illness or trauma, the adult brain retains some ability for regeneration and compensation [90]. These interventions have primarily be en utilized with individuals with minor cognitive impairment and with individuals with mild to moderate dementia [91].

Cognitive stimulation utilizes a range of activities aimed at the general enhancement of cognitive abilities, while cognitive training involves guided learning and repetition related to a set of tasks designed to improve particular areas of cognitive function, such as memory, orientation, attention, language, and executive function [90]. Positive effects of cognitive stimulation and training typically are modest at best with improvements limited to the specific activity that is being practiced and rehearsed [90–93]. Some studies do show longer term benefit related to general cognitive functioning and personal well-being, but many of these studies suffer from methodological concerns [92, 93]. Typically, there is little evidence to support that cognitive stimulation and training results in clinically significant improvements in mood, behavior, or performance of activities of daily living [90, 92, 93].

Emotion-Oriented interventions

Emotion-oriented interventions consist of techniques and strategies designed to address patients' emotional needs through the use of empathy, reassurance, distraction and/or guided interactions that elicit and emphasize positive emotions. The three most common emotion-oriented interventions include reminiscence, validation therapy, and simulated presence [76]. Reminiscence therapy encourages the discussion of past events, experiences, and relationships with other people. Reminiscence can occur in a dyad or in a group setting and utilizes items such as photographs, newspapers, and personal items that are likely to elicit discussion and positive emotions. While research involving reminiscence and life review among individuals with dementia has been limited, there is some evidence that reminiscence improves mood, quality of life, and well-being [76, 94–96]. Reminiscence is most effective for BPSD when activities are individualized [97]. Shared, common experiences are less likely to have a positive impact on mood and well-being [96, 97].

Validation therapy focuses on the acceptance of the patient's emotions and their perceived reality. Validation therapy is the opposite of reality orientation and has been more effective among individuals with more severe cognitive impairment [76]. Validation therapy has not been rigorously tested and the findings related to efficacy are mixed [76, 91]. Simulated presence therapy is based on personal attachments and relationships and typically involves the use of recorded voices or videography of close relatives and friends of the individual with dementia. Additionally, dolls and stuffed animals have also been used as substitutes for caring for children and cherished pets. Goals for simulated presence typically involve adherence to medications or treatments, performance of activities of daily living, and minimizing resistance to care and other behavioral symptoms [98]. Research related to simulated presence therapy is rare, poorly designed and results are mixed [76, 98, 99]. There is no convincing evidence that simulated presence therapy is effective in the management of behavioral symptoms and in some instances there have been worsening of behavioral symptoms among some individuals with dementia [76].

Physical Activity and Exercise

Exercise and physical activity interventions have been widely studied among individuals with dementia in community and long term care settings [53, 100–104]. Common physical activities and exercise that are used with individuals with dementia include walking, dancing, resistance exercises, swimming, Tai Chi, and yoga. Additionally, for individuals with more severe cognitive impairment and/or frailty, increasing mobility through ambulation, wheel chair self-propulsion, chair exercises, dancing, physically active games, and active participation in functional activities are also commonly used.

Physical inactivity has been associated with more frequent and more severe agitated behaviors among older adults with dementia [105, 106]. Promoting optimum level of patient physical activity and active participation in functional activities could decrease the risk of behavioral symptoms while simultaneously optimizing function [62, 107]. Even for those with severe cognitive impairment, use of cueing, gesturing, pantomime, and hand over hand care reduces fear and resistance to care and also promotes functional independence and physical activity [108]. While this physical, functional and behavioral approach has been tested in isolated care tasks such as dressing [109], bathing [63], and mouth care [62], little work has been done that integrates this approach across all activities of daily living and actually measures both functional and behavioral outcomes with the goal of improving function and decreasing behavioral symptoms.

While there are some studies that have demonstrated improvements in behavioral symptoms among individuals with dementia through the use of exercise, physical activity, and active participation in functional activities [53, 100, 102, 110, 111], overall, the findings are mixed. Improvements in physical function, mood, sleep, and decreased caregiver burden are more common positive findings with the implementation of exercise and physical activity interventions [76, 91, 100, 103, 106, 112].

Behavioral Education and Training Interventions

Behavioral education and training interventions encompass a wide variety of management techniques including functional analysis of specific behaviors, token economies, communication training, establishment of routines, behavioral modification, and individualized behavioral reinforcement strategies [76]. Most behavioral interventions are focused on training caregivers to effectively interpret the behaviors of individuals with dementia through identifying and resolving an unmet need or a stressor, and/or adapting the caregiver's response to the patient's behavior [76, 77]. Behavioral education and training interventions have been widely studied and show promise in improvements in BPSD and decreasing caregiver stress [62, 76, 77, 91, 107, 113]. Although this is not a comprehensive list, Table 3

Table 3 Caregiver interaction strategies that minimize behavioral symptoms [78, 114, 115]

Caregiver interaction strategy	Rationale
Use simple words and phrases when giving directions	Minimizes the impact of receptive aphasia
Resist the urge to talk too much; cue and role model desired behaviors	Minimizes the impact of receptive aphasia and decreases an over-stimulating environment
Speak in a lower pitch for individuals with hearing loss	For individuals with sensorineural healing loss, lower pitched sounds are easier to hear than high pitched sounds
Be patient and give patients time to respond to questions	Minimizes the impact of receptive aphasia and response delay
Engage patients in talking about pleasant events before attempting to involve them in the care task at hand	Use familiar objects, older photographs, favorite music which may assist in normalizing the environment and the interaction
Avoid overwhelming the patient with several caregivers at one time	Too many caregivers increases environmental stimulation and may be perceived by the patient as a threat
Avoid reasoning and rationalizing	Memory loss, deficits in executive functioning, and decreased insight into cognitive deficits leads to inability to process reality orientation and rationalizing
Actively involve the patient in his/her own care activities	Physical assistance with care is perceived as a threat that often results in a fear, fight or flight response [41], resistance to care and other behavioral symptoms

offers simple suggestions for caregivers that may help to optimize the caregiver's interaction with individuals with dementia.

While caregiver knowledge about behavioral assessment, interpretation and management are essential, educational interventions alone are unlikely to result in improvements in BPSD [116]. Knowledge, in addition to caregiver motivation, coaching, practice and support over time are necessary to decrease BPSD and caregiver stress [63]. Additionally, intervention delivery is highly dependent on the knowledge and skill of the interventionist.

Implementing Non-pharmacological Interventions: A Step Approach

Step 1: Assessment of the Environment and Caregiver Support Network

Prior to implementing non-pharmacological interventions to manage behavioral symptoms for individuals with dementia, it is helpful to critically appraise the environment and potential sources of support for the caregiver(s). For example, is there safe access to the outdoors that could be used for walking and exercise? Does the home or institutional setting have resources or supplies that are needed for sensory stimulation or reminiscence activities? Additionally, it is important to identify potential sources of support for both the patient and the caregiver. For example, having the patient attend a nearby medical adult day program provides structured activities and opportunities for the patient, but also much needed respite for the caregiver. In a long term care facility, are direct care workers given a reasonable amount of time to complete assignments and incorporate non-pharmacological approaches in their care practices? Is the administration of the long term care facility supportive of non-pharmacological approaches to dementia care?

Step 2: Establishing a Philosophy of Care that Supports Non-pharmacological Interventions

The success of any intervention designed to minimize behavioral symptoms of individuals with dementia depends on the caregivers' receptiveness to learn new care techniques and strategies and on their motivation to use these new techniques routinely [117–121]. The first step in implementing non-pharmacological interventions is to strengthen the caregivers' self-efficacy (their beliefs in their own ability to implement non-pharmacological approaches) and outcome expectations (their beliefs in the benefits of non-pharmacological approaches) [122]. Caregivers will need an educational introduction to the different types of non-pharmacological interventions and should be given strategies on how they can implement them in their setting and situation. Caregivers should learn about the potential benefits of implementing non-pharmacological interventions, such as, improved BPSD and quality of life for the patient and decreased caregiver burden, decreased risk of injury, and increased satisfaction with the caregiving role for both family and direct care workers.

Step 3: Describe the Behavior and Assess Underlying Cognition and Physical/Functional Capabilities

In order to develop appropriate behavioral care goals, a comprehensive assessment should be completed to determine the underlying capabilities, strengths, and personal preferences of the individual with dementia. Strategies for the assessment of cognition, function, behavior, were discussed earlier in this chapter and measurement tools are described in Table 2. An accurate and detailed description of the target behavior is necessary in order to rule out complicating medical problems and to select and implement an appropriate non-pharmacological management plan.

Step 4: Set Individualized and Behavioral Goals

Non-pharmacological interventions should be individualized, person-centered and encourage activities that are familiar and consistent with the individual's past life experiences. Long term memory and routine activity and behavioral patterns are preserved until later stages of dementia. Knowing the patient's previous routines, experiences, and preferences can be used to motivate him/her to participate in individualized non-pharmacological interventions. For example, an individual who has always loved animals may respond positively to animal assisted therapy, and a former athlete may enjoy engaging in exercise and physical activities. In additional to providing familiar and comfortable experiences, patients can also benefit from trying activities or interactions that are new and different. For example, a patient who has infrequently engaged in physical activity may enjoy a lively movement group with peers. Or a spouse, who was rarely involved with grocery shopping, may take pleasure in shopping and packing groceries with his spouse.

Step 5: Ongoing Mentoring and Monitoring

It is important to recognize that implementing non-pharmacological interventions is challenging, and that all caregivers require ongoing support and encouragement. In addition to believing in the potential positive benefits of non-pharmacological approaches, caregivers must begin to have confidence in their ability to understand behavioral symptoms and implement non-pharmacological interventions. While skills training and education is helpful, caregivers should receive positive feedback and be applauded for any and all attempts to utilize non-pharmacological strategies.

Conclusion

Due to potential risks associated with pharmacological management of BPSD, non-pharmacological interventions are recommended as the primary intervention for individuals with dementia. While there are methodological concerns regarding some non-pharmacological interventions, their minimal risk to patients and evidence of efficacy particularly among behavioral education and training and physical activity/exercise, provides justification for their continued use. Future research should focus on larger randomized controlled trials, and testing the

efficacy of these interventions when implemented in real world settings by front-line caregivers in community and institutional settings.

References

1. Sadak TI, Katon J, Beck C, Cochrane BB, Borson S. Key neuropsychiatric symptoms in common dementias: prevalence and implications for caregivers, clinicians, and health systems. Res Gerontol Nurs. 2014;7(1):44–52.
2. Desai AK, Schwartz L, Grossberg GT. Behavioral disturbance in dementia. Curr Psychiatry Rep. 2012;14(4):298–309.
3. Schneider LS, Dagerman KS, Insel P. Risk of death with atypical antipsychotic drug treatment for dementia: meta-analysis of randomized placebo-controlled trials. JAMA. 2005;294(15):1934–43.
4. Huybrechts KF, Gerhard T, Crystal S, Olfson M, Avorn J, Levin R, et al. Differential risk of death in older residents in nursing homes prescribed specific antipsychotic drugs: population based cohort study. BMJ. 2012;344, e977.
5. Schneider LS, Tariot PN, Dagerman KS, Davis SM, Hsiao JK, Ismail MS, et al. Effectiveness of atypical antipsychotic drugs in patients with Alzheimer's disease. N Engl J Med. 2006;355(15):1525–38.
6. Kales HC, Kim HM, Zivin K, Valenstein M, Seyfried LS, Chiang C, et al. Risk of mortality among individual antipsychotics in patients with dementia. Am J Psychiatry. 2012;169(1):71–9.
7. Sterke CS, van Beeck EF, van der Velde N, Ziere G, Petrovic M, Looman CWN, et al. New insights: dose–response relationship between psychotropic drugs and falls: a study in nursing home residents with dementia. J Clin Pharmacol. 2012;52(6): 947–55.
8. Galik E, Resnick B. Psychotropic medication use and association with physical and psychosocial outcomes in nursing home residents. J Psychiatr Ment Health Nurs. 2012;15.
9. Tolson D, Rolland Y, Andrieu S, Aquino J-P, Beard J, Benetos A, et al. International Association of Gerontology and Geriatrics: a global agenda for clinical research and quality of care in nursing homes. J Am Med Dir Assoc. 2011;12(3):184–9.
10. Alzheimer's Association Expert Advisory Workgroup on NAPA. Workgroup on NAPA's scientific agenda for a national initiative on Alzheimer's disease. Alzheimers Dement. 2012;8(4):357–71.
11. Mitka M. CMS seeks to reduce antipsychotic use in nursing home residents with dementia. JAMA. 2012;308(2):119–21.
12. Rabins P, Blacker D, Rovner B, Rummans T, Schneider L, Tariot P, et al. Treatment of patients with Alzheimer's disease and other dementias [Internet]. American Psychiatric Association; 2007

[cited 2014 Sep 7]. Available from: http://psychia-tryonline.org/content.aspx?bookid=28&sectionid=1679489

13. Lyketsos CG, Colenda C, Beck C, Blank K, Doriaswamy M, Kalunian D, et al. Principles of care for patients with dementia resulting from Alzheimer disease [Internet]. American Association of Geriatric Psychiatry; 2006 [cited 2014 Sep 7]. Available from: http://www.aagponline.org/index.php?src=news&submenu=Tools_Resources&srctype=detail&category=Position%20Statement&refno=35

14. Centers for Medicare and Medicaid Services. Partnership to improve dementia care in nursing homes: antipsychotic drug use in nursing homes trend update [Internet]. 2014. Available from: https://www.ascp.com/sites/default/files/National%20Partnership%20to%20Improve%20Dementia%20Care%20-%20Updated%20Trends.pdf

15. Lemay CA, Mazor KM, Field TS, Donovan J, Kanaan A, Briesacher BA, et al. Knowledge of and perceived need for evidence-based education about antipsychotic medications among nursing home leadership and staff. J Am Med Dir Assoc. 2013;14(12):895–900.

16. Cohen-Mansfield J, Jensen B, Resnick B, Norris M. Knowledge of and attitudes toward nonpharmacological interventions for treatment of behavior symptoms associated with dementia: a comparison of physicians, psychologists, and nurse practitioners. Gerontologist. 2012;52(1):34–45.

17. Morgan DG, Cammer A, Stewart NJ, Crossley M, D'Arcy C, Forbes DA, et al. Nursing aide reports of combative behavior by residents with dementia: results from a detailed prospective incident diary. J Am Med Dir Assoc. 2012;13(3):220–7.

18. Etters L, Goodall D, Harrison BE. Caregiver burden among dementia patient caregivers: a review of the literature. J Am Acad Nurse Pract. 2008;20(8):423–8.

19. Kolanowski A, Fick D, Frazer C, Penrod J. It's about time: use of nonpharmacological interventions in the nursing home. J Nurs Scholarsh. 2010;42(2):214–22.

20. Seitz DP, Brisbin S, Herrmann N, Rapoport MJ, Wilson K, Gill SS, et al. Efficacy and feasibility of nonpharmacological interventions for neuropsychiatric symptoms of dementia in long term care: a systematic review. J Am Med Dir Assoc. 2012;13(6):503–6.e2.

21. Alzheimer's Association. Alzheimer's disease facts and figures. Alzheimer's Association: Chicago, IL; 2014.

22. Fauth EB, Gibbons A. Which behavioral and psychological symptoms of dementia are the most problematic? Variability by prevalence, intensity, distress ratings, and associations with caregiver depressive symptoms. Int J Geriatr Psychiatry. 2014;29(3):263–71.

23. Moorhouse P, Rockwood K. Vascular cognitive impairment: current concepts and clinical developments. Lancet Neurol. 2008;7(3):246–55.

24. Connolly B, Fox SH. Treatment of cognitive, psychiatric, and affective disorders associated with Parkinson's disease. Neurotherapeutics. 2014;11(1):78–91.

25. Borroni B, Agosti C, Padovani A. Behavioral and psychological symptoms in dementia with Lewy-bodies (DLB): frequency and relationship with disease severity and motor impairment. Arch Gerontol Geriatr. 2008;46(1):101–6.

26. Onyike CU, Sheppard J-ME, Tschanz JT, Norton MC, Green RC, Steinberg M, et al. Epidemiology of apathy in older adults: the Cache County Study. Am J Geriatr Psychiatry. 2007;15(5):365–75.

27. Ishizaki J, Mimura M. Dysthymia and apathy: diagnosis and treatment. Depress Res Treat. 2011;2011:893905.

28. Mortby ME, Maercker A, Forstmeier S. Apathy: a separate syndrome from depression in dementia? A critical review. Aging Clin Exp Res. 2012;24(4):305–16.

29. Tagariello P, Girardi P, Amore M. Depression and apathy in dementia: same syndrome or different constructs? A critical review. Arch Gerontol Geriatr. 2009;49(2):246–9.

30. Politis AM, Vozzella S, Mayer LS, Onyike CU, Baker AS, Lyketsos CG. A randomized, controlled, clinical trial of activity therapy for apathy in patients with dementia residing in long-term care. Int J Geriatr Psychiatry. 2004;19(11):1087–94.

31. Steinberg M, Shao H, Zandi P, Lyketsos CG, Welsh-Bohmer KA, Norton MC, et al. Point and 5-year period prevalence of neuropsychiatric symptoms in dementia: the Cache County Study. Int J Geriatr Psychiatry. 2008;23(2):170–7.

32. Howard R, Ballard C, O'Brien J, Burns A. Guidelines for the management of agitation in dementia. Int J Geriatr Psychiatry. 2001;16(7):714–7.

33. Voyer P, Verreault R, Azizah GM, Desrosiers J, Champoux N, Bédard A. Prevalence of physical and verbal aggressive behaviours and associated factors among older adults in long-term care facilities. BMC Geriatr. 2005;5:13.

34. Schreiner AS. Aggressive behaviors among demented nursing home residents in Japan. Int J Geriatr Psychiatry. 2001;16(2):209–15.

35. Volicer L, Van der Steen JT, Frijters DHM. Modifiable factors related to abusive behaviors in nursing home residents with dementia. J Am Med Dir Assoc. 2009;10(9):617–22.

36. Bidzan L, Bidzan M, Pąchalska M. Aggressive and impulsive behavior in Alzheimer's disease and progression of dementia. Med Sci Monit. 2012;18(3):CR182–9.

37. Cohen-Mansfield J, Thein K, Marx MS, Dakheel-Ali M, Murad H, Freedman LS. The relationships of environment and personal characteristics to agitated behaviors in nursing home residents with dementia. J Clin Psychiatry. 2012;73(3):392–9.

38. Tak S, Sweeney MH, Alterman T, Baron S, Calvert GM. Workplace assaults on nursing

assistants in US nursing homes: a multilevel analysis. Am J Public Health. 2010;100(10):1938–45.

39. Menne HL, Bass DM, Johnson JD, Primetica B, Kearney KR, Bollin S, et al. Statewide implementation of "reducing disability in Alzheimer's disease": impact on family caregiver outcomes. J Gerontol Soc Work. 2014;57(6–7):626–39.

40. Kong E-H. Agitation in dementia: concept clarification. J Adv Nurs. 2005;52(5):526–36.

41. Maren S. Building and burying fear memories in the brain. Neuroscientist. 2005;11(1):89–99.

42. Volicer L, Bass EA, Luther SL. Agitation and resistiveness to care are two separate behavioral syndromes of dementia. J Am Med Dir Assoc. 2007;8(8):527–32.

43. Mahoney EK, Hurley AC, Volicer L, Bell M, Gianotis P, Hartshorn M, et al. Development and testing of the Resistiveness to Care Scale. Res Nurs Health. 1999;22(1):27–38.

44. García-Alberca JM, Lara JP, Cruz B, Garrido V, Gris E, Barbancho MÁ. Sleep disturbances in Alzheimer's disease are associated with neuropsychiatric symptoms and antidementia treatment. J Nerv Ment Dis. 2013;201(3):251–7.

45. Kim S-S, Oh KM, Richards K. Sleep disturbance, nocturnal agitation behaviors, and medical comorbidity in older adults with dementia: relationship to reported caregiver burden. Res Gerontol Nurs. 2014;27:1–9.

46. Stern Y, Tang MX, Albert MS, Brandt J, Jacobs DM, Bell K, et al. Predicting time to nursing home care and death in individuals with Alzheimer disease. JAMA. 1997;277(10):806–12.

47. Lyketsos CG, Steinberg M, Tschanz JT, Norton MC, Steffens DC, Breitner JC. Mental and behavioral disturbances in dementia: findings from the Cache County Study on Memory in Aging. Am J Psychiatry. 2000;157(5):708–14.

48. Steele C, Rovner B, Chase GA, Folstein M. Psychiatric symptoms and nursing home placement of patients with Alzheimer's disease. Am J Psychiatry. 1990;147(8):1049–51.

49. Mohamed S, Rosenheck R, Lyketsos CG, Schneider LS. Caregiver burden in Alzheimer disease: cross-sectional and longitudinal patient correlates. Am J Geriatr Psychiatry. 2010;18(10):917–27.

50. Matsumoto N, Ikeda M, Fukuhara R, Shinagawa S, Ishikawa T, Mori T, et al. Caregiver burden associated with behavioral and psychological symptoms of dementia in elderly people in the local community. Dement Geriatr Cogn Disord. 2007;23(4):219–24.

51. McKenzie G, Teri L, Pike K, LaFazia D, van Leynseele J. Reactions of assisted living staff to behavioral and psychological symptoms of dementia. Geriatr Nurs. 2012;33(2):96–104.

52. Lekan-Rutledge D, Palmer MH, Belyea M. In their own words: nursing assistants' perceptions of barriers to implementation of prompted voiding in long-term care. Gerontologist. 1998;38(3):370–8.

53. Teri L, Gibbons LE, McCurry SM, Logsdon RG, Buchner DM, Barlow WE, et al. Exercise plus behavioral management in patients with Alzheimer disease: a randomized controlled trial. JAMA. 2003;290(15):2015–22.

54. Teri L, Huda P, Gibbons L, Young H, van Leynseele J. STAR: a dementia-specific training program for staff in assisted living residences. Gerontologist. 2005;45(5):686–93.

55. Alexopoulos GS, Abrams RC, Young RC, Shamoian CA. Cornell scale for depression in dementia. Biol Psychiatry. 1988;23(3):271–84.

56. Kørner A, Lauritzen L, Abelskov K, Gulmann N, Marie Brodersen A, Wedervang-Jensen T, et al. The Geriatric Depression Scale and the Cornell Scale for depression in dementia. A validity. Nord J Psychiatry. 2006;60(5):360–4.

57. Marin RS, Biedrzycki RC, Firinciogullari S. Reliability and validity of the Apathy Evaluation Scale. Psychiatry Res. 1991;38(2):143–62.

58. Cohen-Mansfield J. Conceptualization of agitation: results based on the Cohen-Mansfield Agitation Inventory and the Agitation Behavior Mapping Instrument. Int Psychogeriatr. 1996;8:309–15.

59. Cohen-Mansfield J, Marx M, Rosenthal A. A description of agitation in a nursing home. J Gerontol. 1989;44:M77–84.

60. Algase DL, Antonakos C, Yao L, Beattie ERA, Hong G-RS, Beel-Bates CA. Are wandering and physically nonaggressive agitation equivalent? Am J Geriatr Psychiatry. 2008;16(4):293–9.

61. King-Kallimanis B, Schonfeld L, Molinari VA, Algase D, Brown LM, Kearns WD, et al. Longitudinal investigation of wandering behavior in Department of Veterans Affairs nursing home care units. Int J Geriatr Psychiatry. 2010;25(2):166–74.

62. Jablonski RA, Kolanowski A, Therrien B, Mahoney EK, Kassab C, Leslie DL. Reducing care-resistant behaviors during oral hygiene in persons with dementia. BMC Oral Health. 2011;11:30.

63. Mahoney EK, Trudeau SA, Penyack SE, MacLeod CE. Challenges to intervention implementation: lessons learned in the Bathing Persons with Alzheimer's Disease at Home study. Nurs Res. 2006;55(2 Suppl):S10–6.

64. Seitz DP, Adunuri N, Gill SS, Gruneir A, Herrmann N, Rochon P. Antidepressants for agitation and psychosis in dementia. Cochrane Database Syst Rev. 2011;(2):CD008191.

65. Wang LY, Borisovskaya A, Maxwell AL, Pascualy M. Common psychiatric problems in cognitively impaired older patients: causes and management. Clin Geriatr Med. 2014;30(3):443–67.

66. Folstein MF, Folstein SE, McHugh PR. Mini-mental state" A practical method for grading the cognitive state of patients for the clinician. J Psychiatr Res. 1975;12(3):189–98.

67. Nasreddine ZS, Phillips NA, Bédirian V, Charbonneau S, Whitehead V, Collin I, et al. The

Montreal Cognitive Assessment, MoCA: a brief screening tool for mild cognitive impairment. J Am Geriatr Soc. 2005;53(4):695–9.

68. Rabins P, Steele C. A scale to measure impairment in severe dementia and similar conditions. Am J Geriatr Psychiatry. 1996;4(3):247–51.

69. Tinetti ME. Performance-oriented assessment of mobility problems in elderly patients. J Am Geriatr Soc. 1986;34(2):119–26.

70. Mahoney FI, Barthel DW. Functional evaluation: the Barthel Index. Md State Med J. 1965;14:61–5.

71. Resnick B, Boltz M, Galik E, Wells C. Physical capability scale: psychometric testing. Clin Nurs Res. 2013;22(1):7–29.

72. Resnick B, Galik E, Boltz M. Basic physical capability scale: psychometric testing with cognitively impaired older adults. Am J Alzheimers Dis Other Demen. 2014;29(4):326–32.

73. Cummings JL, Mega M, Gray K, Rosenberg-Thompson S, Carusi DA, Gornbein J. The Neuropsychiatric Inventory: comprehensive assessment of psychopathology in dementia. Neurology. 1994;44(12):2308–14.

74. Kong E-H, Evans LK, Guevara JP. Nonpharmacological intervention for agitation in dementia: a systematic review and meta-analysis. Aging Ment Health. 2009;13(4):512–20.

75. Nazir A, Unroe K, Tegeler M, Khan B, Azar J, Boustani M. Systematic review of interdisciplinary interventions in nursing homes. J Am Med Dir Assoc. 2013;14(7):471–8.

76. O'Neil MEME, Freeman MM, Christensen VV, Telerant RR, Addleman AA, Kansagara DD. A systematic evidence review of non-pharmacological interventions for behavioral symptoms of dementia. Washington, DC: Department of Veterans Affairs; 2011.

77. Ayalon L, Gum AM, Feliciano L, Areán PA. Effectiveness of nonpharmacological interventions for the management of neuropsychiatric symptoms in patients with dementia: a systematic review. Arch Intern Med. 2006;166(20):2182–8.

78. Eggenberger E, Heimerl K, Bennett MI. Communication skills training in dementia care: a systematic review of effectiveness, training content, and didactic methods in different care settings. Int Psychogeriatr. 2012;2:1–14.

79. Cruz J, Marques A, Barbosa A, Figueiredo D, Sousa LX. Making sense(s) in dementia: a multisensory and motor-based group activity program. Am J Alzheimers Dis Other Demen. 2013;28(2):137–46.

80. Cohen-Mansfield J, Marx MS, Dakheel-Ali M, Thein K. The use and utility of specific nonpharmacological interventions for behavioral symptoms in dementia: an exploratory study. Am J Geriatr Psychiatry. 2014;26.

81. Ho S-Y, Lai H-L, Jeng S-Y, Tang C-W, Sung H-C, Chen P-W. The effects of researcher-composed music at mealtime on agitation in nursing home residents with dementia. Arch Psychiatr Nurs. 2011;25(6):e49–55.

82. Hammar LM, Emami A, Götell E, Engström G. The impact of caregivers' singing on expressions of emotion and resistance during morning care situations in persons with dementia: an intervention in dementia care. J Clin Nurs. 2011;20(7–8):969–78.

83. Gray SG, Clair AA. Influence of aromatherapy on medication administration to residential-care residents with dementia and behavioral challenges. Am J Alzheimers Dis Other Demen. 2002;17(3):169–74.

84. Friedmann E, Galik E, Thomas SA, Hall PS, Chung SY, McCune S. Evaluation of a pet-assisted living intervention for improving functional status in assisted living residents with mild to moderate cognitive impairment: a pilot study. Am J Alzheimers Dis Other Demen. 2014;11.

85. Majić T, Gutzmann H, Heinz A, Lang UE, Rapp MA. Animal-assisted therapy and agitation and depression in nursing home residents with dementia: a matched case–control trial. Am J Geriatr Psychiatry. 2013;21(11):1052–9.

86. Nordgren L, Engström G. Effects of dog-assisted intervention on behavioural and psychological symptoms of dementia. Nurs Older People. 2014;26(3):31–8.

87. Edwards NE, Beck AM, Lim E. Influence of aquariums on resident behavior and staff satisfaction in dementia units. West J Nurs Res. 2014;17.

88. Maseda A, Sánchez A, Marante MP, González-Abraldes I, Buján A, Millán-Calenti JC. Effects of multisensory stimulation on a sample of institutionalized elderly people with dementia diagnosis: a controlled longitudinal trial. Am J Alzheimers Dis Other Demen. 2014;29(5):463–73.

89. Anderson K, Bird M, Macpherson S, McDonough V, Davis T. Findings from a pilot investigation of the effectiveness of a snoezelen room in residential care: should we be engaging with our residents more? Geriatr Nurs. 2011;32(3):166–77.

90. Spector A, Orrell M, Hall L. Systematic review of neuropsychological outcomes in dementia from cognition-based psychological interventions. Dement Geriatr Cogn Disord. 2012;34(3–4):244–55.

91. Olazarán J, Reisberg B, Clare L, Cruz I, Peña-Casanova J, Del Ser T, et al. Nonpharmacological therapies in Alzheimer's disease: a systematic review of efficacy. Dement Geriatr Cogn Disord. 2010;30(2):161–78.

92. Aguirre E, Woods RT, Spector A, Orrell M. Cognitive stimulation for dementia: a systematic review of the evidence of effectiveness from randomised controlled trials. Ageing Res Rev. 2013;12(1):253–62.

93. Woods B, Aguirre E, Spector AE, Orrell M. Cognitive stimulation to improve cognitive functioning in people with dementia. Cochrane Database Syst Rev. 2012;(2):CD005562.

94. Blake M. Group reminiscence therapy for adults with dementia: a review. Br J Community Nurs. 2013;18(5):228–33.

95. Serrani Azcurra DJL. A reminiscence program intervention to improve the quality of life of long-term care residents with Alzheimer's disease: a randomized controlled trial. Rev Bras Psiquiatr. 2012;34(4):422–33.

96. Van Bogaert P, Van Grinsven R, Tolson D, Wouters K, Engelborghs S, Van der Mussele S. Effects of SolCos model-based individual reminiscence on older adults with mild to moderate dementia due to Alzheimer disease: a pilot study. J Am Med Dir Assoc. 2013;14(7):528.e9–13.

97. Subramaniam P, Woods B. The impact of individual reminiscence therapy for people with dementia: systematic review. Expert Rev Neurother. 2012;12(5):545–55.

98. Zetteler J. Effectiveness of simulated presence therapy for individuals with dementia: a systematic review and meta-analysis. Aging Ment Health. 2008;12(6):779–85.

99. O'Connor CM, Smith R, Nott MT, Lorang C, Mathews RM. Using video simulated presence to reduce resistance to care and increase participation of adults with dementia. Am J Alzheimers Dis Other Demen. 2011;26(4):317–25.

100. Thuné-Boyle ICV, Iliffe S, Cerga-Pashoja A, Lowery D, Warner J. The effect of exercise on behavioral and psychological symptoms of dementia: towards a research agenda. Int Psychogeriatr. 2012;24(7):1046–57.

101. McCurry SM, Pike KC, Vitiello MV, Logsdon RG, Larson EB, Teri L. Increasing walking and bright light exposure to improve sleep in community-dwelling persons with Alzheimer's disease: results of a randomized, controlled trial. J Am Geriatr Soc. 2011;59(8):1393–402.

102. Neville C, Henwood T, Beattie E, Fielding E. Exploring the effect of aquatic exercise on behaviour and psychological well-being in people with moderate to severe dementia: a pilot study of the Watermemories Swimming Club. Australas J Ageing. 2014;33(2):124–7.

103. Forbes D, Thiessen EJ, Blake CM, Forbes SC, Forbes S. Exercise programs for people with dementia. Cochrane Database Syst Rev. 2013;(12): CD006489.

104. Guzmán-García A, Hughes JC, James IA, Rochester L. Dancing as a psychosocial intervention in care homes: a systematic review of the literature. Int J Geriatr Psychiatry. 2013;28(9):914–24.

105. Scherder EJA, Bogen T, Eggermont LHP, Hamers JPH, Swaab DF. The more physical inactivity, the more agitation in dementia. Int Psychogeriatr. 2010;22(8):1203–8.

106. Christofoletti G, Oliani MM, Bucken-Gobbi LT, Gobbi S, Beinotti F, Stella F. Physical activity atten-uates neuropsychiatric disturbances and caregiver burden in patients with dementia. Clinics (Sao Paulo). 2011;66(4):613–8.

107. Beck CK, Vogelpohl TS, Rasin JH, Uriri JT, O'Sullivan P, Walls R, et al. Effects of behavioral interventions on disruptive behavior and affect in demented nursing home residents. Nurs Res. 2002;51(4):219–28.

108. Chalmers JM. Behavior management and communication strategies for dental professionals when caring for patients with dementia. Spec Care Dentist. 2000;20(4):147–54.

109. Beck C, Heacock P, Mercer SO, Walls RC, Rapp CG, Vogelpohl TS. Improving dressing behavior in cognitively impaired nursing home residents. Nurs Res. 1997;46(3):126–32.

110. Rolland Y, Pillard F, Klapouszczak A, Reynish E, Thomas D, Andrieu S, et al. Exercise program for nursing home residents with Alzheimer's disease: a 1-year randomized, controlled trial. J Am Geriatr Soc. 2007;55(2):158–65.

111. Galik EM, Resnick B, Gruber-Baldini A, Nahm E-S, Pearson K, Pretzer-Aboff I. Pilot testing of the restorative care intervention for the cognitively impaired. J Am Med Dir Assoc. 2008;9(7):516–22.

112. Galik E, Resnick B, Hammersla M, Brightwater J. Optimizing function and physical activity among nursing home residents with dementia: testing the impact of function focused care. Gerontologist. 2014;54(6):930–43.

113. Cohen-Mansfield J, Thein K, Marx MS, Dakheel-Ali M, Freedman L. Efficacy of nonpharmacologic interventions for agitation in advanced dementia: a randomized, placebo-controlled trial. J Clin Psychiatry. 2012;73(9):1255–61.

114. Burgio LD, Allen-Burge R, Roth DL, Bourgeois MS, Dijkstra K, Gerstle J, et al. Come talk with me: improving communication between nursing assistants and nursing home residents during care routines. Gerontologist. 2001;41(4):449–60.

115. Frank EM. Effect of Alzheimer's disease on communication function. J S C Med Assoc. 1994; 90(9):417–23.

116. Davison TE, McCabe MP, Visser S, Hudgson C, Buchanan G, George K. Controlled trial of dementia training with a peer support group for aged care staff. Int J Geriatr Psychiatry. 2007;22(9):868–73.

117. Norton M, Allen R, Lynn Snow A, Michael Hardin J, Burgio L. Predictors of need-driven behaviors in nursing home residents with dementia and associated certified nursing assistant burden. Aging Ment Health. 2010;14(3):303–9.

118. Rogers JC, Holm MB, Burgio LD, Hsu C, Hardin JM, McDowell BJ. Excess disability during morning care in nursing home residents with dementia. Int Psychogeriatr. 2000;12(2):267–82.

119. Resnick B, Galik E, Gruber-Baldini A, Zimmerman S. Perceptions and performance of function and

physical activity in assisted living communities. J Am Med Dir Assoc. 2010;11(6):406–14.

120. Resnick B, Petzer-Aboff I, Galik E, Russ K, Cayo J, Simpson M, et al. Barriers and benefits to implementing a restorative care intervention in nursing homes. J Am Med Dir Assoc. 2008;9(2):102–8.

121. Resnick B, Simpson M, Galik E, Bercovitz A, Gruber-Baldini A, Zimmerman S, et al. Making a difference: nursing assistants' perspectives of restorative care nursing. Rehabil Nurs. 2006;31(2):78–86.

122. Bandura A. Self-efficacy: the exercise of control. New York: WH Freeman Company; 1997.

Experience and Perspective of the Primary Care Physician and Memory Care Specialist

Catherine A. Alder, Michael A. LaMantia,
Mary Guerriero Austrom, and Malaz A. Boustani

Dementia in all its forms is complex and can be challenging to manage. Most patients will experience a gradual decline in both cognition and function, but the rate of decline and the range of symptoms vary widely from person to person, presenting challenges to detection, diagnosis and disease management [1].

Care models developed and tested over the last three decades provide a significant evidence

C.A. Alder, JD, MSW, LSW (✉)
Aging Brain Care, Eskenazi Health,
720 Eskenazi Avenue, Fifth Third Bank Building,
2nd Floor, 46202 Indianapolis, IN 46202, USA
e-mail: calder@iupui.edu

M.A. LaMantia, MD, MPH
Indiana University Center for Aging Research,
Indianapolis, IN, USA

Regenstrief Institute, Inc., Indianapolis, IN, USA

M.G. Austrom, PhD
Department of Psychiatry, Indiana University School
of Medicine (IUSM), Indianapolis, IN, USA

Outreach, Recruitment and Education Core, Indiana
Alzheimer's Disease Center, Indiana University
School of Medicine (IUSM), Indianapolis, IN, USA

Office for Diversity and Inclusion, Indiana University
School of Medicine (IUSM), Indianapolis, IN, USA

M.A. Boustani, MD, MPH
Indiana University Center for Aging Research,
Indianapolis, IN, USA

Regenstrief Institute, Inc., Indianapolis, IN, USA

Center for Health Innovation and Implementation
Science, Indiana University School of Medicine
(IUSM), Indianapolis, IN, USA

base for recognition, diagnosis and management of dementia [2]. Yet despite widespread agreement on the need for timely detection [3, 4] and the elements of best-practice care models [2], the current health care system falls short in all phases of care delivery. Symptoms often go unrecognized, diagnosis is made late or missed altogether, and care management is frequently less than ideal [3, 5, 6, 8]. The current practice environment is simply unable to accommodate the essential components of an effective dementia care program due to multiple barriers that interfere with both timely identification and effective intervention. Examining these barriers is the first step in redesigning the practice environment to assimilate and support evidence-based care for dementia.

While the majority of dementia patients are found in primary care, both the primary care physician and the memory care specialist play critical roles in the dementia care delivery system. Understanding the challenges and perspective of both practitioners is key to improving the experience and health outcomes of both patients and their informal caregivers.

The United States is facing a critical shortage of geriatrics-trained health care providers to care for the rapidly growing population of older Americans [9]. Therefore, most patients with dementia will continue to be cared for in primary care settings where as many as two-thirds of dementia cases remain unrecognized [3, 10]. Even when dementia is recognized, most patients and caregivers receive sub-optimal care [6]. These poor outcomes are the result of multiple deficits and constraints in the health care delivery system that together impede the timely detection and diagnosis of dementia and the provision of quality care.

The purpose of this paper is twofold: (1) to examine the challenges to recognizing, diagnosing, and treating dementia in both primary and specialty care and (2) to provide a review of our local response to these barriers.

Barriers in Primary Care

Quality dementia care includes timely detection and diagnosis followed by effective care management. Multiple factors affect both the diagnostic and care management practices of primary care physicians including failure of the patient and caregiver to report symptoms, deficits in physician training and assessment tools, lack of time and resources, and physician attitudes and values that can negatively influence both communication with patients and physician priorities [5, 11, 12].

Failure of Patient and Caregiver to Report Symptoms

Diagnosis of dementia begins with assessment of the signs and symptoms reported by the patient and family to the physician. Symptoms of dementia, especially in the early stages of the disease, are often subtle and intermittent and therefore can be very difficult to recognize [13]. While some patients want to discuss their symptoms with their physician and look to health care providers for help managing their cognitive difficulties [7], others hide or minimize their symptoms because of concern about the stigma of being labeled with dementia and how this label might affect their independence, ability to access insurance, and relationships with family and friends [14]. Still other patients may be asymptomatic, unaware of their cognitive symptoms, or misinterpret their cognitive symptoms to be the result

of normal aging [5]. Caregivers may also fail to detect or recognize the importance of the patients' cognitive symptoms; or they may choose not to report symptoms in an effort to protect the patient from the potentially negative consequences of the dementia diagnosis [5]. Finally, both patients and caregivers often choose to remain silent simply because, in the absence of a cure or disease altering medications, they believe nothing can be done to help [5]. As a result, in many cases the burden is on the physician to detect and assess symptoms of cognitive impairment based on interactions with the patient during a typical primary care visit.

Deficits in Physician Training and Diagnostic Tools

Unfortunately, many primary care physicians believe their training has been inadequate to prepare them to detect and diagnose dementia, particularly early in the disease process [5]. They have difficulty recognizing cognitive symptoms and, even when symptoms are detected, they often do not appreciate their significance [5]. In particular, physicians lack basic knowledge about what cognitive changes are consistent with "normal" aging and what changes suggest the possibility of dementia. Others may be able to distinguish normal aging from dementia, but lack knowledge about dementia sub-types and the reversible causes of dementia [5]. Physicians also express concern about the lack of access to comprehensive, clinically practical assessment tools [5]. Although there are many tools designed to monitor symptoms of dementia through caregiver report, most are too lengthy for use in the clinical setting [15]. Other tools can be administered quickly, but assess only a limited range of symptoms [15]. Furthermore, cost is another factor that affects access to clinical assessment tools. Tools that are limited in scope can still be helpful in the primary care environment, but such tools may be practically unavailable as a result of licensing fees charged by the copyright holders.

As a result of these deficits in training and resources, primary care physicians worry about the negative consequences of misdiagnosing a patient. Many avoid making an early diagnosis, choosing to pursue a "wait and see approach" until the disease progresses and the diagnosis is more certain [5]. Finally, despite widespread lack of confidence in their ability to detect symptoms and diagnose dementia, many primary care physicians express even less confidence in their ability to manage the needs of dementia patients and their caregivers after a diagnosis is made.

Co-morbidities

Most older adults suffer from multiple chronic diseases. As a result, depression, hypertension, diabetes, visual impairment, hearing impairment, and cardiovascular disease are commonly comorbid with dementia [16]. Depending on the number and severity of these other health conditions, the patient's cognitive symptoms may not be assigned the highest priority, even when recognized. Primary care physicians often focus their time and attention on these other conditions while the cognitive impairment is moved to the end of the list of concerns to be addressed [11]. This approach not only fails to recognize the importance and consequences of the dementia, but also fails to appreciate the impact of the dementia on the patient's other medical conditions. Cognitive impairment complicates management of the other diseases because it interferes with the patient's ability to accurately report symptoms, adhere to the prescribed medication regimen and otherwise comply with the plan of care. Therefore, failure to take the dementia into account can have serious consequences for the patient's health.

Time

Lack of time is another barrier contributing to missed diagnoses and poor quality of care. As chronic diseases have become more prevalent, the time required to care for patients with these conditions has increased dramatically. National practice guidelines provide recommendations for comprehensive management of these diseases, but there are simply not enough hours in the day to deliver all the recommended health care services required by these guidelines [17]. The time required to provide care for the ten most prevalent chronic conditions alone is now greater than the time available to primary care physicians for delivery of all clinical services [17]. As physicians struggle to deliver quality care to all of their patients, the amount of time that can be devoted to any one patient is limited. The typical primary care appointment is a 15-min visit. Given such time constraints, it is hardly surprising that symptoms of dementia often go unrecognized. Yet even when physicians suspect that there may be a problem with cognition, time constraints remain a serious barrier to further investigation [11]. Assessment tools require time to administer and that means less time available for addressing other medical concerns [11]. Finally, time constraints continue to be a problem for effective care management after diagnosis. Dementia care is complex, intensive and time consuming. Behavioral and mood problems are common in dementia and the related psychosocial needs of the caregiver require comprehensive and detailed discussion in order to develop an effective plan of care. The typical 15-min appointment simply cannot accommodate these critical conversations [18].

Lack of Evidence to Support Dementia Screening

In an effort to improve early detection and diagnosis, a wide range of clinicians, researchers and advocates have recommended routine screening for dementia in primary care [19]. In 2011, the Centers for Medicare and Medicaid Services (CMS) brought the issue of screening to the forefront by providing beneficiaries with a new benefit called the "Annual Wellness Visit", which includes detection of cognitive impairment (although screening is not explicitly recommended) [3]. However, notwithstanding the push for early detection, both physicians and policy makers remain uncertain about the benefits of dementia screening and many are concerned about potential harms. In 2003 and again in 2014, the United States Preventive Services Task Force (USPSTF) reviewed the evidence regarding the benefits and harms of dementia screening in primary care and concluded "that the current evidence is insufficient to assess the balance of benefits and harms of screening for cognitive impairment" and "more research on the harms of screening is needed" [8]. Recognizing the need to offer effective interventions to patients who screen positive, the USPSTF further concluded that "research on new interventions that address the changing needs of patients and families and interventions that clearly have an effect on the long-term clinical course of mild to moderate dementia are also critically needed" [8]. Given that the current evidence base does not support formal dementia screening, symptom recognition remains critical to early diagnosis.

Physician Attitudes and Values

Physician attitudes and values also play a role in unrecognized symptoms, missed diagnosis and sub-optimal care [5, 11]. Unfortunately, deficits in training and experience with dementia play a role in shaping the beliefs and principles that help guide the physician's communication with patients and families and decisions about priorities for care.

Some physicians believe that a patient who is aware enough to express concern about his or her own cognition is probably fine—simply one of the "worried well"—while the family's concern is much more likely to be indicative of a problem [11]. These physicians tend to minimize concerns expressed by the patient, while more aggressively pursuing those raised by the family [11]. However, the reality is that while some patients with cognitive complaints are simply experiencing the signs of normal aging, others have in fact identified the earliest symptoms of dementia. When the physician discounts the patient's concerns, the patient may either feel dismissed or be left with a false assurance that everything is fine.

Lack of effective interventions and/or lack of access to these interventions may also influence a primary care provider's attitude about the need for early detection and diagnosis [5, 11]. Currently, there are no treatments available to alter the course or prognosis of dementia [20]. While psychosocial interventions have been proven to help with behavioral symptoms and improve the quality of life for both patients and their caregivers, these interventions are not widely available. Lack of time and interdisciplinary teams make it impossible to provide these evidence-based interventions absent major restructuring of the primary care practice environment [18, 21]. Furthermore, many providers practice in communities lacking the resources needed to assist patients with dementia and their caregivers [11, 18, 21]. Even when these resources are available, physicians are often uninformed or poorly connected to the agencies providing them [18, 21]. Without access to community-based organizations capable of providing education and services to these complex patients, physicians are left feeling they have little to offer. Taken together, these factors can cause primary care physicians not only to question the value of early detection and diagnosis, but also to adopt a belief that diagnosis, especially in the early stages of the disease, causes more harm than good [5, 11]. As a result, they may opt to delay diagnosis even for patients who already exhibit some evidence of impairment [5, 11].

Legal Requirements

In addition to the barriers within the primary care system, legal requirements aimed at broader societal concerns also have an effect on dementia care. Dementia poses a serious risk to driving safety. Virtually all states have established policies related to identifying potentially impaired drivers, but most states provide for *voluntary* physician reporting [22]. A few states, however, mandate physicians to report their patients with dementia to the state's department of motor vehicles [22]. Although compulsory reporting is designed to protect public safety, it is not necessarily effective at preventing dementia patients from driving [22]. Patients with dementia may have little or no insight into their impairment and may not be capable of understanding the consequences of the loss of licensure [22]. If the family is unwilling or unable to step in to prevent the patient from driving, the patient may continue to do so at even greater risk to public safety due to the loss of insurance. Furthermore compulsory reporting has profound implications for the confidentiality of the patient-physician relationship [22]. Patients inclined to seek medical help for cognitive symptoms may be deterred from doing so out of fear of losing their independence; patients who are reported after seeking help may feel betrayed and terminate the relationship with the physician. In the end, these patients and their families will be left without the help they need to manage this devastating disease.

Considering the multiple barriers to quality dementia care faced by primary care physicians described above, it is no wonder that care for these patients within the current system of primary care is less than optimal. However, primary care represents only half of the story. Specialty physicians also play an important role in dementia care and face their own unique challenges in providing effective care to these patients and their informal caregivers.

Barriers in Specialty Care

While memory care specialists can help ease the burden of dementia on the primary care system, specialists face their own obstacles to effective dementia management. Multiple factors impede the specialists' ability to provide quality care to patients and caregivers.

Shortage of Memory Care Specialists

A fundamental constraint of specialty care is the limited number of specialists available. This shortage translates to longer and longer wait times for patients to be evaluated. Currently the

number of physicians with specialized training in geriatrics is insufficient to serve the number of older adults needing care; that deficit is growing as the number of geriatricians continues to decline while the population of older adults is rapidly increasing [23]. Furthermore, the number of nurses, social worker and pharmacists specializing in geriatrics is also lacking [23–25]. Neurologists and psychiatrists, particularly geriatric psychiatrists are also in short supply, further limiting access to both memory and behavioral care services [18]. As a result, many primary care physicians feel obliged to manage these patients on their own despite feeling ill-prepared to do so [18].

Even when specialists are available, primary care physicians may be reluctant to refer their patients for consultation if they perceive that the patient stands to benefit little or not at all from the referral. The potential benefit depends on a number of factors including the patient's willingness to accept the referral, the patient's social support, the range of services being offered by the specialist, and system incentives for continuing to manage the patient within primary care.

Patient's Acceptance

Obviously there is no benefit to making a referral if the patient refuses to go. A patient may refuse to see a specialist because of the same worries that interfere with patients seeking help from the primary care physician—i.e., the stigma of being labeled with dementia and how this label might affect their independence, access to insurance, and relationships with family and friends [14]. But even if the patient agrees to the referral, a number of factors may limit the value of the specialty consultation.

Lack of Social Support

Because the cognitively impaired patient will not be a reliable source of information about medical history or current symptoms, the specialty physician must rely on the presence of a knowledgeable and reliable caregiver to provide information relevant to the diagnosis. If the patient doesn't have such a caregiver, then the specialist may not have enough information about the patient's history to make the diagnosis. Even when the diagnosis is not in question, the cognitively impaired patient will likely have difficulty understanding the diagnosis and/or be unable to follow through on the plan of care. In such cases, the referral has questionable value.

Lack of Follow-Up Services in Specialty Care

In the current care delivery system, there is an important difference in both the function and the focus of the specialty physician compared to the primary care physician. The primary care physician is charged with providing comprehensive care that takes into account all aspects of the patient's health; the specialist, on the other hand, focuses on just one aspect or one problem area. When a patient is referred to a specialist for a problem, the specialist is charged with evaluating the problem and making a diagnosis. Once the diagnosis is made, the specialist will do one of two things. The specialist may communicate recommendations to the patient and to the primary care physician with the expectation that those recommendations will be integrated into the patient's comprehensive care plan and managed within the primary care system. Alternatively, the specialist may continue to follow the patient to implement, monitor, and modify the plan of care as needed over time. However, not all memory care specialists have the ability to offer ongoing care and the diagnosis alone is likely to be of little or no benefit to a dementia patient. Some primary care physicians have expressed frustration at the lack of actionable recommendations from the specialist. Calling attention to the problem without offering a workable solution is not helpful to the referring physician or the patient. Furthermore, given the limited time and resources, the primary care physician most likely cannot meet the needs of the dementia patient and caregiver in the current primary care environment.

Volume-Based Incentives

Even when the memory care specialist is able to assume responsibility for ongoing care management, the primary care physician may choose not to make the referral. In many primary care systems, physicians are compensated based on the number of patients seen in the clinic. This type of compensation structure incentivizes primary care physicians to manage dementia within the primary care setting. However, volume-based systems often fail to take into account the complexity of the patients being seen. In such cases these physicians may actually be motivated to refer their dementia patients because caring for them is so time intensive.

While the typical memory care practitioner does not face the time constraints experienced by primary care physicians, there are multiple other barriers to effective care management including lack of resources and system dysfunctions around communication and care coordination.

Lack of Resources

Evidence-based models developed over the last two decades utilize multi-disciplinary teams to provide long term management of the patient's symptoms and the related caregiver stress [2]. However, most memory care specialists do not have access to a multi-disciplinary work force. Even when clinical teams are providing support, they often lack the specialized knowledge and experience necessary to provide effective dementia care. Furthermore, as is the case for many primary care physicians, many specialists practice in communities lacking the resources needed to support the care of these complex patients.

Lack of Communication and Care Coordination

Another barrier to the effectiveness of the memory care specialist is poor coordination of care among all providers involved in caring for the patient with dementia. While fragmented care is common in our health care system, it is particularly perilous for the dementia patient because, as previously discussed, the cognitive impairment has implications for all aspects of the patient's health. Therefore, in order to be effective, the memory care provider must operate within the broader context of the patient's comprehensive plan of care. Communication and collaboration among all providers, as well as the family caregiver, is critical to developing a workable plan of care that takes into account not only the patient's medical needs, but also the cognitive limitations of the patient and the social supports available to address those limitations.

Reimbursement System

Finally, broader systemic issues in the health care delivery system may also impede the quality of dementia care in both the primary care and specialty care settings. The current system of medical reimbursement simply does not provide the incentives to facilitate appropriate management of dementia. The system promotes volume-based activities rather than encouraging innovative models of care that reduce cost [26, 27]. Acute care utilization events, while costly to the payer, generally represent income to the provider. In addition, reimbursement principles fail to take into account the complex care needs of dementia patients and their caregivers. As a result, many services deemed necessary in the evidence-based models do not meet Medicare's criteria for a billable service (Table 1) [27].

We have described multiple barriers to effective dementia care from the perspective of both the primary care physician and the memory care specialist. While the picture is somewhat discouraging, understanding these barriers is the critical first step in redesigning the practice environment to accommodate and support the essential components of effective models of dementia care.

Solutions

During the past few decades, scientists have developed several new and innovative models to address the needs of patients with dementia and

Table 1 Barriers to detection, diagnosis and quality care for Dementia

Failure of patient or caregiver to report cognitive symptoms
Deficits in physician training
Lack of clinically practical, comprehensive assessment tools
Co-morbid conditions
Lack of time
Lack of evidence to support Dementia screening
Physician attitudes and values
Compulsory reporting of Dementia patients to department of motor vehicles
Shortage of memory care specialists
Lack of social support for patient or caregiver
Lack of follow-up services in specialty care
Misaligned reimbursement incentives
Lack of community resources
Poor communication among providers
Lack of care coordination

their caregivers [2]. Clinical trials have demonstrated the effectiveness of these models in improving health outcomes and quality of care [28]. These models offer a blueprint for modifying the primary care environment to accommodate evidence-based interventions for dementia [10]. In addition, they extend the delivery of care beyond the clinic into the homes and communities of patients and their caregivers [10]. Finally, they emphasize person-centered collaborative care delivered by a multi-disciplinary team and coordinated across multiple providers, agencies, and settings.

A review of these models reveals a number of common recommendations and guidelines for best practices in dementia care including the following [2]:

- Perform a full diagnostic evaluation (including evaluation for reversible causes and potential contributing factors).
- Educate the patient and family about the diagnosis, prognosis, and available treatment options (including a discussion about goals of care).
- Periodically assess and track the patient's symptoms and the related caregiver stress.

- Consider cognition enhancing drugs and continuously assess for cognitive side effects of prescription and non-prescription medications.
- Identify and address depression, psychoses, behavioral disturbances and safety concerns.
- Identify and treat disability from comorbid conditions.
- Design and deliver person-centered non-pharmacological interventions (including care coordination, self-management skills training, modification of physical environment, and referral to community resources) aimed at reducing the physical and psychological burden of both the patient and the caregiver.
- Measure and track identified outcomes using tools available to all providers and modify the intervention as necessary in response to these outcomes and changing goals of care.
- Utilize interdisciplinary care across the course of the disease including end/late stage disease and palliative care and hospice care.

But despite the evidence that these components have been effective in improving outcomes, these models have not been widely adopted because of the barriers in the current system of health care delivery described above. The translation of these research models into real world clinical programs will require broad restructuring of the practice environment including integration of multi-disciplinary teams and, most likely, a new payment/reimbursement system. Bringing these models to scale will require development of an innovative new work force trained to deliver care beyond the limits of the traditional clinic setting. This work force cannot be limited by the shortage of clinical professionals and instead must include paraprofessional and nonprofessional workers who possess the core qualities and skills necessary for caregiving and are trained in the best practices of quality dementia care.

With the population of older adults with dementia expected to triple by the year 2050 [20, 29], the need to develop, test, and implement innovative health care service delivery and payment models is urgent.

Acknowledgments The project described was supported by Grant Number 1C1CMS331000-01-00 from the Department of Health and Human Services, Centers for Medicare & Medicaid Services. The contents of this publication are solely the responsibility of the authors and do not necessarily represent the official views of the US Department of Health and Human Services or any of its agencies. MG Austrom is also supported in part by the Indiana Alzheimer's Disease Center funded by NIA P30AG10133.

References

1. Grand JH, Caspar S, Macdonald SW. Clinical features and multidisciplinary approaches to dementia care. J Multidiscip Healthc. 2011;4:125–47. doi:10.2147/jmdh.s17773.
2. Callahan CM, Sachs GA, Lamantia MA, Unroe KT, Arling G, Boustani MA. Redesigning systems of care for older adults with Alzheimer's disease. Health Aff (Millwood). 2014;33(4):626–32. doi:10.1377/hlthaff.2013.1260.
3. Cordell CB, Borson S, Boustani M, Chodosh J, Reuben D, Verghese J, et al. Alzheimer's Association recommendations for operationalizing the detection of cognitive impairment during the Medicare Annual Wellness Visit in a primary care setting. Alzheimers Dement. 2013;9(2):141–50. http://dx.doi.org/10.1016/j.jalz.2012.09.011.
4. Institute of Medicine Committee on Quality of Health Care in, A. Crossing the quality chasm: a new health system for the 21st century. Washington, DC: National Academies Press; 2001. Copyright 2001 by the National Academy of Sciences. All rights reserved.
5. Bradford A, Kunik ME, Schulz P, Williams SP, Singh H. Missed and delayed diagnosis of dementia in primary care: prevalence and contributing factors. Alzheimer Dis Assoc Disord. 2009;23(4):306–14. doi:10.1097/WAD.0b013e3181a6bebc.
6. Chodosh J, Mittman BS, Connor KI, Vassar SD, Lee ML, DeMonte RW, et al. Caring for patients with dementia: how good is the quality of care? Results from three health systems. J Am Geriatr Soc. 2007;55(8):1260–8.doi:10.1111/j.1532-5415.2007.01249.x.
7. Chodosh J, Sultzer DL, Lee ML, Hahn TJ, Reuben DB, Yano EM, et al. Memory impairment among primary care veterans. Aging Ment Health. 2007;11(4):444–50. doi:10.1080/13607860601086272.
8. Moyer VA. Screening for cognitive impairment in older adults: U.S. preventive services task force recommendation statement. Ann Intern Med. 2014;160(11):791–7. doi:10.7326/m14-0496.
9. Cottingham AH, Alder C, Austrom MG, Johnson CS, Boustani MA, Litzelman DK. New workforce development in Dementia care: screening for "caring": preliminary data. J Am Geriatr Soc. 2014;62(7):1364–8. doi:10.1111/jgs.12886.

10. Boustani M, Sachs G, Callahan C. Can primary care meet the biopsychosocial needs of older adults with Dementia? J Gen Intern Med. 2007;22(11):1625–7. doi:10.1007/s11606-007-0386-y.

11. Boise L, Camicioli R, Morgan DL, Rose JH, Congleton L. Diagnosing dementia: perspectives of primary care physicians. Gerontologist. 1999;39(4): 457–64.

12. Chodosh J, Berry E, Lee M, Connor K, DeMonte R, Ganiats T, et al. Effect of a Dementia Care Management Intervention on Primary Care Provider Knowledge, Attitudes, and Perceptions of Quality of Care. J Am Geriatr Soc. 2006;54(2):311–7. doi:10.1111/j.1532-5415.2005.00564.x.

13. Heneka MT, O'Banion MK. Inflammatory processes in Alzheimer's disease. J Neuroimmunol. 2007;184(1–2):69–91. doi:10.1016/j.jneuroim.2006.11.017.

14. Fowler NR, Boustani MA, Frame A, Perkins AJ, Monahan P, Gao S, et al. Effect of patient perceptions on dementia screening in primary care. J Am Geriatr Soc. 2012;60(6):1037–43. doi:10.1111/j.1532-5415. 2012.03991.x.

15. Monahan PO, Boustani MA, Alder C, Galvin JE, Perkins AJ, Healey P, et al. Practical clinical tool to monitor dementia symptoms: the HABC-Monitor. Clin Interv Aging. 2012;7:143–57. doi:10.2147/CIA. S30663.

16. Marventano S, Ayala A, Gonzalez N, Rodriguez-Blazquez C, Garcia-Gutierrez S, Forjaz MJ. Multimorbidity and functional status in community-dwelling older adults. Eur J Intern Med. 2014;25(7):610–6. doi:10.1016/j.ejim.2014.06.018.

17. Ostbye T, Yarnall KS, Krause KM, Pollak KI, Gradison M, Michener JL. Is there time for management of patients with chronic diseases in primary care? Ann Fam Med. 2005;3(3):209–14. doi:10.1370/afm.310.

18. Hinton L, Franz C, Reddy G, Flores Y, Kravitz R, Barker J. Practice constraints, behavioral problems, and Dementia care: primary care physicians' perspectives. J Gen Intern Med. 2007;22(11):1487–92. doi:10.1007/s11606-007-0317-y.

19. Borson S, Frank L, Bayley PJ, Boustani M, Dean M, Lin PJ, et al. Improving dementia care: the role of screening and detection of cognitive impairment. Alzheimers Dement. 2013;9(2):151–9. doi:10.1016/j. jalz.2012.08.008.

20. Alzheimer's Association. 2014 Alzheimer's disease facts and figures. Alzheimers Dement. 2014;10(2):e47–92.

21. Apesoa-Varano EC, Barker JC, Hinton L. Curing and caring: the work of primary care physicians with dementia patients. Qual Health Res. 2011; 21(11):1469–83. doi:10.1177/1049732311412788.

22. Berger JT, Rosner F, Kark P, Bennett AJ. Reporting by physicians of impaired drivers and potentially impaired drivers. The committee on bioethical issues of the medical society of the state of New York. J Gen Intern Med. 2000;15(9):667–72.

23. Kovner CT, Mezey M, Harrington C. Who cares for older adults? Workforce implications of an aging society. Health Aff (Millwood). 2002;21(5):78–89.

24. Alliance EW. Geriatrics workforce shortage: a looming crisis for our families. Washington, DC: Eldercare Workforce Alliance; 2012.

25. Health, U. D. o., & Services, H., Health Resources and Services Administration. The registered nurse population: initial findings from the 2008 national sample survey of registered nurses. Merrifield, VA: US Department of Health and Human Services–Health Resources and Services Administration; 2010.

26. Colla CH. Swimming against the current—what might work to reduce low-value care? N Engl J Med. 2014;371(14):1280–3. doi:10.1056/NEJMp1404503.

27. French DD, LaMantia MA, Livin LR, Herceg D, Alder CA, Boustani MA. Healthy aging brain center improved care coordination and produced net savings. Health Aff (Millwood). 2014;33(4):613–8. doi:10.1377/hlthaff.2013.1221.

28. Gitlin LN, Belle SH, Burgio LD, Czaja SJ, Mahoney D, Gallagher-Thompson D, et al. Effect of multicomponent interventions on caregiver burden and depression: the REACH multisite initiative at 6-month follow-up. Psychol Aging. 2003;18(3):361–74. doi:10.1037/0882-7974.18.3.361.

29. Hebert LE, Beckett LA, Scherr PA, Evans DA. Annual incidence of Alzheimer disease in the United States projected to the years 2000 through 2050. Alzheimer Dis Assoc Disord. 2001;15(4):169–73.

Community Mobility and Dementia: The Role for Health Care Professionals

Nina M. Silverstein, Anne E. Dickerson, and Elin Schold Davis

Introduction

Most people do not think about how they get around their communities when they need or want to go somewhere. We are accustomed to the convenience of the personal automobile and the spontaneity it offers being available 24/7. For example, we may have specific destinations in mind and then spontaneously add or subtract destinations from our intended route with little effort or concern for the implications. However, the freedom of movement that comes with the privilege of a driver's license is in jeopardy when a person is identified as "unsafe" to drive because of a cognitive impairment. Of all the losses experienced when living with dementia, for a driver, the loss of freedom and independence associated with driving cessation is described by clients and families as tragic, catastrophic, and isolating, and elicits quotes such as "I'd rather be told I have cancer." About 60–70 % of Americans with

N.M. Silverstein, PhD (✉)
University of Massachusetts Boston,
Boston, MA, USA
e-mail: nina.silverstein@umb.edu

A.E. Dickerson, PhD, OTR/L, FAOTA
East Carolina University, Greenville, NC, USA
e-mail: dickersona@ecu.edu

E. Schold Davis
American Occupational Therapy Association,
Bethesda, MD, USA
e-mail: escholddavis@aota.org

dementia live in the community [1]; and about 40 % of persons with dementia continue to drive following diagnosis [2]. The question is not simply whether individuals with dementia should or should not drive, but "when" cessation is enforced as driving skills predictably worsen with the progression of the disorder [3]. Hunt et al. [4] reported on 207 media reports of lost drivers with dementia over a 10-year period and noted that 70 drivers were not found, 32 were found dead, and although 116 were found alive, 35 had sustained an injury [4].

At a certain point, which may be years past the initial diagnosis, it becomes clear to all (except perhaps the driver) that cessation of driving is inevitable. In fact, most often family members see the problems of the diminishing abilities to execute critical driving skills in the form of speed of response, flexibility of thinking, problem solving, and frustration tolerance as first indicators of a problem prior to the diagnosis. This is a challenge to individuals and their family members because there may not be any understanding of the safety implications associated with these errors "anyone could make." Furthermore, there often is not a formal diagnosis because many older adults only see a primary care physician who may not use a formal diagnosis, so errors do not become part of the larger picture of function. This is a very important point for the primary care health provider. In the case of dementia, these early indicators are not benign, and we must be vigilant to not explain them away. An example

© Springer International Publishing Switzerland 2016
M. Boltz, J.E. Galvin (eds.), *Dementia Care*, DOI 10.1007/978-3-319-18377-0_9

may be getting lost while driving, particularly in an area that should be familiar. In fact, it is one of the first warning signs that indicate investigation into cognitive processes or diagnostic evaluation is needed.

Usually, at the early stage of the disease process, individuals are likely not connected to services and supports. In the case of transportation and particularly driving, this has implications for everyone, including the public. Accordingly, drivers are not identified as "patients" and family members do not consider themselves "caregivers." This puts the individual, family and community at risk by not intervening early with support, education and opportunities to intervene in order to extend driving years if possible, but more importantly, promote mobility and participation outside the home whenever possible with other methods of transportation. There are stakeholders beyond the individual and family members that have an active role in the transition from driver to passenger. If we embrace the concept that "mobility" is the desired outcome rather than working toward "giving up the keys," stakeholders can contribute to a more positive message and benefit the older adult, the family, and the public.

Stakeholder Perspectives

As an activity, driving is highly valued, even by those with significant medical impairments like stroke [5]. For the older adult, driving is an over-learned task. Consequently for individuals with beginning dementia, it can be easily accomplished in familiar environments. From the driver's perspective, the activity of driving is not difficult, their skills remain unchanged, and therefore it is not seen as a problem activity for the individual.

Driving and cessation of driving is a topic that is critical issue for older adults and emotional for those stakeholders needing to make determinations for fitness-to-drive. Moreover, stakeholders (e.g., licensing authorities, health care providers, families, drivers) have diverse information and perspectives about this topic making the subject not necessarily about facts and decision points, but about how best to manage a process of transition from community

independence to maintenance of dignity and self-worth in a shrinking world.

It is imperative that health care professionals consider the perspectives of the various stakeholders when addressing the issue of driving and community mobility for persons with dementia. It is important to understand, but not always obvious, that the role, duties and relationship of individuals to the person with dementia may include confrontation or interdependencies when it comes to changes in transportation behaviors, and this may confound their perspectives. Especially consider the perspective of the adult child. Even in the best of family relationships, there are roles, duties, and interpersonal relationships that are interwoven and complex. As we know, individual perspectives drive interest, study, action and follow through. The adult child, who has the best interest of their parent with beginning dementia may have a surprising response about cessation of driving. Juggling conflicting perspectives, the son or daughter may be thinking, "if he stops driving then I need to leave work to drive him," "mom depends on him," "he'll never agree to stop-this will be war." This results in the key supporters or caregivers becoming effectively paralyzed in the decision of how to act. A frequent example is the adult son or daughter expressing concern about their parent's ability to maintain finances and take over budgeting, but when it comes to transportation, the adult child chooses, intentionally or unintentionally, to ignore the discussion about driving because of the possibility of becoming the taxi service for mom and/or dad.

The key point for the reader about driving of older adults with cognitive impairment, you cannot assume nor be surprised by the actions or expressed perspective of any one individual or stakeholder in a particular role. A common occurrence and example of a stakeholder not related to family members, but evokes the emotions of important roles in families is the police officer who stops a vehicle because of a safety concern but decides to not issue a ticket because "she [the driver] reminded me of my grandmother." In this case, the emotional conflict of causing anxiety to the older adult in addition to the significant financial burden to the senior on limited resources overrides the safety issue for

Table 1 Indication or "warning signs" of possible Alzheimer's disease and how these deficits may affect driving and/or the use of transportation options

Warning signs or indicators	Examples affecting driving	Examples affecting use of transportation options
Memory loss	May forget the destination; may be at risk if stop to try to remember in an unsafe place (e.g., turn lane, middle of intersection not remembering which way to turn)	Cannot remember ride time or appointment
Difficulty performing tasks	Comes upon a stalled vehicle or accident and cannot negotiate how to get around or a new route to destination	Has a problem making transit arrangement
Problems with language	Unable to understand signs or nonverbal behavior of other drivers	Unable to communicate with driver
Disorientation to time/place	May get lost easily and cannot find their way home	Gets lost after transit drop-off
Poor or decreased judgment	Cannot safely judge: when to merge with other traffic, gaps between vehicles to make a turn, what to do at a complex interaction (flashing arrows or two lane turn)	Has difficulty paying fares or making change
Abstract thinking	Unable to plan another route if there is an accident, construction, or road closure	Unable to navigate route changes
Misplacement of things	Forgets where vehicle is parked	Leaves belongings in vehicle
Changes in mood/behavior	Becomes agitated when other vehicles honk for the person to move over or make a turn sooner	Becomes agitated for no apparent reason
Changes in personality	Refuses to give up driving even when problems pointed out; upset when confronted with driving discussion	Becomes suspicious of driver
Loss of initiative	Will keep driving (even when not sure where s/he is going) instead of stopping and asking for help	Does not want to get in or out of vehicle

the conscientious officer, who may be convinced it will not happen again. When in fact, one of the "best" warning signs for family members is a ticket from a law enforcement officer as it is relatively "objective," and hopefully not wait for a crash which is often a crisis.

Warning signs inherently mean that the person who is "warned" should act. The literature offers a growing array of warning signs for unsafe driving behaviors alerting stakeholders to the risk the individual with dementia poses to him/herself and others when driving (see Table 1). Unfortunately, barriers to the conversations about driving risk are often described relative to those stakeholders who might do the warning. "Physicians fear losing patients if they report," "families do not want to sever/disturb relationships," and "practitioners fear liability if they discuss the issue." Most of the literature reports the cost of evaluation as a significant barrier, rarely mentioning or even recognizing the cost of injury or death in balance. The responsibility to recognize, report and act is a virtual "hot potato" in the driving community.

In many cases, the unstated plan is the hope that someone else will act [6].

The older population (age 65+) numbered 43.1 million in 2012 representing 13.7 % of the U.S. population [7]. With the recognition of the relationship between age and its accompanying health care issues that may impact critical driving skills, the driving stakeholder and advocacy groups have worked hard to (1) identify needs, (2) develop educational resources, and (3) build training programs in order to provide services that address the concern of the medically compromised driver, who by definition place themselves and their communities at risk. These resources have included identifying pathways of service to the professionals and/or community services to assist drivers and their families. In fact, defining the issue and describing what needs to be done has been admittedly, the easier phase. The motivation as well as "whom" should act is more complicated and complex. With that in mind, we will describe the conflicting roles and perspectives of the people involved. Figure 1 illustrates the

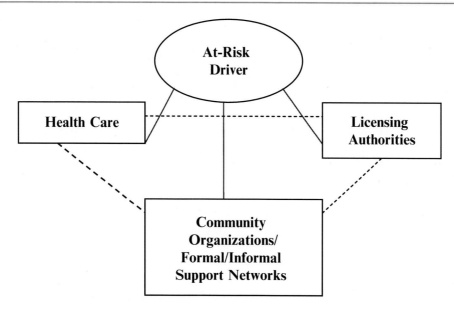

Fig. 1 Shift toward a public health paradigm sharing scope of responsibility. *Source*: Adler and Silverstein [8]

numerous stakeholders frequently involved in the driving decision.

The "driver-at-risk" is the **patient or client** with dementia (or suspected of having signs of early dementia) who is at the heart of this discussion. As noted in previous chapters, the disease itself erodes an individual's capability for insight, self-reflection and sound judgment. So the person him or herself is the least capable to act or advocate on his or her own behalf at the times when critical decisions are made, including the decision when to retire from driving. The goal for the client should be aimed to raise awareness and done early in the process, so that ideally, a "willingness" to comply with recommendations to reduce or eventually stop driving can be made at a time when understanding the implications are possible. Resources can include review of warning signs, a checklist of alternative methods of transportation, contracts by family members to reveal "when it is time," and worksheets that show how to balance the cost of an automobile versus alternative methods of transit. The client should be shown information about transportation options early enough in the course of this progressive disease to successfully plan and be a part of the action that will need to occur. In the best scenario, the individual makes known his or her wishes,

complies with restrictions when driving is deemed unsafe and avails him or herself of alternatives to stay mobile. This is the ideal goal, yet not achieved for varied reasons.

The **family** is comprised of related persons. Assumptions may be made that they are close both geographically and emotionally attached to the individual diagnosed with dementia. The family who is positioned, willing, and equipped to provide strong support offers options and potential for a more desired outcome by the treatment team. However, many adult children of older adults are geographically dispersed. Moreover, even when family members reside near or with the person with dementia, the family member may not be available or willing to assist the medically-at-risk driver who has to cease driving. Even with the rich description of resources for screening, evaluation, expert consult and planning, the family is often overburdened and reeling from just the reality of dealing with the disease process. Transportation mode change, particularly denying access to the driver's vehicle to enforce the loss of driving privileges, may be the first duty that marks a family member's role transition to the one of "caregiver."

Transportation is a critical instrumental activity of daily living (IADL) and if the individual no longer drives, the responsibility lands squarely on the family. The shift in everyday responsibilities that dependence in transportation brings impacts all members on the family when a driver with dementia gives up the keys. Healthcare providers and licensing agencies may be ill advised if they rely on the family to report warning signs or driving concerns. As illustrated, some family members have varying investments in the ability for the medically-at-risk driver to continue driving or not. In addition to busy adult children, the current cohort of older women may be less likely to drive and may be dependent on the spouse with dementia. If you take away his driving abilities away, you have restricted the spouse's ability to get where she wants and needs to go. For the driving decision, the family often becomes the default party who is left with both making the decision about driving, enforcing the decision (i.e., taking the keys and car away), and then having to provide the transportation for every need of the family member. Families describe this role as heartbreaking and impossible (Schold Davis, Personal Communications nd). As concerned and committed primary health care providers, it is important to acknowledge the conflicting roles of family members. In addition, recognizing the realities as well as offering the family members information on methods to cope should be part of the responsibilities of the provider. It takes a skillful family member to be a gatekeeper and loved one simultaneously. Family members understand how to offer support and reminders. However imposing restrictions, particularly when it is in opposition to the individual's wishes, requires the determination and support that is often too difficult for even the best of family relationships.

Driving cessation support groups [9] and resources [10] have been developed in recent years to assist with the transition from driver to passenger [11–13]. These interventions are targeted toward family members to help them effectively communicate with medically-at-risk drivers throughout the process of driving cessation [14]. The reality, however, is that few *supportive, dementia-friendly transportation alternatives* exist that would fully address the challenges of maintaining mobility and participation for the non-driver with dementia.

The **Physician** (or primary health care provider). The general assumption by patients, families and the larger society is that the physician will know, and will take responsibility to inform the medically-at-risk client when it is time to stop driving. This assumption is flawed on two levels. First, although the physician is skilled in evidence-medical symptoms, understands the course of this progressive disease, and understands the complexities of operating a motor vehicle, most physicians are not trained in assessment of driving nor is there any accepted valid tool easily applied to determine the answer in the physician's office. Thus, unless the client is moderately or severely demented, most physicians do not know when it is time to cease driving. Second, physicians often have to give clients "bad" news, but more often than not, there is a pill or strategy offered that gives the patient hope to confront the problem. In most communities, the physician does not have the knowledge of any strategies to offer clients or family members for continued community mobility and engagement in daily living.

Nevertheless, the physician's role is critical as patients (and families) look to their physician for guidance about this important instrumental activity of daily living (IADL). Although the physician is not skilled to assess driving per se, if it becomes clear that the client is having difficulty with higher level activities such as managing bills, medication compliance, managing their appointments, the health care provider should consider the person's safety risk in activities such as cooking, bathing, or driving. The difference between activities such as managing their medication, cooking or bathing and driving is that if the person exceeds the risk, the harm will likely only be to the client; while with driving, the harm could potentially be to others. Thus, primary health care practitioners need to ask themselves "Would I want this client to drive down the street where my children or grandchildren play?" It is not for the physician to have to always make the decision, although sometimes it is clear, but it is important to know when it is time to get driving assessed by experts in this practice area.

In 2003, with a revision in 2010, the National Highway Traffic Safety Administration (NHTSA) funded the AMA to develop a *Physician's Guide for Assessing and Counseling Older Drivers* [15, 16]. This *Guide* offers evidence-based information about the changes associated with aging in the areas of concern (i.e., vision, physical ability and cognition), offers a description of a brief screening tool to assess for driving risk, discusses evidence about the medical conditions most associated with driving risk, explains how driver rehabilitation specialists are the specialty service for assessment of driving and reviews each state's licensing guidelines and reporting obligations. In addition to the guide, NHTSA worked with the AMA to develop an online training for physician. The training offers written resources that support physicians working together with their healthcare team to build a network of services and resources that support planning and offer options for families and patients along the declining path of dementia. In many states the physician is the key healthcare provider to report unsafe drivers to the licensing authority. Informed physicians should use the best evidence-based screening tools, and refer appropriate candidates for either an IADL evaluation by an occupational therapist if several IADL tasks appear impaired or a comprehensive driving evaluation by an occupational therapy/driving rehabilitation specialist, adhere to state reporting and licensing guidelines, and communicate decisions from planning to driving cessation.

All **Healthcare professionals** who interact with a person diagnosed with dementia have a role in driving and community mobility, as driving is the "enabler" for participation and engagement in daily life. In fact, the diverse and complex responsibilities require a team of healthcare professionals.

Healthcare professionals working with clients in their earliest stages have the opportunity to put driving "on the table" as a valued IADL that requires careful consideration and planning, much like planning for housing and finances. Screening tools may assist with identifying those at risk. Education and planning are critical components to *frame* driving as a *transitional process* and not a life altering, abrupt and devastating "on the spot" mandate. Resources and toolkits are available to support and encourage healthcare professionals to provide education and early intervention through support groups (see AARP and The Hartford Insurance resources on the reference list). It is important to bring persons with dementia and their families together in order to access resources and become empowered to take an active role in their own driving decisions that affect the safety of the individual, their family and the community.

The **community stakeholders** most important to this discussion are the authorities that make the actual licensing decisions. Unlike the popular belief that driving is a person's "right," it is actually a legal privilege. The legal determination for an individual's privilege to drive/not drive is solely within the jurisdiction of the state driver licensing authority. Health care providers, including physicians, are often asked to make recommendations to the licensing authority but the final decision is the licensing authority's alone.

Thus, as health care professionals, it is important to know the licensing and renewal policies in your location as they vary from state to state. In a few states, physician reporting of medical conditions that may impact critical driving skills is mandatory, while in most states, reporting is voluntary. Chapter 8 of the AMAs *Physician's Guide to Assessing and Counseling Older Drivers* contains a state-by-state review of state-specific policies.

Many states licensing authorities have Medical Advisory Boards (MAB). Implied by the name, this is a group of individuals who assist in the decision making process for the individuals with medical conditions. Unfortunately, there is such great variation in the function and composition of those boards across the country, there is not a lot that can be said in general about the MABs. When utilized, MABs can plan a critical role in making decisions related to driving by individuals with medical conditions that significantly impair their critical driving skills.

In NHTSA's recently released five-year plan December 2013, they included recommendations for state Medical Advisory Boards. While the overall responsibility is for processing medically-related concerns, NHTSA encourages MAB recommendations to move from just determining the pass/fail to including recommendations for re-evaluations for progressive disorders and/or geographic restrictions (e.g., restricted highway driving or a mileage restriction) for persons facing changes from a degenerative disease such as dementia. While certain restrictions work, for example no night driving for glaucoma, there is no consensus among researchers for driving restrictions for the driver with dementia. We believe restricted licenses are not appropriate for the driver with dementia. Since memory is the hallmark of dementia, by the time restrictions are necessary, the person with dementia will likely not remember the restriction and thus, possibly endangering his or herself and unaware passengers.

Law Enforcement Officers have been recognized as important partners in addressing the issue of identifying at-risk drivers. Most adult drivers recognize unsafe behaviors on the road. These clearly include the distracted driver who is texting, talking on the cell phone, eating, or just not paying attention to events on the road. In fact, we know that drivers who are texting are the most dangerous, especially when it is a young person who is often speeding and talking with his or her friends. In contrast, the person with cognitive challenges is not using the phone, but generally working hard to concentrate on the road to manage the quickly changing environment. The difference is the momentarily distracted driver usually can recover quickly, process the information and take quick action. The individual with dementia is typically driving slower, cannot process quickly, and has difficulty taking action, which is why the police officer pulls the older adult over for indecision in an intersection or missing the stop sign.

As mentioned previously, it has been recognized that many police officers, and especially state highway patrol officers, are empathic to older drivers and may not ticket. When in reality, the ticket could be the "red flag" signaling it is time for family members to act. In order to educate and counteract this tendency to not acknowledge impaired driving due to cognition, the National Highway Traffic Safety Administration (NHTSA) has developed law enforcement training modules for state and local

law enforcement. Many states law enforcement agencies have used the information to develop their own training tools and are working in hand with licensing authorities to directly refer citizens they stop and see are impaired to the licensing authorities. Two examples of these strategies include: (1) In 2011, each of North Carolina's state highway patrol officers received a "cue card" with information about how to observe and determine if the motorists had a cognitive impairment [17], and (2) California has developed a slick version of a mini-mental exam for their law enforcement officers that has been useful in the development of tools by other municipalities.

Law Enforcement in a growing number of communities have also been actively involved in the Silver Alert® program designed to assist in finding cognitively-impaired persons who become lost while driving.

The **Judicial** system as a partner to assist in driving decisions has yet to be fully utilized. In one example, the American Occupational Therapy Association worked with Administrative Law Judges to develop resources that included recommendations to consider the comprehensive driving evaluation when data gathering prior to making decisions about the medically-at-risk older driver. Another example from the state of Florida, a court used creative sentencing where the decision to cancel the license of an older driver with early dementia was accompanied by required sessions to learn effective use of community mobility alternatives (i.e., the bus) to both ensure mobility but also reduce the chances that the driver would resume driving unlicensed for lack of any known option to get around. Such examples are important avenues to both pursue and develop. The Judicial Factsheets can be accessed on the AOTA website www.aota.org

The Process of Awareness and Transition from Driver to Passenger

While in some situations, an at-fault crash or acute situation may hasten driving cessation, recognizing warning signs and beginning the transition from driver to passenger earlier in the

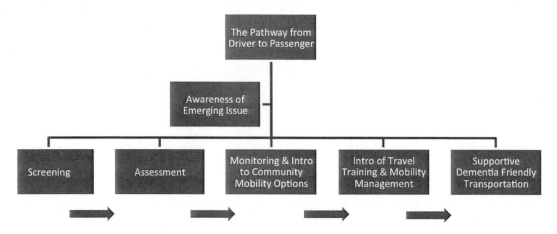

Fig. 2 Community mobility continuum: the pathway from driver to passenger. *Source*: Adapted from Silverstein [18]

disease process undoubtedly offers the best outcomes for all. Figure 2 depicts the continuum representing the transition from the driver's seat to the passenger's seat. The transition is not always a linear one, especially in cases where a condition may be temporary. For example, an acute issue like a hip fracture might temporarily cause driving cessation and the need for supportive transportation or a medication change may exacerbate confusion that resolves with time. However, for the individual with dementia, the progression does eventually end up with the need for supportive transportation. Understanding the continuum can help health care professionals identify the triggers or "red flags" for referring patients for specialized driving assessment and when to develop a mobility plan that includes all transportation options, while always reassuring patients and their family members that the important outcome is mobility, regardless of transportation mode.

There are several educational resources that are helpful in increasing an individual and family member's awareness of critical driving skills. In the earliest stages, the "red flags" or warning signs include getting lost in familiar areas, taking longer to travel to and from destinations, unexplained scrapes and dents on the vehicle or other concerns that might arise informally. Any of these occurrences might suggest the need to offer the client a screening for driving. The Hartford

Guides, *We Need to Talk* and *At the Crossroads: Driving & Dementia* are helpful resources to begin informal conversations about driving safety and concerns about driving skills. The former provides opening topics for general discussion such as a checklist of areas of concern (i.e. other drivers honking at you, driving too fast or too slow, or being confused at highway exits); a worksheet for determining the cost of operating a vehicle; and a "getting there" worksheet to consider how an individual can get to needed or desired destinations without driving oneself. The latter guide considers the special issues of a driver with dementia and includes a non-binding agreement with the doctor that families may refer to later in the disease process and states that the individual agrees to stop driving when he or she is no longer able to drive safely and may inflict harm to him or herself or to others. Both of these resources were developed based on research work done by the MIT Age Lab, backed by qualitative research in the field. Additionally they are written **for the client** rather than the professional and are shipped free of charge for professionals to distribute freely. Several are available in multiple languages at: http://www.thehartford.com/mature-market-excellence/publications-on-aging

Awareness of the Problem When there is beginning awareness of driving issues by family members or others, it is time to do a screening, regardless of the driver's perception. One method of screening is the self-administered tools which can be done with a family member or friend.

In a general sense, the word *screening* refers to obtaining and reviewing data to determine the need for evaluation. It precedes formal assessment. For example, schools have vision screenings for children and parents are alerted if their child may need to see an optometrist. Screening for driving is more complex and can range from simple visual acuity screens to computer tools that screen for cognition. There are multiple types of self-screening tools. Self-screening is when the individual obtains and reviews data to determine the need for an evaluation. Two examples of self-administered screening tools are *Roadwise Review*® and the *Driving Decisions Workbook. Roadwise Review*® was developed by the American Automobile Association (AAA) and can be done online or by requesting a CD-ROM from an AAA club. It provides an indication of an individual's performance on several physical and mental tasks that are used for driving, although caution should be exercised in placing too much emphasis on self-screening as there is not strong research evidence between screening outcomes of Roadwise Review and driving evaluations [19].

A different type of screening tool is *The Driving Decisions Workbook* that was developed by researchers at the University of Michigan Transportation Research Institute ([20]; available online or download). Although it is self-administered and gives the individual feedback for making decisions, the main purpose of the workbook is to increase awareness of age-related changes that may impact safe driving.

Proxy screening is when an individual obtains and reviews data to determine the need for evaluation of another person. Several tools have been developed that include proxy screening (in the form of checklists and decision trees) in response to needs expressed by spouses or other family caregivers who want to know **when** to address driving in their family member's progression of the disease. One example of a proxy-screening tool used for the driver with dementia is the *Fitness to Drive Screening (FTDS)* Measure [21].

It is a web-based tool that allows the caregivers and/or family members to rate their observations by responding to descriptions of 54 driving skills. Using an item response theory model of analysis (Rasch analysis) of these observations, the program generates a rating profile that classifies the driver into one of three categories with recommendations offered for those who might be considered at risk (http://fitnesstodrive.phhp.ufl.edu). Although the FTDS has significant research behind its development [22–24], it is not a diagnostic assessment tool and should only be used to identify driving difficulties and raise family/caregiver awareness. Screening tools identify what difficulties are of importance which offer information to the experts who then are skilled to do in-depth evaluations.

In addition to self-screening and proxy screening, a health care professional might do a screening, which may be referred to as an *evaluator screening*. In this case, a professional skilled in specific screening tools obtains and reviews data to determine the need for evaluation for a specific individual. When a health care provider, skilled in the use of the tool, uses a screening tool that is similarly used as self or proxy screens, it is important to understand that with the training or expertise, the screen tool may be more discriminate and/or useful to the expert, especially if based on observation. A good example is a simple brake reaction timer. Although the physical action of simple reaction time is not linked to any driving outcome in the literature [25], when the person with dementia has difficulty understanding the directions and the evaluator has seen many other persons perform appropriately with the same screening tool, the expertise might gain a more accurate view of impairment over others who are purely looking at the reaction time.

Ultimately, screening is seen as the conduit to determine, in the case of this chapter, whether the individual with dementia needs further evaluation to assess their fitness-to-drive. There are also several levels and definitions of driver evaluations as further described in the Appendix. If the results of the screening tool warrants, an assessment is the next step. In some cases, if the individual has other issues with complex IADLs, a formal assessment of safety with all IADLs by an occupational therapist might be useful. The professional would consider what activities are valued by the client and what environmental supports can be used to continue those valued activities. In the case of driving and community mobility, the *comprehensive driving evaluation* might be the next step on the community mobility continuum. The comprehensive driving evaluation consists of an array of clinical assessment tools to evaluate visual, cognitive, physical, and perceptual abilities including an on-road component (this will be further described below).

It is important to note that a diagnosis of Alzheimer's disease or a related dementia does not necessarily imply that a person should cease driving immediately. The decision of when to stop driving should be based on functional performance, not just on diagnosis or chronological age. However, it is very important to understand that the standard road test at the state licensing authority is not a sufficient assessment of fitness-to-drive in persons with dementia. The mechanics of operating a vehicle are likely an overlearned task that the driver may perform without error especially if the examiner is cueing the driver with single commands. This next section will expand on the issue and process of driving evaluations.

Driving Evaluation for Individuals with Dementia

Who administers a driving evaluation depends on the setting, state of residency, and qualifications of evaluators. As discussed previously, in each state, there is a licensing authority with a driving test or evaluation for at least their novice drivers; usually a structured system with results in a pass or fail outcome. How each state system deals with medical conditions also vary significantly. Some licensing authorities refer drivers with complex medical conditions directly to driver rehabilitation specialists who then provide individualized clinical and on-road evaluations while others have specific MABs, as described earlier. What is important for health care practitioners as well as consumers to understand about driving

evaluations is that the service, resources, and consequences of options are vastly distinct between the licensing authorities and driver rehabilitation specialists. Just like an eye exam, there are different outcomes from the school nurse's eye screening, the optometrist, and the ophthalmologist. Importantly, the implications for each of these options are the difference in approaches to assessment, not just simply the cost.

Health care professionals trained to administer a specialized driver evaluation are driver rehabilitation specialists (DRS) or occupational therapists with specialized education in driving and community mobility. A lower percentage are driving instructors that have undergone the specialized training. Regardless, driver rehabilitation specialists (DRS) are professionals with specialized training who plan, develop, coordinate, or implement driving rehabilitation services for individuals with disabilities [26]. As of 2014, there are about 600 DRS in the United States and approximately 80 % of the DRS are occupational therapists. Assessment starts with clinical measures conducted in the office setting then followed by a behind-the-wheel (BTW) or on-road assessment. Two national organizations maintain databases of DRS in North America. The AOTA has a listing of occupational therapists that have specialized training in driving rehabilitation (www.aota.org/olderdriver) and the *Association of Driver Rehabilitation Specialists (ADED)* is the professional organization dedicated specifically to driver rehabilitation across all disciplines and maintains a database of its members for the public (www.aded.net).

A comprehensive driving evaluation completed by a DRS typically includes a clinical assessment component and the "in context" component or on-road assessment. The clinical assessment usually starts with an interview to gather the client's medical and driving histories. Then comprehensive assessment of the individual's physical, cognitive, visual, and perceptual skills and abilities are performed using a diverse set of tools [62]. Depending on the outcome of the clinical evaluation, the on-road component follows. The usual pattern of the on-road is starting in a quiet parking lot or neighborhood, progressing to low traffic, intersections, and then busy streets and/or highway. The comprehensive driving evaluation can take from 2 to 5 h depending on the client and selected assessment tools. The on-road component typically lasts at least 45–60 min with the clinical component from 1 to 3 h. Outcomes from the comprehensive driving evaluation include recommendations to: (1) continue to drive with no restrictions, (2) drive with restrictions (e.g., no nighttime driving, limit speed or distance, no highway), (3) periodic review in cases of progressive diseases, (4) retirement from driving, and/or (5) assistance with community mobility. Presently, assistance with community mobility is inconsistent. It can range from a handout with local transportation to the development of a mobility plan that coordinates with resources in the community, with the former being more common. There is a push for DRSs to develop more beyond just driving evaluation and training with adaptive equipment in specialized vehicles to assist with the development of community options for the older adults with dementia [63]. However, although theoretically the DRS should follow through with community mobility, there are compelling reasons for other health care professionals to address this final component. First, a DRS is trained in driver rehabilitation including assessment tools, behind the wheel maneuvers and techniques, adaptive equipment for the vehicles, and training of clients. Community mobility other than driving expands that skill set significantly and although the DRS probably can offer valuable information, it will not be their service strength. Second, there is a limited number of DRSs in some areas so that there are waiting lists for evaluation services, thus it makes economic and efficacy sense not to have the DRS fulfill the community mobility component. Finally, the most compelling argument is that when an individual receives the recommendation from the DRS that cessation of driving is necessary, the client does not welcome (in fact often refuses) further conversation about transportation alternatives. For many DRS programs the best plan for assistance with community mobility would be a referral to another health care provider more knowledgeable and skilled in

assisting with that transition such as a Mobility Manager, a social worker or case worker that can help an individual figure out available and appropriate options that will be discussed further later on in this chapter.

For best practice it is a more practical and effective process if the individual with dementia and family work through a transition process over time with primary healthcare providers. One important development has been the *Assessment of Readiness for Mobility Transition (ARMT)* [13] developed by a team of educators and researchers to assess an individual's awareness and readiness in planning the mobility transition needed for all older adults. This clinical tool uses an interview and questions to characterize four types of emotional/attitudinal categories about mobility and offers strategies for each of the categories. In the ideal situation, when an older adult becomes more medically compromised with decreased cognitive abilities, the physician would screen their client, recognize the need for specialized assessment, and refer the client to a driving rehabilitation specialist to determine their level of risk. However, there are many reasons that the ideal situation does not occur. As the number of older adults grows, people with beginning dementia may not recognize (or want to admit) their slow decline in driving performance. Further, compensatory mechanisms to drive slower and avoid high traffic situations, self-limitations lauded as good strategies for the older adult, may prolong an older adults' driving life. However, in the case of a driver with dementia, it may actually be putting them at risk for getting lost or involved in crashes because they are driving beyond their cognitive capabilities, especially if a critical event occurs.

The question then is what is the solution to the issue? How can at-risk older drivers and in particular, medically-at-risk drivers get evaluated appropriately for either, (1) goals and strategies to remain driving with limited risk, or (2) if necessary, retire from driving, but be able to find alternative means of meeting their transportation needs [27]. It is unlikely the state licensing authorities have or will ever have the funding to build the manpower to fully meet the needs.

Further, politically, states will be hard pressed to institute screening measures perceived to be prejudicially age-based. However, the more compelling problem is describing the skill set needed to appropriately evaluate fitness-to-drive of individuals with complex medical issues.

When considering individuals with beginning or mild dementia, the issue is how to determine when their *strategic level* skills are impaired so that he or she can no longer compensate by modifying or restricting their driving to avoid making a dangerous decisions at the *tactical* or *operational* levels [28]. These terms—strategic, tactical, and operational—are originally derived from Michon's Hierarchy of Driving Behaviors [29]. *Operational* is the driver's ability to perform the physical actions of steering the wheel, moving the gears, and pressing the accelerator or brake. These are the actions that are overlearned and habitual so that the action of performance is automatic. *Tactical* is the driver executes the maneuvers in order to complete the trip. The environment requires the driver's response within rules; are typically learned and practiced; and used frequently in the driving situation (e.g., maintaining lane position, obstacle avoidance, gap acceptance, obeying traffic signals, turning). The *strategic* level defines the general planning of a trip, including trip goals, route, and modal choice with the associated costs and risks involved. It also includes the ability to adapt plans when necessary, such as changing a route due to an accident or construction, needing to make an unexpected stop (e.g., use a bathroom), a change in trip's goals, or seeking help if lost. When the individual is so impaired that the operational and tactical skills are impaired, it is not a difficult determination through clinical testing or an on-road assessment. The much more difficult scenario is determining at what level of strategic impairment is putting the individual and/or public at risk. If the individual with mild dementia is operationally and tactically "fit" to drive to a few select places during non-rush hours, is that not a positive move to prolong aging-in-place? However, if the usual route is blocked because of the city cutting trees for right away of power lines, and forces the individual to turn on a less

familiar street, does he or she have enough strategic abilities to negotiate an alternative route home? This complex level of evaluation requires a skilled professional, who understands the intricacies of a disease process and differentiating the levels of abilities of that individual at their present level of the disease process.

The main point here is the understanding that it takes a skilled professional to evaluate fitness-to-drive for individuals with early dementia. The individual with early dementia, who still has intact operational driving behaviors and all or most of their tactical, may perform well on a "driving test" due to its structure, such as the road test that may accompany license renewal where an individual responds to one-on-one cues like, "turn left"… "turn right.". However, he or she may in fact, be in danger if there are limitations in their strategic abilities and, for example, they may not be able to figure out a way home if a regular driving route has been altered unexpectedly.

Addressing Driving Risk Within IADL Tasks

The risk factor of driving needs to be framed as any other complex instrumental task of daily living (IADL) that has some level of risk. Healthcare practitioners, and in particular, occupational therapists routinely evaluate safety risk of their clients for independent living, cooking, handling their finances, managing medication, shopping, and others. Occupational therapists should also understand the importance of community mobility and be able to help individuals make a smoother transition from driving to using other forms of transportation, maintaining their autonomy, independence, and sense of self-worth. While general occupational therapists and other health care practitioners know our ability to move about our community affects the quality of our lives, occupational therapists trained in driver rehabilitation understand the critical demands of driving. They have the skills to evaluate an individual's overall ability to operate a vehicle safely, and, where appropriate, to provide rehabilitation to strengthen skills used in driving. In order to

Occupational Therapy Intervention:
Evidence, Clinical Judgment, and Risk

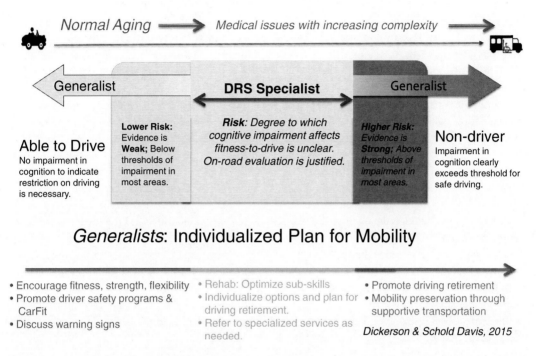

Fig. 3 Framework for occupational therapy judgment on fitness-to-drive

meet the needs of the growing population, the key is to integrate the generalists and specialists roles and skill sets to effectively address the driving continuum.

It is clear from research, that normal aging per se is not the reason individuals cannot continue to drive [30]. It is the medical issues, including and particularly cognitive impairment that puts drivers at risk. Figure 3 illustrates an occupational therapy framework for using an occupational therapist's clinical judgment to determine fitness to drive based on evidence and risk [31]. A general practice occupational therapist routinely evaluates cognition, visual-perception, and motor skills and has expertise to determine if an individual's impairment exceeds the threshold for driving safely. This framework illustrates that only when the degree to which the impairment affects fitness to drive is unclear, is an on-road evaluation or full evaluation by a specialist is justified. Additionally, occupational therapists can begin to assist older

adults in planning and building options for community mobility at the early stages of dementia or other progressive disorders. Planning for the transition to non-driving that will eventually occur can assist clients and their families in a more positive and constructive process over time, instead of what is too often the case, a sudden and highly disruptive event such as a crash. If the recommendation is for periodic re-assessment, then monitoring the clients' driving habits and behaviors is important. A more detailed description that health care providers can use to distinguish the type of services needed for an older adult is provided in the Appendix.

Evidence supports this framework. Specifically, in a study to compare an IADL evaluation to the outcome of a driving evaluation [32], results suggested using an IADL assessment predicted who would fail or pass the driving evaluation. Drivers (N=47), ranging from healthy volunteers to clients (referred by physicians or the state DMV) received comprehensive driving evaluations and the Assessment of Motor and Process Skills (AMPS [33]). The AMPS evaluates an individual's ability to organize and execute a complex IADL (e.g., preparing a salad, making a bed, brewing coffee with eggs and toast, preparing a tuna salad sandwich) that is familiar to the client. The evaluator scores the performance on two universal taxonomies of skill items that yield interval level data. The data are compared to the outcome of the driving evaluation, which was categorized as failed, restricted or passed. All participants who scored higher on both the motor and process scales, passed the on-road assessment. Conversely, participants who scored low on both the motor and process scales, almost all failed the on-road assessment. Interesting, although the clients who passed the test tended to be younger, a one way ANOVA demonstrated no significance between age and outcome $(F(2.43)=2.014, p=0.146)$ supporting driving outcome is based on performance and not chronological age.

In a more recent research of drivers recovering from stroke, Stapleton [34] examined why all 48 drivers who completed a comprehensive driving examination "passed" the on-road component. In his qualitative study with occupational therapists, evaluators, and physicians, it appeared that the occupational therapists only referred to the driving evaluator when the individual was "ready" for the evaluation, that is, when it was most likely that the individual would pass the exam. Although more research is needed, this study supports the perspective that observations of clients performing other complex IADL can generalize their expert clinical observation to the activity of driving.

Accepting the assumption that general practice occupational therapists should be the first line of providers for determining fitness-to-drive, the American Occupational Therapy Association joined in a cooperative agreement with the National Highway Traffic Safety Administration (NHTSA) called the *Gaps and Pathways Project* with implementation dates from July, 2012 to June, 2015. This project's overall aim was to build and expand programs to address driving as a means of community mobility. Specifically, the

project objectives included (1) identifying the gaps for delivering best practice services, (2) improving direct service to older drivers through general practice occupational therapy practitioners and driver rehabilitation specialists, and (3) equip practitioners through education, training, and understanding the best pathways of referrals. Not every driver rehabilitation program needs to have a full range of services, but each program might have a screening program and/or have the knowledge and access of *pathways for referrals* so that the older adult is getting the right level service by the right provider at the right time. One of the outcomes of this project is the *Spectrum of Driver Services: Right Services for the Right People at the Right Time* (Appendix) [35]. This Table illustrates the range and diversity of services for older drivers. It specifically identifies the service providers educational background, credentials, and expected outcomes, providing consumers, referral sources, healthcare providers, and other stakeholders with the information in refer to the right people to the right service at the right time [35, p. 177].

Monitoring Drivers with Dementia

Monitoring has been greatly enhanced by the ability to instrument an individual's personal vehicle. While some technologies already may be used to monitor persons with dementia in their vehicles such as *Comfort Zone®* [59], a location mapping service device available through the Alzheimer's Association, the range of behaviors important to monitor that are critical to the progression of Alzheimer's disease have currently just been measured in research. Eby et al. [36] used in-vehicle technology to monitor driving behaviors of persons with memory loss in naturalistic driving for over a month and compared their behaviors to drivers without cognitive impairment. The memory loss group was found to have significantly restricted driving space relative to the comparison group. They drove shorter distances, to fewer destinations, and avoided freeways and most restricted driving to daytime. This study is the first to show, using objective measures of driving, that drivers with memory loss restrict their driving space. At the same time, the memory loss group (which had been previously cleared by an DRS as safe to drive) drove as safely as the comparison group. Few safety-related behavioral errors were found for either group. Wayfinding problems were rare among both groups, but the memory loss group was significantly more likely to get lost.

While the use of a range of monitoring instruments in naturalistic driving would be ideal, currently, monitoring encompassing asking the individual to return for a specialized driving reassessment within a specified interval of time, usually from 6 months to a year. Research shows that about 30–40 % of drivers with dementia are likely to continue driving for 3–4 years past diagnosis [37].

The clear message in this chapter is that eventually the individual with dementia is going to need to cease driving. As such, the best time to start with the introduction of other transportation options is from the very beginning of the diagnosis. This would allow the individual to learn about the services when they are perhaps still able to adapt to new travel modes and allows them to retire from driving in a more measured and dignified manner. Transportation options are part of the *Family of Transportation Services* that Burkhardt [38] notes as a concept that was developed in Sweden by Ståhl [39] and emphasizes that both public and private modes are needed. This includes automotive travel, walking, public transit, service routes, paratransit operations (including taxis and agency services), escorted or assisted transportation, and emergency services are needed to respond to community mobility challenges [38, p. 221]. As previously stated, Eby et al. [36] noted that driving space becomes restricted. The implications of that reduced driving space suggest that trips to certain destinations and at particular times of day may be lessened. Unfortunately, a consequence of reduced trips could lead to depression [40] or increased social isolation [41]. A needed intervention is to help medically-at-risk drivers and their family members reframe the impending loss of driving to an opportunity to enhance mobility. A message that readers should take away from this Chapter is that mobility is the outcome. Driving is just one mode in the family of transportation services. Concepts critical to developing a mobility plan are *travel training* and *mobility management*.

Travel Training teaches persons with disabilities and older adults how to use public transit. People with memory loss who have been driving all their adult lives and may have rarely, if at all, tried public transportation are not likely (or later in the disease process, able) to stop driving and hop on a bus. The impairments in critical driving skills are likely to be similar reasons for not being able to safely navigate public transportation. While travel training in the general population is short-term, travel training for persons with dementia may need a different model that goes beyond learning how to use a specific mode of transit and includes a travel buddy or additional supports that cue the environment.

Mobility Management is a strategic approach, generally by a professional, to optimize mobility to meet daily needs. The mobility manager can assist the individual and family member with understanding the different modes of transportation and the levels of assistance available to get to the desired destination. There are efforts to expand this service in both private and public domains. However, in the public domain, budget cuts are so massive in the area of services for older adults, this new service, although needed, is barely growing and only in a few venues. In terms of the private sector, there may be small pockets of services, but with no national recognition.

The final frame in the continuum described in Fig. 2 is not yet a reality in many communities across the United States and in other countries. Transportation options are not yet fully senior-friendly, let alone dementia-friendly and offering needed levels of assistance. Understanding what the ten warning signs of dementia mean for transportation provision is a critical step toward meeting the community mobility needs of this heretofore underserved, invisible population. Table 1 presented earlier in this chapter, illustrates the warning signs of Alzheimer's disease and the potential impact on transportation options.

Providing Alternative Transportation Options

To address safety and mobility for the person with dementia, driving cannot be looked at in isolation of instrumental activities of daily living and community engagement. The impetus for developing Table 1 was to illustrate why persons with cognitive impairment who are assessed as no longer safe to drive are not likely to safely navigate public or paratransit. That is, reasons for impairments in critical driving skills are likely to be similar to reasons why an individual may not be able to stop driving and then use other means of transit. The cognitive demand may be too high for keeping track of and dispensing fares; watching for transit stops; and reaching desired destinations, both external and internal as in a specific doctor's office in a building. In discussing discharge planning, Silverstein and Maslow [42] note the importance of reviewing a patient's driving history and making a determination if driving skills should be assessed and monitored post hospitalization. They further state that plans for community mobility options should be discussed if driving cessation is necessary.

Potential Strategies

Silverstein conducted 32 interviews in 2012 with public officials/lead agency staff members, transportation providers and university researchers in transportation and aging who were asked to share their knowledge, experiences, and opinions related to the topic [64]. Interviewees were shown an earlier version of Table 1 [60] (without the impact on driving skills noted) and asked to imagine a transportation option that would satisfy the needs of persons with cognitive impairment. They were asked to keep in mind the level of support available in how transportation is provided: curb to curb, door to door, door through door, hand to hand/chair to chair, stay at the destination, and escort/companion/attendant. The following are selected comments that best illustrate the themes that emerged from this qualitative study relevant to dementia.

Characterizing the need as a "caregiver model of transportation," one respondent stated:

> Well, obviously the volunteer driver program is a big part of addressing this need, quite a bit. Because it is more one-on-one. It is a caregiver model. Someone picks you up and waits with you…that's not what ADA services [were] built to do. And I think that's the reason why caregivers do so much transportation. (Policy leader)

Consistency is critical for the person with dementia:

> We made sure that we had the same driver on the day that this person went to his daycare. We had the bus kept at a consistent temperature, we had him sit in the same place. Even if we had to ask someone to move, this person sat in the same place every time he got on the bus. And we were able to take him successfully, then for a long time after that. (Transportation provider)

Specific ideas for strategies tried or proposed related to passengers with cognitive impairment in order to make the transportation for effective, efficient, successful for the company and the client:

> I envision some sort of travel training specific to clients or individuals with dementia…It really is a travel buddy, whether it's somebody who can show me if I'm capable of traveling independently, early on … showing me how to do it. And doing it enough times so that I become comfortable. And then as the disease progresses, that would evolve into escorted transportation. (Policy leader)
>
> Use of telephone and electronic reminders (cell phones)—creative use of cell phones as cuers…A robo call—the driver can use his radio to call the dispatcher to say, 'Can you please call Mrs. Smith and tell her I'll be there in about 2-5 minutes' so that she can get herself ready, prepared. (Transportation provider)
>
> Use travel aids like pictures, written descriptions for the driver. Like, there might be something specific that the family might want us to know about such as having a card on him that has the address and phone number of his destination. (Transportation provider)

These examples illustrate the value of strategies that directly support persons with dementia to better age-in-place in their communities. Public and paratransit today fall short of implementing universal design that is inclusive of persons with cognitive impairment. As health professionals tackle the transition to driving cessation, please help families learn their options and advocate for better options in communities where options are limited.

Driving Assessment and Current Research: No One Test Fits All

The two main questions pursued by researchers when considering driving with dementia are: (1) when does the individual become unsafe, and (2) what is the best method of screening to identify those individuals. These two questions have been examined over the last 20 years resulting in some definitive answers. Systematic reviews of the literature [43–45] are consistent in supporting the statement that *individuals with moderate or severe dementia should not drive*. Although there may be differences in how the severity of dementia is categorized, significant dementia is easily assessed with familiar cognitive assessments like the Mini Mental Status Exam (MMSE®) (e.g., below 18 on MMSE indicates moderate dementia [46]) or other similar cognitive screening tools.

Unfortunately, it is individuals with undiagnosed, early or mild dementia that pose the dilemma for physicians and families. The MMSE does not correlate with "on-road" performance, especially when the scores for the individual are in the upper range (e.g., 24 or above). This underscores the critical point that cognitive screening tools do **not** predict whether someone is "safe" to drive. In fact, there is strong agreement that one single screening or assessment tool is not adequate for use with medically-at-risk drivers [19, 25, 47, 48]. This is primarily due to the complexity of the driving task requiring integration of multiple sensory, perceptual, cognitive, and motor skills, as discussed previously. The task of driving cannot be delegated to measurement of "discrete" skills of visual acuity, neck range of motion, leg strength, sensation of feet, reaction time and cognitive processing speed. To appraise the environment, consider what action to take in a few seconds, and negotiate a 3,000 pound motor vehicle in the complexity of a dynamic roadway environment takes the integration of all the discrete skills to drive "safely." These skills are overseen by our *executive functioning*, a relatively recent umbrella term used to explain the management of cognitive functions. Thus, it is unreasonable to expect one assessment tool to be able to capture the full range of variables that underlie fitness-to-drive [47]. More importantly, properties of assessment tools only apply to the research conditions under which they are tested [49]. Therefore, outcomes for individuals with stroke, for example, cannot be generalized to a sample of individuals with dementia.

There is already evidence that for the assessment of driving, there will likely be a battery of tools used for specific diagnoses rather than a single instrument. For example, in a study on Parkinson's Disease [21], the Useful Field of View® (UFOV) [50] and the Rapid Pace Walk were found as potentially promising assessment tools, as they best predicted road test outcomes for individuals with Parkinson's disease. However, in a more recent systematic review, only the UFOV, Trail Making Tests A and B [51], Rey-Osterrieth Complex Figure Test, and contrast sensitivity were most closely linked [52], though not strongly. More large population based studies are needed to determine which assessments provide the best evidence for Parkinson's disease and many other diagnoses, including dementia.

Seeking to find a functionally-based screening tool for dementia, Carr et al. [53] compared measures of visual, motor, and cognitive functioning to the on-road assessment for 99 older adults with dementia. Their best predictive model with 85 % accuracy was using an eight-point interview (e.g., AD-8 Dementia Screening Tool), a clock drawing, and the time to complete either the Trail Making Test A or the Snellgrove Maze [54] test. Interestingly, visual and motor functioning was not associated with road test failure, distinctly different from the findings of screenings for Parkinson's Disease. This supports the concept of different screening and assessment for different diagnoses.

Continuing their work, Carr et al. [55] compared cognitively intact (N=24) and demented drivers (N=124) on the AD-8, the Short Blessed Test, and caregiving rating on functional tasks. Not surprisingly, impairments in activities of daily living, caregiver ratings and the brief cognitive screening were the best correlates of impaired road test performance, although more studies are needed. Another interesting finding was that drivers with dementia demonstrated more abnormal driving behaviors. However, these subnormal driving behaviors did not reach the level to be able to predict failure of the road test, demonstrating the problem with identifying when and how the driver with dementia becomes unsafe [55]. This is consistent with all other evidence that indicates individuals with dementia consistently make more errors and demonstrate poorer on-road performance but their on-road performance does not always rise to the level of being "unsafe." Complicating the issue is the fact that individuals at the level of mild dementia are often able to pass an on-road driving evaluation when the testing is completed in a familiar area, with simple one-on-one cued directions (e.g., turn right, go straight, turn left) that do not require quick processing (e.g., yielding onto a highway) or new information that requires executive functioning (e.g., negotiating around an accident or a new roundabout). This is explained by the fact that driving is an overlearned activity, performed with "motor memory" to steer, brake, and accelerate, and years of following the same "rules" of the road (e.g., stopping at a stop sign, staying in the lines). However, as previously mentioned, everyday traffic is not always predictable and any change in the environment can easily confuse a person with compromised cognitive abilities. Thus, specialized assessment at the "mild" and "very mild" levels of dementia (with regular re-evaluation) is necessary in order to ensure that the individual with dementia can manage the task of driving under most circumstances, not just ideal conditions.

Driving Simulation

An interactive driving simulator is a computer-controlled environment that represents selected aspects of the driving experience considered to be representational of real-world driving and allows objective measurements of users' responses to designed driving tasks and scenarios. The interactive component allows the users' responses to influence subsequent events within the simulation

program through accelerator, brake, and steering components. There is a wide range of simulators, from desktop computer programs with one screen to the total immersion, sitting in a motor vehicle with wide screen projection of a driving scene. Despite the diversity, for functional clinical use, there are a handful of models that have been designed and developed specifically for the use with clients. In addition to the decrease in technology costs, companies have worked hard to develop ready-made systems for therapists to literally "put in the key and use." Most of the systems have developed a way to report the findings in clinical terms rather than *engineer speak* that has been used in the past. Specifically, the systems have evolved from the therapists or researchers needing to develop their own scenarios (i.e., individualized driving *runs* that unfold with designed events) and determine how to evaluate the behaviors and outcomes, to reporting programs that document critical errors and response times. With increasing development and use of driving simulators, there is beginning evidence for the efficacy of using driving simulators for both assessment and intervention in driver rehabilitation.

Just as with the on-road evaluations, research evidence shows that individuals with dementia consistently make more errors and demonstrate poorer performance on simulators [44, 45, 56]. A major advantage of simulation is the ability to purposefully put at-risk drivers into situations that demand quick action. These critical incidents can be programmed on a simulator that never could be done on a real roadway (e.g., a child running onto the road, possible head-on collisions). Thus, therapists can evaluate driving competencies that include the individual's ability to avoid risk while keeping them safe from actual danger. Using this strategy in a pilot study, Dickerson and Davis (2014) evaluated the performance on three different critical incidents with nine older adults who were considered at-risk through self-referred, family referred, or referred by a physician. The simulator experience included (1) orientation to the simulator through familiarization runs, (2) "driving" two standard scenarios with critical incidents (e.g., scenarios that required specific actions to avoid collisions), (3) additional training on drives, and (4) completed the same two standard scenarios with an additional scenario to include a third critical incident. After each scenario, the participant was asked how many errors he or she had made and to evaluate their safety on the drive. When compared to the average score of four trained observers, it was the participants with diagnosed cognitive impairment that were the most significantly different. In several cases, even when the driver crashed in a head-on collision, he or she still rated themselves as a *safe driver*. The results of this pilot study are inconclusive and not generalizable due to the small sample. However, the data clearly showed the variability of older adults' performance and the lack of correlations between objective measures and subjective perceptions for individual older drivers. This study also reinforces experienced clinicians' knowledge that there is tremendous variation between the individual with dementia ability to reflect and truly understand their actual driving capacity, which underscores the necessity for careful screening and assessment that is performance based, not dependent on self report. Naturally, one could argue that the driving simulator is significantly different from driving one's own vehicle. Nevertheless, the simulator does require integration of more driving skills than pen and pencil tasks frequently used to evaluate driving performance.

Unfortunately, driving simulators will not be the panacea for determining fitness-to-drive for dementia for a number of reasons. First, the issue of simulator adaptation disorder or simulator sickness is significant for older adults. Although there are multiple theories to explain its occurrence, in general, because of the incongruity of the moving road on the screens and the motionlessness of the seating, older adults often have severe motion sickness type symptoms and cannot use the simulator. Second, for seniors, face validity of the simulator is low [43], although when asked if the simulator would be helpful to identify safety risk with individuals that have significant medical problems, the same respondents indicated that they thought it might be helpful.

Overall, driving simulators show promising results for the translation of performance measures or "errors" measured on an interactive driving simulator to on-road performance (see [57]). However, with the wide variety of simulator technology, careful study and interpretation is required when applying research data between the different models and outcome measures for individual clients. As with the current state of research on-road assessment, large-scale studies are needed because of the wide variance of technology and other issues.

Conclusion

Health care professionals are well-positioned to have "the conversation," counsel, and advise patients with dementia and their care partners about medical conditions that impact critical driving skills. Alzheimer's disease and related dementias are such medical conditions. The health care professional should be aware of available screening and assessment tools such as those described in this chapter, but more importantly, should identify driver rehabilitation specialists in their communities and appropriately refer to such specialists when warranted. And the next time a patient with dementia is in your office, ask the question, "how did you get here today?"

Appendix

Spectrum of Driver Services: Right Services for the Right People at the Right Time

A description consumers and health care providers can use to distinguish the type of services needed for an older adult.

Spectrum of Driver Rehabilitation Program Services

A description consumers and health care providers can use to distinguish the services provided by driver rehabilitation programs which best fits a client's need.

	Community-based education		Medically based assessment, education, and referral		Specialized evaluation and training
Program type	Driver safety programs	Driving school	Driver screen	Clinical IADL evaluation	Driver rehabilitation programs (includes driver evaluation)
Typical providers and credentials	Program specific credentials (e.g. AARP and AAA Driver Improvement Program).	Licensed driving instructor (LDI) certified by state licensing agency or Dept. of Education.	Health care professional (e.g., physician, social worker, neuropsychologist).	Occupational therapy practitioner (generalist or driver rehabilitation specialist[a]). Other health professional degree with expertise in instrumental activities of daily living (IADL).	Driver rehabilitation specialist[a], certified driver rehabilitation specialist[b], occupational therapist with specialty certification in driving and community mobility[c].
Required Provider's knowledge	Program specific knowledge. Trained in course content and delivery.	Instructs novice or relocated drivers, excluding medical or aging conditions that might interfere with driving, for purposes of teaching/training/refreshing/updating driving skills.	Knowledge of relevant medical conditions, assessment, referral, and/or intervention processes. Understand the limits and value of assessment tools, including simulation, as a measurement of fitness to drive.	Knowledge of medical conditions and the implication for community mobility including driving. Assess the cognitive, visual, perceptual, behavioral and physical limitations that may impact driving performance. Knowledge of available services. Understands the limits and value of assessment tools, including simulation, as a measurement of fitness to drive.	Applies knowledge of medical conditions with implications to driving. Assesses the cognitive, visual, perceptual, behavioral and physical limitations that may impact driving performance. Integrates the clinical findings with assessment of **on-road** performance. Synthesizes client and caregiver needs, assist in decisions about equipment and vehicle modification options available. Coordinates multidisciplinary providers and resources, including driver education, health care team, vehicle choice and modifications, community services, funding/payers, driver licensing agencies, training and education, and caregiver support.

Typical services provided	(1) Classroom or computer based refresher for licensed drivers: review of rules of the road, driving techniques, driving strategies, state laws, etc. (2) Enhanced self-awareness, choices, and capability to self-limit.	(1) Enhance driving performance. (2) Acquire driver permit or license. (3) Counsel with family members for student driver skill development. (4) Recommend continued training and/or undergoing licensing test. (5) Remedial programs (e.g., license reinstatement course for teens/adults, license point reduction courses).	(1) Counsel on risks associated with specific conditions (e.g., medications, fractures, post-surgery). (2) Investigate driving risk associated with changes in vision, cognition, and sensory-motor function. (3) Determine actions for the at-risk driver. • Refer to IADL evaluation, driver rehabilitation program, and/or other services. • Discuss driving cessation; provide access to counseling and education for alternative transportation options. (4) Follow reporting/referral structure for licensing recommendations.	(1) Evaluate and interpret risks associated with changes in vision, cognition, and sensory-motor functions due to acute or chronic conditions. (2) Facilitate remediation of deficits to advance client readiness for driver rehabilitation services. (3) Develop an individualized transportation plan considering client diagnosis and risks, family, caregiver, environmental and community options and limitations. • Discuss resources for vehicle adaptations (e.g., scooter lift). • Facilitate client training on community transportation options (e.g., mobility managers, dementia-friendly transportation). • Discuss driving cessation. For clients with poor self-awareness, collaborate with caregivers on cessation strategies. • Refer to driver rehabilitation program. (4) Document driver safety risk and recommended intervention plan to guide further action. (5) Follow professional ethics on referrals to the driver licensing authority.	Programs are distinguished by complexity of evaluations, types of equipment, vehicles, and expertise of provider. (1) Navigate driver license compliance and basic eligibility through intake of driving and medical history. (2) Evaluate and interpret risks associated with changes in vision, cognition, and sensory-motor functions in the driving context by the medically trained provider. (3) Perform a comprehensive driving evaluation (clinical and on-road). (4) Advises client and caregivers about evaluation results, and provides resources, counseling, education, and/or intervention plan. (5) Intervention may include training with compensatory strategies, skills, and vehicle adaptations or modifications for drivers and passengers. (6) Advocates for clients in access to funding resources and/or reimbursement. (7) Provide documentation about fitness to drive to the physician and/or driver-licensing agency in compliance with regulations. (8) Prescribe equipment in compliance with state regulations and collaborate with mobility equipment dealer[d] for fitting and training. (9) Present resources and options for continued community mobility if recommending driving cessation or transition from driving. Recommendations may include (but not restricted to): (1) drive unrestricted; (2) drive with restrictions; (3) cessation of driving pending rehabilitation or training; (4) planned re-evaluation for progressive disorders; (5) driving cessation; (6) referral to another program.
Outcome	Provides education and awareness.	Enhances skills for healthy drivers.	Indicates risk or need for follow-up for medically at-risk drivers.	Determines fitness to drive and provides rehabilitative services.	Determines fitness to drive and provides rehabilitative services.

[a] *DRS* Health professional degree with specialty training in driver evaluation and rehabilitation

[b] *CDRS* Certified driver rehabilitation specialist-credentialed by ADED (Association for Driver Rehabilitation Specialists)

[c] *SCDCM* Specialty certified in driving and community mobility by AOTA (American Occupational Therapy Association)

[d] Quality approved provider by NMEDA (National Mobility Equipment Dealers Association)

Driver Rehabilitation Programs Administers comprehensive driving evaluation to determine fitness to drive and/or provides rehabilitative services

Program type	Basic	Low tech	High tech
Levels of program and typical provider credentials	Provider is a driver rehabilitation specialist (DRS)[a] with professional background in occupational therapy, other allied health field, driver education, or a professional team of CDRS or SCDCM with LDI[e]	Driver rehabilitation specialist[a], certified driver rehabilitation specialist[b], occupational therapist with specialty certification in driving and community mobility[c], or in combination with LDI *Certification in driver rehabilitation is recommended as the provider for comprehensive driving evaluation and training*	Driver rehabilitation specialist[a], certified driver rehabilitation specialist[b], occupational therapist with specialty certification in driving and community mobility[c] *Certification in Driver Rehabilitation is recommended as the provider for comprehensive driving evaluation and training with advanced skills and expertise to complete complex client and vehicle evaluation and training*
Program service	Offers comprehensive driving evaluation, training and education May include use of adaptive driving aids that do not affect operation of primary or secondary controls (e.g. seat cushions or additional mirrors) May include transportation planning (transition and options), cessation planning, and recommendations for clients as passengers	Offers comprehensive driving evaluation, training and education, with or without adaptive driving aids that affect the operation of primary or secondary controls, vehicle ingress/egress, and mobility device storage/securement. May include use of adaptive driving aids such as seat cushions or additional mirrors At the low tech level, adaptive equipment for primary control is typically mechanical. Secondary controls may include wireless or remote access May include transportation planning (transition and options), cessation planning, and recommendations for clients as passengers	Offers a wide variety of adaptive equipment and vehicle options for comprehensive driving evaluation, training and education, including all services available in a LOW TECH and Basic programs. At this level, providers have the ability to alter positioning of primary and secondary controls based on client's need or ability level High tech adaptive equipment for primary and secondary controls includes devices that meet the following conditions (1) capable of controlling vehicle functions or driving controls, and (2) consists of a programmable computerized system that interfaces/integrates with an electronic system in the vehicle
Access to driver's position	Requires independent transfer into OEM[d] driver's seat in vehicle	Addresses transfers, seating and position into OEM[d] driver's seat. May make recommendations for assistive devices to access driver's seat, improved positioning, wheelchair securement systems, and/or mechanical wheelchair loading devices	Access to the vehicle typically requires ramp or lift and may require adaptation to OEM driver's seat. Access to driver position may be dependent on use of a transfer seat base, or clients may drive from their wheelchair. Provider evaluates and recommends vehicle structural modifications to accommodate products such as ramps, lifts, wheelchair and scooter hoists, transfer seat bases, wheelchairs suitable to utilize as a driver seat, and/or wheelchair securement systems

Typical vehicle modification: primary controls: gas, brake, steering	Uses OEM[d] controls	Primary driving control examples (A) mechanical gas/brake hand control (B) left foot accelerator pedal (C) pedal extensions (D) park brake lever or electronic park brake (E) steering device (spinner knob, tri-pin, C-cuff)	Primary driving control examples (in addition to low tech options) (A) powered gas/brake systems (B) power park brake integrated with a powered gas/brake system (C) variable effort steering systems (D) Reduced diameter steering wheel, horizontal steering, steering wheel extension, joystick controls (E) reduced effort brake systems
Typical vehicle modification: secondary controls	Uses OEM[d] controls	Secondary driving control examples (A) remote horn button (B) turn signal modification (remote, crossover lever) (C) remote wiper controls (D) gear selector modification (E) key/ignition adaptions	Electronic systems to access secondary and accessory controls Secondary driving control examples (in addition to low tech options) (A) remote panels, touch pads or switch arrays that interface with OEM[b] electronics (B) wiring extension for OEM[d] electronics (C) powered transmission shifter

[a] DRS Health professional degree with specialty training in driver evaluation and rehabilitation
[b] CDRS Certified driver rehabilitation specialist-credentialed by ADED (Association for Driver Rehabilitation Specialists)
[c] SCDCM Specialty certified in driving and community mobility by AOTA (American Occupational Therapy Association)
[d] OEM-original equipment installed by manufacturer. Reference: NMEDA Guidelines http://www.nmeda.com
[e] LDI-licensed driving instructor

References

1. Alzheimer's Association. Alzheimer's disease facts and figures. Alzheimers Dement. 2014;10(2). Available from: http://www.alz.org/downloads/Facts_Figures_2014.pdf.

2. Adler G, Rottunda S. The driver with dementia: a survey of physician attitudes, knowledge, and practice. Am J Alzheimers Dis Other Dement. 2011;26(1):58–64. doi:10.1177/1533317510390350.

3. Adler G, Rottunda S, Bauer M, Kuskowski M. Driving cessation and AD: issues confronting patients and family. Am J Alzheimers Dis. 1999;15:212–16.

4. Hunt LA, Brown AE, Gilman IP. Drivers with dementia and outcomes of becoming lost while driving. Am J Occup Ther. 2010;64(2):225–32.

5. Dickerson AE, Reistetter T, Gaudy J. The perception of the meaningfulness and performance of instrumental activities of daily living from the perspectives of the medically-at-risk older adult and their caregiver. J Appl Gerontol. 2013;32:749–64.

6. Silverstein NM, Murtha J. Driving in Massachusetts: when to stop and who should decide? Paper 31. Gerontol Inst Publ.; 2001. Available from: http://scholarworks.umb.edu/gerontologyinstitute_pubs/31

7. Administration on Aging. A profile of older Americans: 2013. Administration for Community Living, U.S. Department of Health and Human Services. http://www.aoa.gov/Aging_Statistics/Profile/2013/docs/2013_Profile.pdf. Retrieved 9 Oct 2014.

8. Adler G, Silverstein NM. At risk drivers with Alzheimer's disease: recognition, response, and referral. Traffic Inj Prev. 2008;9(4):299–303.

9. Dobbs BM, Harper IA, Woo A. Transitioning from driving to driving cessation: the role of specialized driving cessation support groups for individuals with dementia. Top Geriatr Rehabil. 2009;25(1):73–86.

10. Stern RA, D'Ambrosio LA, Mohyde M, Carruth A, Tracton-Bishop B, Hunter JC, et al. At the crossroads: development and evaluation of a dementia caregiver group intervention to assist in driving cessation. Gerontol Geriatr Educ. 2008;29(4):363–82.

11. National Highway Traffic Safety Administration. Driving transitions education: tools, scripts, and practice exercises. DOT HS 811 152; 2009. Available from: http://www.nhtsa.gov/DOT/NHTSA/Traffic%20Injury%20Control/Articles/Associated%20Files/811152.pdf

12. Croston J, Meuser T, Berg-Weger M, Grant E, Carr DR. Driving retirement in older adults with dementia. Top Geriatr Rehabil. 2009;25(2):154–62.

13. Meuser T, Berg-Weger M, Chibnall JT, Harmon AC, Stowe JD. Assessment for readiness for mobility transition (ARMT). J Appl Gerontol. 2013;32(4):484–507.

14. D'Ambrosio LA, Coughlin J, Mohyde M, Carruth A, Hunter JC, Stern RA. Caregiver communications and the transition from driver to passenger among people with dementia. Top Geriatr Rehabil. 2009; 25(1):33–42.

15. Wang CC, Kosinski CJ, Schwartzberg JG, Shanklin AV. Physician's guide to assessing and counseling older drivers. Washington, DC: National Highway Traffic Safety Administration; 2003.

16. Carr DB, Schwartzberg JG, Manning L, Sempek J. Physician's guide to assessing and counseling older drivers. 2nd ed. Washington, DC: National Highway Traffic Safety Administration; 2010.

17. Dickerson AE, Overton B. Cue cards: help for the state highway patrol? In: Gerontological Society of American annual scientific meeting; 21 Nov 2011; Boston, MA.

18. Silverstein NM. No longer in the driver's seat: current need and future vision for community mobility options. In: Proceedings of the senior safe mobility summit; 26 Oct 2006; Newport Beach, CA.

19. Bédard M, Weaver B, Darzin P, Porter NM. Predicting driving performance in older adults: we are not there yet! Traffic Inj Prev. 2008;9:336–41.

20. Eby DW, Molnar LJ, Shope JT. Driving decisions workbook. No. UMTRI-2000-14. University of Michigan, Ann Arbor: Transportation Research Institute, Social and Behavioral Analysis Division; 2000.

21. Classen S, Witter DP, Lanford DN, Okun MS, Rodriguez RL, Romrell J, et al. Usefulness of screening tools for predicting driving performance in people with Parkinson's disease. Am J Occup Ther. 2011; 65:579–88.

22. Classen S, Winter SM, Velozo CA, Bédard M, Lanford D, Brumback B, et al. Item development and validity testing for a safe driving behavior measure. Am J Occup Ther. 2010;64(2):296–305.

23. Classen S, Wen PS, Velozo C, Bédard M, Winter SM, Brumback B, et al. Psychometrics of the self-report safe driving behavior measure for older adults. Am J Occup Ther. 2012;66(2):233–41.

24. Classen S, Wang Y, Winter SM, Velozo CA, Lanford DN, Bédard M. Concurrent criterion validity of the safe driving behavior measure: a predictor of on-road driving outcomes. Am J Occup Ther. 2013; 67(1):108–16.

25. Dickerson AE, Meuel BD, Ridenour C, Cooper K. The predictive validity of screening and assessment tools for driving: a systematic review. Am J Occup Ther. 2014;68(6)670–680.

26. Dickerson AE, Schold Davis E. Welcome to the team! Who are the stakeholders? In: McGuire MJ, Schold Davis E, editors. Driving and community mobility: occupational therapy strategies across the lifespan. Bethesda, MD: American Occupational Therapy Association, Inc; 2012. p. 49–77.

27. Dickerson AE. Driving with dementia: evaluation, referral, and resources. Occup Ther Health Care. 2014;28(1):62–76.

28. Dickerson AE. Screening and assessment tools for determining fitness to drive: a review of the literature for the pathways project. Occup Ther Health Care. 2014;28(2):82–121.

29. Michon JA. A critical view of driver behavior models: what do we know, what should we do? New York: Springer; 1985. p. 485–524.

30. Dickerson AE, Molnar LJ, Eby DW, Adler G, Bédard M, Berg-Weger M, et al. Transportation and aging: a research agenda for advancing safe mobility. Gerontology. 2007;47(5):578–90.

31. Dickerson AE. Driving as a valued occupation. Appendix A. In: McGuire MJ, Schold Davis E, editors. Driving and community mobility: occupational therapy strategies across the lifespan. Bethesda, MD: American Occupational Therapy Association, Inc; 2012. p. 417–22.

32. Dickerson AE, Reistetter T, Schold Davis E, Monahan M. Evaluating driving as a valued instrumental activity of daily living. Am J Occup Ther. 2011;65:64–75.

33. Fisher AG. Assessment of motor and process skills, vol. 2. Fort Collins, CO: Three Star Press; 2006.

34. Stapleton T. An exploration of the process of assessing fitness to drive after stroke within an Irish context of practice [unpublished dissertation]. Trinity College; 2012.

35. Lane A, Green E, Dickerson AE, Davis ES, Rolland B, Stohler JT. Driver rehabilitation programs: defining program models, services, and expertise. Occup Ther Health Care. 2014;28(2):177–87.

36. Eby DW, Silverstein N, Lisa M, LeBlanc D, Adler G. Driving behaviors in early stage dementia: a study using in-vehicle technology. Accid Anal Prev. 2012;49:330–7. doi:10.1016/j.aap.2011.11.021.

37. Lloyd S, Cormack CN, Blais K, Messeri G, McCallum MA, Spicer K, et al. Driving and dementia: a review of the literature. Can J Occup Ther. 2001;68(3):149–56.

38. Burkhardt J. Outside the box: new models for transportation partnerships (Chap. 13). In: Coughlin J, D'Ambrosio L, editors. Aging America and transportation personal choices and public policy. New York: Springer; 2012. p. 217–32.

39. Ståhl A. Service routes or low floor buses? Study of travel behaviour among elderly and disabled people. In: Coughlin J, D'Ambrosio L, editors. Aging America and transportation. personal choices and public policy, Chap. 13 (2012). Proceedings of the 8th international conference on transport and mobility for elderly and disabled people; September 1998; Perth, New York: Springer. 269 pp.

40. Ragland DR, Satariano WA, MacLeod KE. Driving cessation and increased depressive symptoms. J Gerontol Ser A Biol Sci Med Sci. 2005;60(3):399–403. doi:10.1093/gerona/60.3.399.

41. Bailey L. Aging Americans: stranded without options. Washington, DC: Surface Transportation Policy Project; 2004. Available from: http://www.transact.org/library/reports_html/seniors/aging.pdf.

42. Silverstein NM, Maslow K, editors. Improving hospital care for persons with dementia. New York: Springer; 2006.

43. Dickerson AE, Schwarga A, Wethington C. Evaluating the use of an interactive driving simulator from the perspective of occupational therapists and older adults. In: Annual conference of the American Occupational Therapy Association; April 2014; Baltimore, MD.

44. Dubinsky RM, Stein AC, Lyons K. Practice parameter: risk of driving and Alzheimer's disease (an evidence based review): report of the quality standards subcommittee of the American academy of neurology. Neurology. 2000;54:2205–11.

45. Iverson DJ, Gronseth GS, Reger MA, Classen S, Dubinsky RM, Rizzo M. Practice parameter update: evaluation and management of driving risk in dementia. Neurology. 2010;74:1316–24.

46. National Highway Traffic Safety Administration and American Association of Motor Vehicle Administrators. Driver fitness medical guidelines. Washington, DC, Arlington, VA; 2009.

47. Bédard M, Dickerson AE. Consensus statements for screening and assessment tools. Occup Ther Health Care. 2014;28(2):127–31.

48. Gamache PL, Hudon C, Teasdale N, Simoneau M. Alternative avenues in the assessment of driving capacities in older drivers and implications for training. Curr Dir Psychol Sci. 2010;9(6):370–4.

49. Streiner DL, Norman GR. Health measurement scales: a practical guide to their development and use. Oxford: Oxford University Press; 2008.

50. Ball K, Owsley C, Sloan ME, Roenker DL, Bruni JR. Visual attention problems as a predictor of vehicle crashes in older drivers. Invest Ophthalmol. 1993;34(11):3110–23.

51. Reitan R. Validity of the trail making test as an indicator of organic brain injury. Percept Mot Skills. 1958;8:271–6.

52. Crizzle AM, Classen S, Uc EY. Parkinson disease and driving: an evidence-based review. Neurology. 2012;79(20):2067–74.

53. Carr D, Barco P, Wallendorf MJ, Snellgrove CA, Ott BR. Predicting road test performance in drivers with dementia. J Am Geriatr Soc. 2011;59:2112–17.

54. Snellgrove C. Cognitive screening for the safe driving competence of older people with mild cognitive impairment or early dementia. Australian Transport Safety Bureau; 2010.

55. Carr D. Caregiver prediction of road test performance. Poster session presented at: Internal conference on Alzheimer's disease (ICAD); 13–18 July 2013; Boston, MA.

56. Frittelli C, Borgheti D, Iudice G, Bonanni E, Maestri M, Tognoni G, et al. Effects of Alzheimer's disease and mild cognitive impairment on driving ability: a controlled clinical study by simulated driving test. Int J Geriatr Psychiatry. 2009;24:232–8.

57. Classen S, Brooks J. Driving simulators for occupational therapy screening, assessment, and intervention. Occup Ther Health Care. 2014;28(2):154–62.

58. AAA Foundation for Traffic Safety. Roadwise Review®. https://www.aaafoundation.org/roadwise-review-online. Retrieved 14 July 2014.

59. Alzheimer's Association. Comfort Zone®. http://www.alz.org/comfortzone/about_comfort_zone.asp. Retrieved 14 July 2014

60. Beverly Foundation. Transportation and dementia. Fact sheet series [Internet]. 2008 [cited 2014 June 25];1(8). Available from: http://beverlyfoundation.org/wp-content/uploads/Fact-Sheet-8-transportation.Dementia.pdf

61. Hartford Insurance. We need to talk: family conversations with older drivers; at the crossroads: driving and dementia; and your road ahead: a guide to comprehensive driving evaluations are free driving safety guides. Available at: http://www.thehartford.com/mature-market-excellence/publications-on-aging. Retrieved 14 July 2014.

62. Dickerson, A.E. (2013). Driving Assessment Tools Used by Driver Rehabilitation Specialists: Survey of Use and Implications for Practice. American Journal of Occupational Therapy, 67, 564–573.

63. Womack, J.L., & Silverstein, N.M. (2012). The Big Picture: Comprehensive Mobility Options. In Maguire, M.J., & Schold Davis, E. (Eds). Driving and Community Mobility, Occupational Therapy Strategies Across the Lifespan. Bethesda: American Occupational Therapy Association Press: 19–48.

64. Silverstein, N., & Turk, K. Students explore supportive transportation for older adults (2015). Gerontology & Geriatrics Education/Routledge Taylor & Francis. DOI:10.1080/02701960.2015.1005289.

Part III

Toward Person-Centered Community-Based Dementia Care

Experiences and Perspectives of Persons with Dementia

Abhilash K. Desai, F. Galliano Desai,
Susan McFadden, and G.T. Grossberg

Introduction

"Dignity for me…is being seen…as me…not as some may believe I have become…" (A person with dementia) ([1], p. 10)

Persons with dementia have innumerable resources of resilience built up over time that they continue to utilize to meet the challenges and tragedy of living with dementia [2]. This is true also for persons in more advanced stages of dementia [3]. Although coming to terms with its irreversibility is an added burden creating negative experiences for persons with dementia, research and clinical experience have shown that many routinely experience positive emotions and

A.K. Desai, MD (✉)
Department of Neurology and Psychiatry, Saint Louis University School of Medicine, St. Louis, MO, USA

Idaho Memory & Aging Center, P.L.L.C.,
Boise, ID, USA
e-mail: drdesai@idahomemorycenter.com

F. Galliano Desai, PhD
Idaho Memory & Aging Center, P.L.L.C.,
Boise, ID, USA
e-mail: alexander122@mac.com

S. McFadden, PhD
Fox Valley Memory Project, Appleton, WI, USA
e-mail: mcfadden@uwosh.edu

G.T. Grossberg, MD
Department of Neurology and Psychiatry, Saint Louis University School of Medicine, St. Louis, Missouri, USA
URL: http://grossbgt.slu.edu

meaningful events in their daily lives [2]. Kitwood [4] and Sabat [5] have highlighted the need to view the person with dementia as someone who may be experiencing cognitive changes but who, in essence, can experience the same feelings, thoughts and responses as we ourselves do. We are in the initial stages of a cultural revolution wherein people with dementia are starting to be recognized and treated as persons and valued members of our human community [6, 7]. Education of healthcare professionals (HCPs), professionals in other fields (e.g., law, finance, retail, business, religion), and lay people has started to alleviate some of the negative impact of dementia diagnosis and disability due to dementia and international efforts supporting dementia-friendly communities and person-centered care practices have accelerated efforts to bring back humanity in caring for persons with dementia [8–10].

In these efforts, the experiences and perspectives of persons with dementia have only just begun to receive the attention they rightly deserve from the research community that has so far been driven by biomedical models of dementia. In this chapter, we will highlight the importance of exploring and understanding the experiences and perspectives of persons with dementia. Based on existing documentary sources in published literature and our own clinical experience, in this chapter we provide descriptions of experiences and perspectives that we believe have significant clinical implications. Respecting the recent call to recognize the social citizenship of the person with dementia and their care partners [11], we consulted with a physician recently diagnosed with dementia as well as another physician whose wife was recently diagnosed with dementia. We wanted to check their perspectives on the ideas presented here. We describe the negative socio-cultural factors that need to be tackled head on, so that perspectives of the person who is living with dementia can play a central role in treatment decisions and in all efforts to improve their quality of life.

Importance of Studying Experiences and Perspectives of Persons with Dementia

The central goal of all treatment approaches and strategies is to improve quality of life (QOL) of persons with dementia and their caregivers. The experiences and perspectives of the person with dementia are important because they directly impact their self-concept and contribute to depressed mood, two factors that affect their quality of life more than cognitive functioning [12]. Furthermore, their attitudes and perspectives may differ from those of their families and HCPs regarding important areas such as brain health [13]. Each experience is unique and complex, as is each person with dementia. The concept of negative and positive experiences of the person with dementia is therefore, at best, an oversimplification. However, the evidence presented of experiences and perspectives of persons with dementia and the wider considerations of their social and cultural factors suggest broad generalizations of experiences and perspectives can have considerable clinical implications.

The Alzheimer's Society has described the current situation well: "Dementia is all too often a fact of life, and no longer out of sight and out of mind. And it requires not just care but also understanding…" [2]. Jokes by comedians about grandma "becoming forgetful" are not funny any more, if they ever were. We believe that research has for too long focused on understanding the neurobiology of dementia and ignored equally important aspects of dementia, the experiences

and perspectives of the person with dementia, or as some say, the "lived experience" and "lifeworld" of dementia [11]. We now know that some persons with dementia even in the advanced stages are able to express their experiences and perspectives about what is important for their QOL [2, 3]. Caregivers and HCPs have frequently expressed frustration that they cannot understand what the person is trying to express, primarily because of deficits in language function. Persons with dementia often stop expressing, withdraw socially and become quiet in order to avoid frustration caused by language deficits. Research on their experiences and perspectives may be able to give voice to those who are silenced by the disease.

Research Methodology

Understanding another person, especially one with dementia is more like an aesthetic judgment than a cognitive action [14]. Thus, research to explore and understand experiences and perspectives of persons with dementia needs to rely more on interpretive phenomenological approaches [15] and other qualitative methods, in addition to the more common use of psychometrically valid and reliable instruments. Experiences and perspectives of persons with dementia have been studied through [1] interviews [2] structured observations (e.g., during dementia care mapping) [3] and through communicative instruments such as "talking mats" and picture cards [2]. Use of tools such as AwareCare and Communi-Care has also been employed to understand experiences and perspectives of persons with advanced dementia [16, 17]. Specific subjective responses such as the experience of hope have been studied using specific tools such as the Heart Hope Index [18]. CORTE guidelines can be utilized to guide research exploring the experiences and perspectives of the person who has dementia [19]. Although many measures of dementia quality of life exist, most were not developed with input from persons with dementia. Movement toward recognition of social citizenship of the person with dementia will, we hope, encourage more researchers to adopt participatory research approaches that employ "active involvement [by persons with dementia] in all aspects of the process, from research design to dissemination" ([6], p. 102).

Negative Experiences

Negative experiences are common, can be potentially life threatening, and often reduce quality of life of people who have dementia as well as their family members and caregivers. We discuss a few in some detail below. Please see Box 1 [20–24] for some other common examples of negative experiences shared by persons with dementia.

Box 1 Examples of Some Common Negative Experiences Expressed by Persons with Dementia

Experience of loss and grief
"When you end up in a situation where you are not able to have a job, you lose your network and friends. You lose your feeling of social cohesion, become a sort of 'social outcast', person on the outside of society and you sit there strong and fit in most ways—except for one thing, your memory loss, and this makes other people unsure." ([22], p. 417)

Experiences of being dismissed
A person with dementia sharing how his complains of memory loss were dismissed by HCPs. "when I went to the doctor to tell her that I knew that I'd got Alzheimer's she just said, —'there is nothing wrong with you'…It didn't worry me…No, because I knew exactly what it was…Oh yes and then I went to Hospital and again they turned round and said, —'there's nothing wrong with you', and I knew there was and it was so frustrating. I don't argue with them because there's no point is there?…I knew very well before because of my father in

law, I researched it for him, so I knew the very beginning signs of it." ([24], p. 6).

"When I tell people about my diagnosis, most are incredulous, dismissing examples of my memory lapses as 'senior moments' and capping them with more serious examples of their own experience. This attitude is not helpful to someone who has struggled to come to terms with their diagnosis." (persons with dementia living in the community) ([20], p. 146).

Experience of lack of direction in one's life
"I had all these Air Force connections. They are less and less tenuous these days. They're still there but not to the same strength. So I think the err, I'm more rudderless. I mean I knew which way I was going. Now I don't know where anything is." ([21], p. 8).

Experiences of struggle with identity
"How can I put the two together? I am the same but I am different" ([22], p. 402)

Experience of dangers of continuing to drive
"I was on my way back home when I found myself driving in the wrong direction on the highway—the police came after me and I managed to avoid the whole thing, and they were very nice to me, but it was a depressing experience. It was the disease, though I was not aware of it at the time." ([23], p. 417)

Experience of fear of social rejection
"Actually, it is not like you give everyone a call…before you know more it is not the time to tell others, but you have no control over what others know about it, and on getting dementia you feel that you have suddenly become a lunatic." ([23], p. 418)

(continued)

Box 1 (continued)
Experience of stress caused by rules and regulations in a care facility
"You're living by their rules and regulations. You have to abide by their rules and regulations and I think that confines everybody in here to those aspects." ([22], p. 399)

Experience of stress caused by care practices that favor safety over dignity
"Christ, if I can't be trusted to go out and have a smoke, then I am over analyzed, or under analyzed perhaps is a better word. Anybody who really knows me knows I don't want to destroy myself in any way, shape or form" ([22], p. 399)

Experience of Fear After Being Given the Diagnosis

A person with dementia sharing his reaction after being diagnosed,

> "It was a shock and it scared me, because I know what is to come and it is quite terrible that I will suddenly turn out to be, ugly as it sounds, 'a second-class citizen." ([23], p. 415).

Clinical Significance

HCPs need to be mindful of the potential serious negative effects of giving a diagnosis of dementia and should try to disclose diagnosis preferably in the presence of a supportive friend or family. HCPs should closely follow up to monitor how well the person with dementia is coping with the diagnosis and their ability to access supportive resources in the community besides help from family and friends (e.g., support groups for early stage dementia, Memory Cafes, supportive spiritual/religious institutions).

Experiences of Despair

> "It is so hopeless…what's the point in continuing to live….only to see yourself become a drooling mess living in a nursing home…" (Mr. B, a patient of the first author who was just diagnosed with mild Alzheimer's disease).

Clinical significance: Experiences of despair are all too common and can lead to the wish to end one's life and even commit suicide. This is the most tragic of all consequences of negative experiences. Although typical care involves giving antidepressants to patients with dementia who share their despair and wish to end their life, psychotherapy (especially interpersonal psychotherapy, dyadic therapy, reminiscence therapy, and meaning-centered psychotherapy rather than cognitive-behavior therapy) may be a more appropriate intervention because the central feature of despair is loss of meaning in life remaining [25–27]. Social support is crucial for persons with dementia to maintain a positive sense of self after diagnosis is given [28]. Peer support can also help reduce and even prevent experiences of despair [29]. It is important to explore perspectives of persons with dementia regarding what "Alzheimer's Disease" or "Dementia" means to them, to their sense of future and their sense of identity. Even more important is for the HCP to take a step back, reflect on his/her own perspective. Many HCPs carry an extremely negative and pessimistic perspective of what it means to have an Alzheimer's disease and related dementias diagnosis and may non-verbally convey such perspectives, potentially harming those with dementia by deepening their experience of despair. HCPs need to develop a more balanced view where they recognize not only the tragedy caused by the dementing condition but also the additional harm—the "excess disability" [30]—caused by stigma. HCPs need to also recognize that there are plenty of positive stories involving persons with dementia and that for some, life may have become paradoxically enriched because of the existential issues raised by the diagnosis of dementia. Furthermore, actively sharing positive stories and perspectives may be the single most effective therapeutic intervention HCPs can employ during appointments with the patient living with dementia.

Experiences of Loss of Dignity

A person with dementia expressed the following after his diagnosis was disclosed to his employer.

> Without consulting with the employee, his employment was terminated and no effort was made to

accommodate his challenges or engage with him directly. "I feel the situation was taken behind closed doors and I don't believe that there were people around those closed doors; it was a case of yes he's got it and we're not prepared to even look for anything" ([31], p. 8).

Clinical significance: Routinely adopting a person-centered dignity conserving model of care at all levels (in outpatient care, hospital care, long-term care) is necessary to adequately address these experiences, as they can often lead to depression and despair. Creating group situations where persons with dementia feel that they are valued members of the group can help mitigate experiences of loss of dignity and value [32]. Another way to enhance the dignity of the person with dementia is through "retrospective dignity experiences" that can happen as the person talks about personal meaningful life-stories, especially in early childhood. "My father produced sausage for most of his life…and he was always happy. There was never a lot of money in our family, but there was kindness and a good spirit…there was love" [person with dementia living in the community] ([1], p. 7) and "My wise mother taught me that money is not everything. It is how we treat one another that is truly important…and that suited me just fine" [person with dementia living in the community] ([1], p. 7).

Abandonment

"I've had a couple of people…you just knew were not comfortable with it [AD]…or with me. And so…It wasn't unkind. You just knew that it just didn't feel good with them" (person with dementia living in the community [33], p. 153).

Many persons with dementia and their care partners comment on the pain of abandonment by friends and family members once a diagnosis of dementia is revealed [34]. Although some relationships are retained after the diagnosis [33], it is common to hear statements like "I want to remember my friend like he was" or "She's just not the same as the person I once knew." In addition, given the high measured levels of religiosity among older adults, it is especially egregious

when this abandonment occurs within faith communities. A woman caring for her husband with dementia had this to say about church friends withdrawing from them:

"Lacking the cognitive abilities to participate in social life or overstepping the unwritten rules of social conventions, one-time friends no longer seek our company. Invitations to dinner at our home, once eagerly accepted are 'postponed' with lame excuses. I learn that I am no longer part of a couple—that honored institution of the church that opens doors for friendship and fellowship. I learn that I am not single either and cannot find solace among the women who complain that the church only has time for those who are married." ([35], pp. 91–92).

In addition to abandonment by friends in a faith community, the person with dementia and their care partners often feel abandoned by their religious leaders. Thibault and Morgan [36] write about how often clergy say "they are too busy or unprepared to do pastoral care for the members with dementia, and they feel uncomfortable visiting members with dementia at home or in locked memory care facilities" (p. 52). In their mixed method study of nursing home residents' perspectives on spiritual support for persons with dementia, Powers and Watson [37] quoted a participant as saying the pastor visits "very seldom. His congregation is very big and he doesn't have time to go visit. Nobody from the church ever comes to visit. It would be nice to have them visit" (p. 65).

Reasons for Negative Experiences

A large part of what people view as the tragedy of dementia is caused by the six horsemen of the apocalypse (e.g., six socio-cultural forces) and consist of [1] ignorance [2] stigma [3] malignant social psychology [4] "war" metaphors for confronting this "epidemic," [5] the "Alzheimerization" of the dialogue to support euthanasia, and last but not the least [6] defining "self" in relation to cognitive function ("I think therefore I am") [4, 5, 38–46]. This was not always the case. The person with dementia was considered a valued member of the community prior to the mid-nineteenth century [47].

We believe the primary reasons for experiences of despair are the socio-cultural factors that interact dynamically with individual factors (e.g., insight, personality, presence of depression, lack of family and friends, inadequate financial resources). The latter need to be addressed using an individualized and contextual approach that takes into account cultural differences [48–50].

Positive Experiences

Positive experiences are also common in persons with dementia and are often under-appreciated or under-recognized by them as well as their friends, families, and HCPs. We discuss some positive experiences below. Please see Box 2 [1, 22–24, 51] for examples of other positive experiences shared by persons with dementia.

Box 2 Examples of Common Positive Experiences Expressed by Persons with Dementia

Experience of hope

"I get the impression that the doctors are… there is a greater awareness now that there are things happening…that doctors are meeting up with conversations on causes. It wasn't here sort of two and a half years ago…but I feel there's an improvement." ([24], p. 12)

"I would say this group [social care groups] is a most invaluable group…because it, it does give a chance…it gives motive for getting out, it gives a feeling at the end that you may have said something useful or done something useful." ([24], p. 10)

"It is very nice for people like me to stay at that daycare center…health personnel there are young, positive and very clever at making us do different things…I am very happy that I have a place there, otherwise I would probably have lain down on the couch again and stayed at home alone all day." ([23], p. 418)

Experience of meaningful moments

"…look out the window right now for example. See the light…the sunshine…and just enjoy it! When I was outside this morning…I walked up to the top of the hill just to enjoy the view…just standing there made me feel good inside…experiences like this are meaningful, powerful,…an important part of life I appreciate very much." ([1], p. 10)

Experience of enjoying group social activities

Peter, a person with dementia sharing why he enjoyed his time in group social activities, "It's like living at my mum's. Everybody's friendly. And I've got four sisters and brothers. So it's a big family. Yes. Yes, a big family. I'm used to lots of people." ([22], p. 401).

Experience of support after disclosing one's diagnosis to one's friends and family

"I didn't want to tell anybody, I don't know why…but it was getting bad and people were reporting me for doing things wrong…then the men at work, the nurses and everybody, when they knew what I had got they were all rallying around. They are quite good." ([51], p. 459).

Experiences reflecting resilience

"I walk with my head held high…it has to do with my sense of dignity. Not easy with this diagnosis…it's challenging…yet I desire to be known a competent individual…just as I always have been." ([1], p. 8)

"…the fact that I have got it [Alzheimer's]…that fact you have got that condition, but, it has never struck me as a kind of, smear or…negative thing…" ([24], p. 7)

"I'm quite happy to have Alzheimer's, there's worse things to have than Alzheimer's…I can cope with it. I wouldn't

(continued)

Box 2 (continued)

like to have other things…I think I'm lucky to have this rather than something worse than this." ([24], p. 7)

"I've found that people here [social care groups] are like me, that aren't sure about what is going on…it makes me feel more saner." ([22], p. 403)

"When you are kind of trapped in a situation where your presence elsewhere isn't possible you have to take what's available and deal with it, and that's what I am having to do." ([22], p. 399)

Experiences representing remarkable intelligence, wisdom, and compassion
"They have limited experience of Alzheimer's or vascular dementia and what have you. I mean, she's an excellent doctor, but she's lacking in certain areas, not her fault, she just doesn't have the time…" ([24], p. 12)

"Because…they can't cater for each person individually. That's not fair on the staff." ([22], p. 404)

Experiences providing insight regarding strategies to improve care practices
"It you look at the kinds of services that care homes and places, they concentrate on food hygiene, how to lift people, how to deal with things that they call aggression, toilet training, there's not much about caring and …I think that's probably the least expensive resource to supply, but people need to be trained and helped to understand why so many of them suffer stress…I think there's a great deal to be done in that respect…" ([24], p. 9)

"You've got the word, awareness…and it's got to be done in simple terminology because general people wouldn't even know what dementia was or what the background was…" ([24], p. 11)

Joy and Gratitude

Many people—both those with and those lacking experience with dementia—would be shocked to discover that there might be positive experiences of dementia. Nevertheless, as McFadden and McFadden [34] note, even in advanced dementia there can be moments of laughter, joy, and love. They described how one daughter noted that she never got so many hugs and kisses from her mother before her dementia. In an interview study of persons with dementia, an African American man commented on his positive experience of gratitude by stating, "When you wake up in the morning, when you thank God for waking up…and then you can say, 'Well what a beautiful day. I'm gonna accomplish a lot today because I'm positive'" ([52], p. 77).

Spiritual Growth and Development

Religion has been described as "an overwhelmingly positive resource" for persons with dementia, particularly African American elders ([52], p. 83). Interviews with 75 persons with dementia showed that faith gave them strength and hope, helped reduce feelings of being alone, promoted a positive attitude, and helped them feel safe. Some even said that regular prayer and scripture reading helped their memory. In addition, faith communities sometimes provide important forms of social support and the scaffolding of regular worship with its music, familiar readings, and prayers. Ethicist Stephen Post noted that "90 % of Americans who are diagnosed with dementia pray" ([53], p. 12), and quoted a man whose dementia was accompanied by what Post called a "spiritual conversion." The man stated:

> Maybe this was to slow me down to enjoy life and to enjoy my family and to enjoy what's out there. And right now, I can say that I'm a better person for it, in appreciation of other people's needs and illnesses, than I ever was when I was working that rat race back and forth day to day. ([53], p. 13)

Making New Friends

As previously noted, the dementia diagnosis can lead to the breaking of social relationships. On the other hand, as more communities are beginning to be intentional about "dementia-friendly" practices, programs, and services, individuals with dementia are gaining opportunities to form meaningful new social relationships. One way is through online self-help networks such as Facebook groups and the Dementia Advocacy and Support Network International (DASNI). A study of users of DASNI found that participation helped them feel a sense of belonging, identity, purpose and value [54].

Memory cafés present another opportunity for persons with dementia and their care partners to make new friends. Despite limited research on the outcomes of memory café participation, communities around the world are establishing these opportunities for stigma-free, enjoyable social interactions with others who are traveling a similar road as they cope with dementia [55].

Perspectives of Persons with Dementia

Understanding the perspectives of the person with dementia is crucial if research, policies, and practice are to be tailored to improve outcomes (e.g., improved QOL, reduced healthcare expenditures). As HCPs begin to understand the perspectives of the person who has dementia, choosing interventions that can improve positive experiences and reduce negative experiences will become clearer. Four most consistent themes that have emerged from the research to date on understanding perspectives of persons with dementia are discussed below.

Supportive Family and Friends

"Quality of life is living with your family—circle of friends and family" [person with dementia living in the community] ([2], p. 17)

Many person with dementia have shared that relationships, being with family and friends is one of the most important factors that promote positive experiences and reduce negative experiences, thereby maintaining and improving their quality of life. This is not surprising as positive relationships with caregivers (family and professional) have been associated with better QOL [56] and when attachment needs are unmet, the person often develops negative emotional states and agitation [57]. HCPs can help family and friends understand the increased importance they now have in the life of person with dementia and provide guidance regarding supportive ways to interact with the person and modify daily activities so that the person with dementia feels included.

Maintaining Independence

"I think it is very important because if you have your own independence then you feel that you are not depending on other people…" ([2], p. 19).

HCPs can from the start emphasize to persons with dementia and family members that there are several approaches and interventions that can help maintain independence of the patient and slow functional decline. Refer to Chapters "Experience and Perspective of the Primary Care Physician and Memory Care Specialist", "Community Mobility and Dementia: The Role for Health Care Professionals", "Home-Based Interventions Targeting Persons with Dementia: What is the Evidence and Where Do We Go from Here?" and "Experiences and Perspectives of Family Caregivers of the Person with Dementia" in this book for more information on approaches and interventions that can help maintain independence of the person with dementia.

Acceptance of the New Normal

"Anybody with…dementia…like a road accident…that person is not going to be the same and the whole family is going to have to change, adjust and develop to the new situation" ([2], p. 26).

HCPs can help the person with dementia and their family members begin the process of coming to terms with the new normal and making adjustments and accommodations in future plans to adapt positively.

Keeping a Sense of Humor

"Oh it is very important to have a laugh… Something that can make you laugh and being made to laugh is very important" ([2], p. 19).

HCPs need to develop skills to use humor in a therapeutic manner during their interactions with the patient with dementia and help the person get in touch with the "lighter side of life."

Narratives, Embodiment, and Sense of Self

"Who will I be in two years…three years…?" (A person with dementia who was a patient of the first author)

Fear of losing one's sense of self is perhaps one of the most distressing aspects of being diagnosed with dementia. The key reason for this is that society imposes its own narratives on the person with dementia, referring to dementia as "a slow unraveling of self." Also, the current culture defines self in relation to cognitive function, and values only those who can speak for themselves. The most tragic outcome of such negative and constricted attitudes is that the person with dementia is considered practically dead to society (e.g., social death). Growing research shows that many people with a dementia diagnosis actively use narratives to maintain a robust sense of self and counter such pejorative assumptions and stereotypes [2, 58]. Through the use of certain narratives (especially autobiographical stories and spiritual reminiscence) a person with dementia is able to find an alternative way of communicating, one that preserves one's sense of self [59–61]. Personal stories from the past are used in conversation to relate to others as well as to self. These stories are commonly told in order to give the listener a sense of who the person with dementia is and in what context the person wants to be viewed. Sharing past memories is a positive and creative way for persons with dementia to imbue past virtues onto the present to help nego-

tiate daily challenges to sense of self. These narratives have the power to give voice to emotions that may otherwise stay hidden. The repetition of autobiographical stories is often viewed as a negative and families and other caregivers often interrupt the person with dementia to remind them that they have already shared their story several times. Mills [62] has suggested that this repetition is a positive and an adaptive aspect of dementia as it helps maintain sense of self. Dynamics of narrative interactions have the potential to move the person who has dementia from being merely receivers (of conversations and care) to active participants in a relationship contributing as much as they receive. Such interactions not only help the person retain a sense of self and self-esteem but more important, give them a sense of being part of a larger family. Conversely, by not giving emphasis to and engagement with narratives, the relationships and sense of self of the person with dementia may begin to weaken.

Although the majority of the persons with dementia attempt to maintain their personal and social identity primarily through narratives, in severe dementia, many may lose all narrative abilities. In these stages, persons with dementia are most at risk of social death. It is important to recognize that selfhood is preserved and expressed as positively and creatively as narratives even in severe dementia [3, 63]. When a person readjusts her necklace so that it can be seen by others, she is expressing her selfhood. In essence, selfhood is an embodied dimension of human existence and no amount of loss of cognitive function can take it away. Such embodied expressions of selfhood can become more apparent to the caregivers if they are fully present and mindful during caregiving. Many caregivers are intuitively aware of the unique aspects of persons in severe stages of dementia and use their relationship with the person with dementia to improve positive experiences for them. AwareCare [16] is a useful tool to promote awareness amongst all caregivers (family and professional) and HCPs regarding expressions of selfhood, reminding them that the person even in severe stages of dementia is very much alive and capable of meaningful life.

Recommendations for Future Research

The clinical significance of understanding the experiences and perspectives of the person with dementia based on research to date highlights the need for detailed contextual and longitudinal evidence in future studies in this area. Although designing studies that explore this area is challenging because of the unique language and other cognitive challenges of persons with dementia, researchers are employing rigorous qualitative analyses of structured observations, interviews with persons with dementia, interviews with their family members, and analyses of focus groups (to name a few) to meet these challenges and produce high quality studies. Some employ multi-method approaches, combining psychometrically valid, reliable scales along with interviews, etc. Occasionally, they employ random assignment to treatment groups. Deeper and richer understanding of these most intimate aspects of the emotional life of persons with dementia will emerge from such high quality studies that begin with the premise that the experiences and perspectives of the person experiencing dementia are as much part of the basic science research on dementia as the study of molecular and genetic determinants of dementia.

Many questions remain. For example, there are virtually no studies available concerning to what extent the experiences and perspectives of the person with dementia can be improved by improving the attitudes of the HCPs and those of their support system, and, or the specific social and psychological factors that may particularly predispose them to experiences of despair. Also important for researchers to address is the question of whether negative experiences and perspectives in persons with dementia are driven more by the presence of a depressive illness than by the influence of stigma and other negative socio-cultural forces. Little evidence exists about how experiences and perspectives of the person with dementia change as dementia progresses. The impact of acetylcholineterase inhibitors (ACEIs) use and the experiences and perspectives of the person with dementia has not been studied and research to date has produced conflicting reports relative to the impact of ACEIs on QOL [64]. Awareness in the person with dementia has received considerable attention in the last decade [65]; awareness in persons with early stage dementia has been associated with reduced self-rated functioning [66]. It will be important to identify and delineate a link between awareness and negative experiences of persons with dementia.

Additional questions include: How are experiences and perspectives different for persons with young-onset dementia (YOD) (onset before age 60) as compared to persons with dementia after age 65? Is the concept of personhood different for YOD compared to late-onset dementia (LOD) [67]? Does functional neuroimaging have any place in studying experiences and perspectives of persons with dementia?

One of the most remarkable findings we have come across during our review of literature is how resilient and resourceful persons with dementia are despite the numerous challenges and losses they experience on a daily basis in the context of culture that stigmatizes them. To us, studying their experiences and perspectives has the potential to not only help eradicate the stigma of dementia but change our very notions of selfhood.

Recommendations for HCP

Research to understand experiences and perspectives of the person with dementia is still in its infancy. Studies to date most likely have captured different phenomena of experiences and perspectives. Hence, our recommendations should be considered preliminary. Based on review of research on experiences and perspectives of persons with dementia, Table 1 [1, 16, 32, 38, 51, 58, 68–84] lists key determinants that need to be addressed in order to improve their QOL. Box 3 lists key resources to increase their positive experiences. The following in our opinion are the seven most important recommendations for HCPs:

Table 1 Determinants of experiences of persons with dementia

Factors	Positive experiences	Negative experiences
Attitude of others and society	Being seen, accepted and recognized by others including one's faith-based community as a valued member of the society Making efforts to understand experiences and perspectives of persons with dementia Expansion of self-identities beyond "person with dementia", "staff", "physician" to "us" and "we" as part of the larger dementia care ecology	Treating persons with dementia as a burden and who has nothing of value to say or contribute to society Dismissing their memory and other cognitive complaints Viewing persons with dementia as less of a person or someone separate from "us" Relegating persons with dementia to margins of social consciousness
Issues around diagnosis	Making early diagnosis routine so that persons with dementia can actively participate in treatment and self-management	HCP[a] avoiding giving a diagnosis and or documenting the diagnosis in their records
Issues around treatment	HCPs sharing positive and uplifting stories of persons living with dementia Involving persons with dementia in discussions about goals of care and choice of treatment options Post-diagnosis support	HCP projecting their own sense of nihilism to convey that the situation is hopeless and nothing can be done to improve QOL[b] of persons with dementia Ignoring persons with dementia during office visits and interacting with their family for care planning
Issues around caregiver support, education and training	Both family and professional caregivers are routinely given accessible, affordable, and high quality respite services, education and training Robust support from local and regional academic organizations and government to provide caregiver support, education and training	HCP managing behavioral and psychological symptoms of dementia with inappropriate or excessive psychopharmacological interventions HCP's lack of knowledge and motivation to promote psychosocial environmental interventions for persons with dementia and their family caregivers
Issues surrounding person-centered care practices	Education intervention for HCPs including primary care providers promoting person-centered responses to persons with dementia HCP are sensitive to lived body experience and nonverbal communication of persons with dementia	Person-Centered care practices being given lip service or used for marketing rather than being embraced as the key aspect of all care practices Forced care of persons with dementia without dialogue amongst team members about ethical issues surrounding forced care
Meaningfulness in daily living	HCPs helping persons with dementia make meaning of the diagnosis and find meaning in daily life HCPs referring persons with dementia for meaning-centered psychotherapy and early-stage support groups when appropriate HCPs encouraging increasing time spent with nature and children by persons with dementia	HCP focusing only on physical health issues during their encounters with the patient Excluding persons with dementia in day to day activities (e.g., family events, religious rituals)
Issues surrounding research	Creating research partnerships with persons with dementia	Focusing only on the positives of being involved in research with inadequate discussion of the potential burdens involvement in research may pose to persons with dementia and their family
Issues around maintaining independence	Improving support for persons with dementia to self-manage medications Valuing dignity over safety Architecture (building design) that supports engagement of persons with dementia both inside and outside the building	Taking driving privileges away from persons with dementia without adequate discussion and support Valuing safety over dignity

(continued)

Table 1 (continued)

Factors	Positive experiences	Negative experiences
Issues around social support	HCPs providing guidance to family and friends of persons with dementia regarding importance of their support and involvement in QOL of Persons with dementia Adult day programs that are accessible and affordable	Having persons with dementia spend much of their time alone or watching television Lack of transportation resources to help persons with dementia maintain their social and spiritual/religious activities
Issues around existential aspects of suffering	Engaging persons with dementia in creative activities such as art, music, and poetry Educating the clergy in modifying religious rituals to accommodate the needs of persons with dementia Routinely utilizing services of chaplain in hospital and other institutional settings	HCP's discomfort with discussions of existential issues raised by diagnosis of dementia

[a]*HCP* Health Care Professional
[b]*QOL* Quality of Life

Box 3 Key Resources for HCPs to Improve Positive Experiences of Persons with Dementia

1. *Insight* is a quarterly educational bulletin produced by the Alzheimer's Society of British Columbia, Canada. The majority of the newsletter content is contributed by persons with dementia.

2. *Alzheimer's from the Inside Out.* Richard Taylor. Baltimore: Health Professions Press; 2006. Richard Taylor, a clinical psychologist diagnosed with Alzheimer's disease, has become a major spokesperson for people with the diagnosis. In this book, he describes what it feels like to have progressive memory loss. Taylor gives lectures all over the world encouraging persons with dementia to "speak up and speak out" about their experiences.

3. *Dementia Care: An Evidence Based Approach.* Editors: Marie Boltz and Jim Galvin. This is the first book that has chapters on experiences and perspectives of persons with dementia as well as a separate chapter on experiences and perspectives of Caregivers, two very important pieces of literature that have been missing in books on Dementia to date.

(continued)

- HCPs need to take patient's concerns related to cognitive decline seriously and not dismiss them as normal part of aging.
- HCPs must routinely strive to have better understanding of the experiences and perspectives of the person with dementia and utilize the understanding to inform care decisions.
- HCPs need to reflect on and discuss their own prejudices regarding living with dementia and on negative experiences shared by persons with dementia (for example, negative experiences mentioned in this chapter) to increase their compassion for them.
- Dementia status alone is not sufficient to conclude that knowledge and history obtained from persons with dementia are unreliable or flawed.
- HCPs need to be aware that the majority of persons with dementia (including those with advanced dementia) can speak for themselves to a much higher degree than usually recognized. It is also important for HCPs to recognize that well-meaning family and friends often give biased or flawed information, especially if the issue is emotionally charged and in this context, experiences and perspectives of persons with dementia are even more important to explore.
- Sharing positive experiences of persons with dementia (for example, ones mentioned in this chapter) with other persons with dementia struggling to cope.

Box 3 (continued)

4. *Psychiatric Consultation in Long-Term Care: A Guide for Health Care Professionals.* Abhilash Desai M.D. and George Grossberg M.D. The Johns Hopkins University Press: Baltimore, MD; 2010. In the chapter titled "Psychosocial and Environmental Interventions" in this book, using several case examples, the authors provide excellent description of various dimensions of person-centered care and its practical application to improve emotional wellbeing of PERSONS WITH DEMENTIA, especially those living in long-term care facilities.

5. *Aging Together: Dementia, Friendship, and Flourishing Communities.* Susan H McFadden and John T McFadden. The Johns Hopkins University Press: Baltimore, MD; 2011. Written by Susan McFadden (a psychology professor) and her husband, John (an ordained minister in the United Church of Christ), this book asserts that all aging baby boomers will be living with dementia, whether they have the diagnosis or friends and family members have it. Unfortunately, persons affected by dementia often report feeling socially isolated. In order to flourish, communities need to find ways to support ongoing, meaningful relationships as people journey into forgetfulness.

6. *The Experience of Alzheimer's Disease; Life through a Tangled Veil.* Steven R Sabat. Blackwell Publications Inc.: Oxford; 2001. In this book, the author emphasizes the importance of looking for "meaning" in the communication of individuals with dementia. The author encourages healthcare professionals to strive to discover and nurture for as long as is possible, the special essence of their clients with dementia.

– HCPs should encourage family and friends of persons with dementia to reflect on and discuss the negative experiences expressed by persons with dementia (for example, ones mentioned in this chapter) to promote compassion for them.

Writing this book chapter has validated much of what we had already come to understand through working with persons with dementia, that HCPs need to join Peter Mittler in his campaign titled "Every Dementia Person Matters", a campaign that can learn a lot from a similar campaign "Every Disabled Child Matters" [20, 85].

Conclusions

Understanding the inner world of persons with dementia is a challenge for family members as well as HCPs because of their language and other cognitive difficulties. Research to date on the experiences and perspectives of persons with dementia has begun to improve our understanding of their inner world and has discovered that dementia is a manageable condition for many of those affected. Research also demonstrates the retained sense of wellbeing and purpose in their interpersonal and intrapersonal world that is conveyed verbally as well as nonverbally (through facial expression and behaviors). Appreciation of this by their family and friends as well as HCPs and sharing of these research findings with the persons who has dementia can bolster efforts to improve their QOL. Research has started to suggest that persons with dementia are experts in what will make their lives more meaningful and happy. HCPs and caregivers need only to develop the skills to follow their lead, understand their language, and create a dementia care ecology that celebrates the individuality, resilience, and creativity of all persons with dementia. This will also humanize care-partnering with persons with dementia and serve as an antidote to the dehumanizing and toxic sociocultural environment that they are currently forced to live in. It is time that HCPs join persons with dementia in moving the rhetoric of "war on dementia" to "working with and for persons with dementia'" in order to make dementia-friendly world a reality.

References

1. Tranvag O, Petersen KA, Naden D. Crucial dimensions constituting dignity experience in persons living with dementia. Dementia. 2014. doi:10.1177/1471301214529783.
2. Williamson T. My name is not dementia: people with dementia discuss quality of life indicators. London: Alzheimer's Society Devon House; 2010.
3. Clare L. Awareness in people with severe dementia: review and integration. Aging Ment Health. 2010; 14(1):20–32.
4. Kitwood T. Dementia reconsidered: the person comes first. Philadelphia, PA: Open University Press; 1997.
5. Sabat R. The experience of Alzheimer's disease: life through a tangled veil. Oxford: Blackwell Publications Inc.; 2001.
6. Bartlett R, O'Connor D. Broadening the dementia debate: towards social citizenship. Portland, OR: The Policy Press; 2010.
7. Beard RL. Advocating voice: organizational, historical, and social milieux of the Alzheimer's disease movement. Sociol Health Illn. 2004;26(6):797–819.
8. Wiersma EC, Denton A. From social network to safety net: dementia-friendly communities in rural northern Ontario. Dementia. 2013. doi:10.1177/1471301213516118.
9. George DR, Stuckey HL, Whitehead MM. How a creative storytelling intervention can improve medical student attitude towards persons with dementia: a mixed methods study. Dementia. 2012;13(3):318–29.
10. Bartlett R, Hick C, Houston A, Gardiner L, Wallace D. Privileging place: reflections on involving people with dementia in a residency. Dementia. 2013. doi:10.1177/1471301213512116.
11. Ashworth A, Ashworth P. The lifeworld as phenomenon and as research heuristic, exemplified by a study of the lifeworld of a person suffering Alzheimer's disease. J Phenomenol Psychol. 2003;34:179–205.
12. Woods RT, Nelis SM, Martyr A, Roberts J, Whitaker CJ, Markova I, Roth I, Morris R, Clare L. What contributes to a good quality of life in early dementia? Awareness and the QoL-AD: a cross-sectional study. Health Qual Life Outcomes. 2014;12:94–104.
13. Beard RL, Fetterman DJ, Wu B, Bryant L. The two voices of Alzheimer's: attitudes toward brain health by diagnosed individuals and support persons. Gerontologist. 2009;49(51):540–9.
14. Hughes JC. 'Y' feel me?' How do we understand the person with dementia? Dementia. 2013;12(3):348–58.
15. Quinn C, Clare L. Interpretive phenomenological analysis. In: Watson R, McKenna H, Cocoman S, Keady J, editors. Nursing research: designs and methods. London: Churchill Livingstone; 2008. p. 375–84.
16. Clare L, Whitaker R, Quinn C, Jelley H, Hoare Z, Woods B, Downs M, Wilson B. AwareCare: development and validation of an observational measure of awareness in people with severe dementia. Neuropsychol Rehabil. 2012;22(1):113–33.
17. Lopez JJB, Bolivar JCC, Perez MS. COMMUNI-CARE: assessment tool for reactions and behaviors of patients with dementia in a multisensory stimulation environment. Dementia. 2014. doi:10.1177/1471301214528346.
18. Hunsaker AE, Terhorst L, Gentry A, Lingler JH. Measuring hope among families impacted by cognitive impairment. Dementia. 2014. doi:10.1177/1471301214531590.
19. Murphy K, Jordan F, Hunter A, Cooney A, Casey D. Articulating the strategies for maximizing the inclusion of people with dementia in qualitative research studies. Dementia. 2014. doi:10.1177/1471301213512489.
20. Mittler P. Journey into Alzheimerland. Dementia. 2011;10(2):145–7.
21. Merrick K, Camic PM, O'Shaughnessay M. Couples constructing their experiences of dementia: a relational perspective. Dementia. 2013. doi:10.1177/1471301213513029.
22. Nowell ZC, Thornton A, Simpson J. The subjective experience of personhood in dementia care settings. Dementia. 2011;12(4):394–409.
23. Johannessen A, Moller A. Experiences of persons with early-onset dementia in everyday life: a qualitative study. Dementia. 2011;12(4):410–24.
24. Sutcliffe CL, Roe B, Jasper R, Jolley D, Challis DJ. People with dementia and carers' experiences of dementia care and services: outcomes of a focus group study. Dementia. 2013. doi:10.1177/1471301213511957.
25. Jones SN. An interpersonal approach to psychotherapy with older persons with dementia. Prof Psychol Res Pract. 1995;26(6):602–7.
26. Moon H, Adams KB. The effectiveness of dyadic interventions for people with dementia and their caregivers. Dementia. 2012;12(6):821–39.
27. Dempsey L, Murphy K, Cooney A, Casey D, O'Shea E, Devane D, Jordan F, Hunter A. Reminiscence in dementia: a concept analysis. Dementia. 2014;13(2):176–92.
28. Lishman E, Cheston R, Smithson J. The paradox of dementia: changes in assimilation after receiving a diagnosis of dementia. Dementia. 2014. doi:10.1177/1471301214520781.
29. Keyes SE, Clarke CL, Wilkinson H, Alexjuk EJ, Wilcockson J, Robinson L, Reynolds J, McClelland S, Corner L, Cattan M. "We're all thrown in the same boat…": a qualitative analysis of peer support in dementia care. Dementia. 2014. doi:10.1177/1471301214529575.

30. Brody EM, Kleban MH, Lawton MP, Silverman H. Excess disabilities of mentally impaired aged: Impact of individualized treatment. Gerontologist. 1971;11(2, Pt. 1):124–133.
31. Chaplin R, Davidson I. What are the experiences of people with dementia in employment? Dementia. 2014. doi:10.1177/1471301213519252.
32. Hochgraeber I, Riesner C, Schoppmann S. The experience of people with dementia in a social care group: case study. Dementia. 2013;12(6):751–68.
33. Harris PB. Dementia and friendship: the quality and nature of the relationships that remain. Int J Aging Hum Dev. 2013;76:141–64.
34. McFadden SH, McFadden JT. Aging together: dementia, friendship, and flourishing communities. Baltimore, MD: The Johns Hopkins University Press; 2011.
35. Barclay A. Psalm 88: living with Alzheimer's. J Relig Disabil Health. 2012;16:88–101.
36. Thibault JM, Morgan RL. No act of love is ever wasted: the spirituality of caring for persons with dementia. Nashville, TN: Upper Room Books; 2009.
37. Powers BA, Watson NM. Spiritual nurturance and support for nursing home residents with dementia. Dementia. 2011;10:59–80.
38. Scholl JM, Sabat SR. Stereotypes, stereotype threat and ageing: implications for the understanding and treatment of people with Alzheimer's disease. Ageing Soc. 2008;28:103–30.
39. Hedman R, Hansebo G, Ternestedt BM, Hellstrom I, Norgerg A. How people with Alzheimer's disease express their sense of self: analysis using Rom Harre's theory of selfhood. Dementia. 2013;12(6):713–33.
40. Johnstone MJ. Metaphors, stigma and the 'Alzheimerization' of the euthanasia debate. Dementia. 2011;12(4):377–93.
41. O'Sullivan G, Hocking C, Spence D. Dementia: the need for attitudinal change. Dementia. 2014;13(4):483–97.
42. Burgener SC, Buckwalter K, Perhounkova Y, Lui MF. The effects of perceived stigma on quality of life outcomes in persons with early-stage dementia: longitudinal findings: part 2. Dementia. 2013. doi:10.1177/1471301213504202.
43. Burgener SC, Buckwalter K, Perkhounkova Y, Lui MF, Riley R, Einhorn CJ, Fitzsimmons S, Hahn-Swanson C. Perceived stigma in persons with early-stage dementia: longitudinal findings: part 1. Dementia. 2013. doi:10.1177/1471301213508399.
44. Innes A, Manthorpe J. Developing theoretical understandings of dementia and their application to dementia care policy in the UK. Dementia. 2012;12(6):682–96.
45. George DR, Whitehouse PJ. The war (on terror) on Alzheimer's. Dementia. 2014;13(1):120–30.
46. Batsch N, Mittelman MS, Alzheimer's Disease International. World Alzheimer report. Overcoming the stigma of dementia. London: Alzheimer's Disease International; 2012.
47. Ballenger J. Self, senility, and Alzheimer's disease in modern America: a history. Baltimore, MD: John Hopkins University Press; 2006.
48. Horning SM, Melrose R, Sultzer D. Insight in Alzheimer's disease and its relation to psychiatric and behavioral disturbances. Int J Geriatr Psychiatry. 2014;29:77–84.
49. De Leo D. Dementia, insight, and suicidal behavior. Crisis. 1996;17(4):147–8.
50. Bird M, Blair A. Clinical psychology and anxiety and depression in dementia: three case studies. Nord Psychol. 2010;62(2):43–54.
51. Clemerson G, Walsh S, Isaac C. Towards living well with young onset dementia: an exploration of coping from the perspective of those diagnosed. Dementia. 2014;13(4):451–66.
52. Sullivan SC, Beard RL. Faith and forgetfulness: the role of spiritual identity in preservation of self with Alzheimer's. J Relig Spiritual Aging. 2014;26:65–91.
53. Post SG. Alzheimer's & grace. First Things. 2004;142:12–4.
54. Clare L, Rowlands JM, Quin R. Collective strength: the impact of development a shared social identity in early-stage dementia. Dementia. 2008;7:9–30.
55. McFadden SH, Koll A. Popular memory cafés in Wisconsin's Fox valley battle social isolation. Gener J Am Soc Aging. 2014;38:68–71.
56. Clare L, Woods RT, Nelis SM, Martyr A, Markova IS, Roth I, Whitaker CJ, Morris RG. Trajectories of quality of life in early-stage dementia: individual variations and predictors of change. Int J Geriatr Psychiatry. 2014;29:616–23.
57. Nelis SM, Clare L, Whitaker CJ. Attachment in people with dementia and their caregivers: a systematic review. Dementia. 2013. doi:10.1177/1471301213485232.
58. Beard RL, Knauss J, Moyer D. Managing disability and enjoying life: how we reframe dementia through personal narratives. J Aging Stud. 2009;23(4):227–35.
59. MacKinlay E. Resistance, resilience, and change: the person with dementia. J Relig Spiritual Aging. 2012;24(1–2):80–92.
60. Bouchard RE, Bannister KA, Anas AP. The dementia narrative: writing to reclaim social identity. J Aging Stud. 2009;23:145–57.
61. Hyden LC, Oruly L. Narrative and identity in Alzheimer's disease: a case study. J Ageing Stud. 2009;23:205–14.
62. Mills MA. Narrative identity and dementia: a study of emotion and narrative in older people with dementia. Ageing Soc. 1997;17:673–98.
63. Kontos PC. Ethnographic reflections on selfhood, embodiment and Alzheimer's disease. Ageing Soc. 2004;24(6):829–49.
64. Hoe J, Katona C, Orrell M, Livingston G. Quality of life in dementia: care recipient and caregiver perceptions of quality of life in dementia: the LASER-AD study. Int J Geriatr Psychiatry. 2007;22:1031–6.

65. Markova IS, Clare L, Whitaker CJ, Roth I, Nelis SM, Martyr A, et al. Phenomena of awareness in dementia: heterogeneity and its implications. Conscious Cogn. 2014;25:17–26.

66. Martyr A, Nelis SM, Clare L. Predictors of perceived functional ability in early-stage dementia: self-ratings, informant ratings and discrepancy scores. Int J Geriatr Psychiatry. 2014;29(8):852–62.

67. Tolhurst E, Bhattacharyya S, Kingston P. Young onset dementia: the impact of emergent age-based factors upon personhood. Dementia. 2014;13(2):193–206.

68. Larner AJ, Hanock P. Are we forcing people with dementia to receive care? Int J Geriatr Psychiatry. 2014;29:767–70.

69. Innes A, Szymczynska P, Stark C. Dementia diagnosis and post-diagnostic support in Scottish rural communities: experiences of people with dementia and their families. Dementia. 2014;13(2):233–47.

70. Dewing J, Dijk S. What is the current state of care for older people with dementia in general hospitals? A literature review. Dementia. 2014. doi:10.1177/1471301213520172.

71. Martin F, Turner A, Wallace LM, Choudhry K, Bradbury N. Perceived barriers to self-management for people with dementia in the early stages. The International Journal of Social Research and Practice 2013; 12(4):481–93.

72. Clare L, Woods RT, Whitaker R, Wilson BA, Downs M. Development of an awareness-based intervention to enhance quality of life in severe dementia: trial platform. Trails. 2010;11:73–81.

73. Quinn C, Anderson D, Toms G, Whitaker R, Edwards RT, Jones C, Clare L. Self-management in early-stage dementia: a pilot randomized controlled trial of the efficacy and cost-effectiveness of a self-management group intervention (the SMART study). Trials. 2014;15:74–82.

74. Fleming R, Goodenough B, Low LF, Chenoweth L, Brodaty H. The relationship between the quality of the built environment and the quality of life of people with dementia in residential care. Dementia. 2014. doi:10.1177/1471301214532460.

75. Tolo AK, Heggestad, Nortvedt P, Slettebo A. Dignity and care for people with dementia living in nursing homes. Dementia. 2013. doi:10.1177/1471301213512840.

76. Robertson JM. Finding meaning in everyday life with dementia: a case study. Dementia. 2014;13(4):525–43.

77. Edwards R, Voss S, Iliffe S. Education about dementia in primary care: Is person-centredness the key? Dementia. 2014;13(1):111–9.

78. Lee SM, Roen K, Thornton A. The psychological impact of a diagnosis of Alzheimer's disease. Dementia. 2014;13(3):289–305.

79. Hafford-Letchfield T. Funny things happen at the Grange: introducing comedy activities in day services to older people with dementia-innovative practice. Dementia. 2012;12(6):840–52.

80. Coaten R, Newman-Bluestein D. Embodiment and dementia-dance movement psychotherapists respond. Dementia. 2013;12(6):677–81.

81. Pavlicevic M, Tsiris G, Wood S, Powell H, Graham J, Sanderson R, Millman R, Gibson J. The 'ripple effect': towards researching improvisational music therapy in dementia care-homes. Dementia. 2013. doi:10.1177/1471301213514419.

82. Guzman-Garcia A, Mukaetova-Ladinska E, James I. Introducing a latin ballroom dance class to people with dementia living in care homes, benefits and concerns: a pilot study. Dementia. 2012;12(5):523–35.

83. Petrescu I, MacFarlane K, Ranzijin R. Psychological effects of poetry workshops with people with early stage dementia: an exploratory study. Dementia. 2014;13(2):207–15.

84. Clark-McGhee K, Castro M. A narrative analysis of poetry written from the words of people given a diagnosis of dementia. Dementia. 2013. doi:10.1177/1471301213488116.

85. Carpenter BD, Kissel EC, Lee MM. Preferences and life evaluations of older adults with and without dementia: reliability, stability, and proxy knowledge. Psychol Aging. 2007;22(3):650–5.

Home-Based Interventions Targeting Persons with Dementia: What Is the Evidence and Where Do We Go from Here?

Laura N. Gitlin, Nancy A. Hodgson, and Scott Seung W. Choi

Introduction

Most persons with dementia live at home either alone or with family over the protracted course of this progressive and terminal condition [1]. This is the case for the over five million persons in the United States (US) as well as the 44 million persons worldwide living with dementia [2, 3].

With disease progression, individuals experience and become at risk for various physical, cognitive, sensorial, behavioral and emotional

L.N. Gitlin, PhD (✉)
Department of Community Public Health, School of Nursing, Johns Hopkins University, Baltimore, MD, USA

Division of Geriatrics and Gerontology, Department of Psychiatry, School of Medicine, Johns Hopkins University, Baltimore, MD, USA

Center for Innovative Care in Aging, Johns Hopkins University, Baltimore, MD, USA
e-mail: lgitlin1@jhu.edu

N.A.Hodgson, PhD, RN
Center for Innovative Care in Aging, Johns Hopkins University, Baltimore, MD, USA

Department of Acute and Chronic Care, School of Nursing, Johns Hopkins University, Baltimore, MD, USA
e-mail: Nhodgson1@jhu.edu

S.S.W. Choi, MA, RN
School of Nursing, Johns Hopkins University, Baltimore, MD, USA
e-mail: schoi51@jhu.edu

decrements due to the condition itself as well as age-associated and comorbid processes [4]. However, these issues typically remain unaddressed in the health care system. Nevertheless, common symptoms and concerns such as pain, sleep disturbances, infections, behavioral symptoms, fall risk, home environmental safety risks, distressed families, are all amenable to intervention and hence improvement [5–7]. The overall quality of life at home for people with dementia is also tenuous. Individuals have many unaddressed needs and spend most days doing little or not being engaged in meaningful activities [5, 8, 9]. The lack of activity in particular, is a persistent concern for families with research showing that inactivity or inappropriate stimulation has negative consequences including increased isolation, dependency, and behavioral and psychological symptoms [10–12].

To date, a comprehensive system of health and human services for persons with dementia as well as clinical treatment guidelines that can address the vicissitudes of this long-term condition do not exist in the United States or worldwide. Further, developing and testing approaches to improve the care, well-being and quality of life for this clinical population has lagged behind other efforts such as the development and testing of caregiver support programs, or the search for a cure and preventive strategies to slow the onset of cognitive decline.

The lack of clinical attention to quality of life and the daily medical, social, psychological, behavioral and physical needs of people with

© Springer International Publishing Switzerland 2016
M. Boltz, J.E. Galvin (eds.), *Dementia Care*, DOI 10.1007/978-3-319-18377-0_11

dementia can be accounted for, in part, to the singular national focus on finding a cure and delaying onset of symptomatology that dominates funded research priorities, the prevailing viewpoint that nothing can be done, and the stigma associated with having dementia as it is a cognitive condition with neuropsychiatric symptoms [13].

Recent and converging developments are promulgating interest in and attention to improving the quality of daily life of persons with dementia living at home. These developments include the fact that a dementia cure is not in near sight, the 2011 passage of the National Alzheimer's Plan Act calling for care planning, early government investments in testing effective caregiver support interventions that also show benefits to persons with dementia and the voices of persons themselves and their family members urging for better care.

Much is known about the supportive interventions that have been designed and tested for family caregivers [14–17]. Also, there are numerous meta-analyses and systematic reviews of non-pharmacologic approaches for persons with dementia [18, 19]. However, previous reviews have either focused on interventions targeting family caregivers themselves [14, 15], include a combination of studies targeting caregivers plus individuals with dementia [20], focus on non-pharmacologic approaches tested mostly with individuals in nursing homes [21], or examine one particular outcome such as functional decline [22]. These reviews overall suggest a growing evidence base supporting the positive benefits of nonpharmacologic approaches in dementia care. However, it is unclear as to the evidence for interventions that target the broad swath of quality of life-related outcomes and which specifically target individuals living at home with dementia. Given the long trajectory of dementia and that most persons live and age at home in their communities with this condition, developing, testing and implementing approaches to improving quality of life related outcomes in the home setting is of utmost importance.

The purpose of this chapter is to provide a systematic review of the extant research on home-based interventions that are designed to improve one or more aspects of the quality of life of individuals living with dementia. Our intent is to evaluate the relative merits and limitations of interventions tested in randomized trials in order to offer suggestions for advancements in this area. Of particular importance is identifying future intervention work that can have clinical applicability for this population. In this review, we sought to answer two basic questions: What home based intervention strategies have demonstrated direct benefits to persons with dementia living at home? What are the key elements of interventions that demonstrate outcomes of clinical importance to persons with dementia? This review is the first to our knowledge to examine existing behavioral intervention research that specifically targets persons with dementia with the express purpose of improving their quality of life at home. Improving quality of life of persons with dementia may involve interventions that directly target the individual, directly target the family caregiver, or which reflect a dyadic or combined approach. We consider all three scenarios in this review.

Conceptual Framework for Identifying Needs and Interventions Along Disease Trajectory

To understand the potential opportunities for intervening with individuals with dementia, Fig. 1 offers a conceptual model that maps disease stage to the known effects of dementia on individuals [23]. It provides a heuristic for identifying and addressing the needs of individuals at each stage of the disease. As such, it also provides a framework for evaluating the disease stage and areas of need addressed by current interventions and those areas that are not addressed for which future efforts could be directed.

Figure 1 suggests that needs emerge early on with the initial onset of symptoms of cognitive impairment and change over the course of the disease. As noted, even in this initial disease stage, persons experience high levels of need for education, care planning, opportunities for engagement in meaningful activities, and assistance with medications. Individuals may also become at increased risk for social isolation and

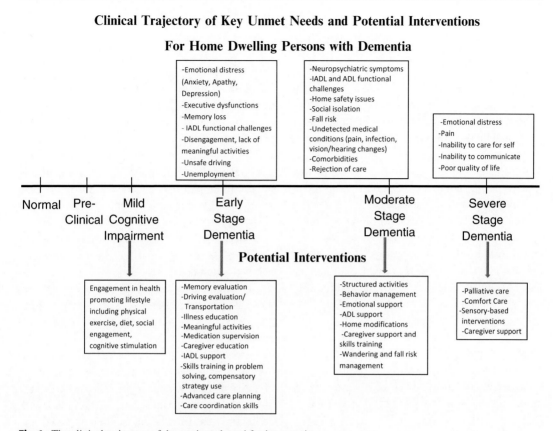

Fig. 1 The clinical trajectory of dementia and need for intervention

unsafe driving. Interventions at this early stage could be designed to involve persons in advanced care planning, use of a range of memory aids, and ways to simplify meaningful activities to promote continued engagement [24]. In the moderate stage, with the increase in functional challenges and neuropsychiatric symptoms such as agitation, rejection of care, or wandering, individuals transition to the need for more structured daily routines and activities and greater oversight. Risk for emotional distress, disengagement, wandering and falls is also heightened at this stage. Interventions that may be effective at this stage could involve home modifications to reduce fall risk and facilitate caregiving, caregiver training in communication and behavioral management strategies, simplification of activities to ensure continued engagement and exercise programs. Lastly, among those at the severe stage of dementia, unmet needs arise due to the person's inability to communicate and their total

dependence on others for meeting daily needs. Interventions for persons in the advanced stage could emphasize a palliative approach focused on comfort care and positive sensory experiences to maximize quality of life.

These needs and known consequences of dementia are practically universal and exist across specific dementia conditions (e.g. Alzheimer's, Vascular, Mixed dementia), and race, ethnic and cultural groups [25].

Intervention Studies Targeting Individuals with Dementia Living at Home

Search Procedures and Results

To examine existing home or community-based interventions that include outcomes specifically targeting individuals with dementia living at home, we used a rapid review process to identify [26] relevant articles. Six electronic databases, MEDLINE (PubMed), CINAHL, Embase, PsycINFO (OVID), Scopus, and Cochrane Database, were searched to identify relevant studies published from database inceptions through July 2014. Search terms and their combination included: condition (dementia, cognitive impairment, or cognitively impaired), study design (randomized controlled trial, clinical trial, random allocation, random assignment, random sampling, or random*), and intervention setting (home care services, home-based, home-delivered, in-home, telephone based, or home care). Additional articles were suggested for inclusion by experts and obtained from reference lists of relevant studies. One of the authors (SC) assessed all titles and abstracts identified by the literature search for relevance.

Potentially relevant articles were then retrieved for full-text review. Each retrieved study was examined along the following criteria to determine eligibility for inclusion in this review: (1) published in a peer-reviewed journal and in English; (2) use of randomized controlled trial design or random allocation of participants to treatment conditions; (3) testing of a nonpharmacological intervention which was provided in the home (face-to-face or telephone) or community setting; (4) inclusion of individuals with a physician diagnosis or caregiver report of any type of dementia; (5) at least one outcome measure related to an aspect of quality of life of the person with dementia.

Likewise, articles were excluded if they had no outcomes related to the person with dementia, if the interventions included pharmacological treatment, drug trials, respite care, or hospice/palliative care, if the interventions occurred outside the home (e.g., at a clinic), if other conditions were present including delirium or schizophrenia, or if outcomes related to the person with dementia were not assessed quantitatively.

Using these criteria, the search yielded an initial set of 1,535 articles. The titles and abstracts were reviewed for relevance which excluded 1,422 non-relevant studies. Then, 113 (7 %) studies were retained for full-text review; this in turn

yielded 40 (35 %) studies that fully met full review criteria. Also, five additional articles were identified through review of reference lists of selected articles, and four other recently published studies were recommended by the primary author. The added literature from reference lists or recommendation had been originally filtered out in the initial search mostly because the publications did not include descriptors of their intervention settings in abstracts or titles. Identifying intervention settings remained a challenge also with the full-text review as some studies were not clear about the setting in which their interventions occur. After full-text review, this resulted in a total of 49 studies that met inclusion criteria and were included in this review (Fig. 2).

Studies included in this review are as follows: those that targeted persons with dementia only and also only reported outcomes for persons with dementia (n=3); those that targeted persons with dementia only but also reported outcomes for both persons with dementia and their family caregivers (n=4); those that targeted family caregivers but also reported outcomes for persons with dementia (n=19); and those that targeted the dyad (caregiver and person with dementia) and report only outcomes for the person with dementia (n=1) and the dyad (n=22). We only summarize the results for those outcomes that are related to persons with dementia in order to understand in-depth the impact of interventions for this clinical population (Fig. 3).

Characteristics of Studies

Table 1 summarizes the essential components of the 49 studies. Shown are only outcomes for persons with dementia that reflected statistically significant between group comparisons. Thus, any one study could have reported other positive changes such as intra-group variations or trends in a positive direction, but these are not considered in this review.

The 49 studies included in this review were conducted in 12 different countries indicating the global recognition of the need for better approaches to dementia care: 28 studies were

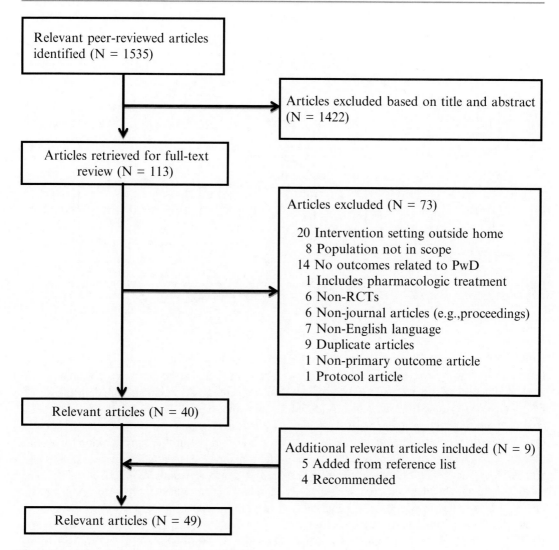

Fig. 2 Search flowchart. *Note*: *PwD* person with dementia

conducted in the US; 5 studies in the United Kingdom, 3 in Finland; 2 studies in Hong Kong, Netherlands, and Taiwan; and 1 study each in Australia, Brazil, France, India, Italy, Peru and Russia. As to participants, across studies, a total of 4,066 persons with dementia were included with the number of participants for any one study ranging from 16 to 642. While disease stage was not reported in 7 (14 %) studies, 5 (10 %) studies targeted individuals at the early disease stage, 13 (27 %) targeted individuals at the mild to moderate

disease stages, 9 (18 %) were at the moderate to severe stage, and 15 (31 %) studies included individuals with a wide range of disease severity from mild to severe. Nevertheless, few studies (e.g. [65]), employed a clinical workup as part of screening for study inclusion so that firm conclusions cannot be drawn concerning the stage of the disease and dementia type represented in study samples (Table 1).

A randomized trial design was required for inclusion in this review. Thus, studies reflected

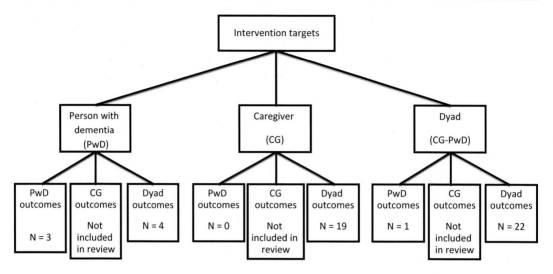

Fig. 3 Number of studies targeting outcomes for persons with dementia. *Note*: *PwD* person with dementia, *CG*
caregiver. For studies of a dyadic focus, only outcomes for PwD are reported

either a Phase II (proof of concept) or Phase III (efficacy) trial with most demonstrating a relatively high level of rigor. Most studies (n=41, 84 %) included two study arms, a treatment and control group condition; whereas 8 (16 %) studies included 3 or more treatment/control groups. The level of blinding to group condition varied with 33 (67 %) using single blinding; this included 31 (63 %) studies in which assessors were blinded and 2 (4 %) studies in which participants were blinded to group allocation. Additionally, 10 (20 %) studies did not use any blinding, and in 6 (12 %) studies, it is not clear whether blinding occurred or not. Only 21 (43 %) studies indicated that some form of treatment fidelity was assessed, although only one study reported an adherence rate to the treatment protocol.

A wide range of outcomes and measures were considered within and across studies with most studies including multiple outcomes. Behavioral symptoms were the most frequently evaluated as an outcome with 27 (55 %) studies; functional status was examined in 17 (35 %) studies; quality of life was examined in 14 (29 %) studies; depression was examined in 12 (24 %) studies, and cognitive status and institutionalization in 8 (16 %) studies. Other study outcomes included health,

anxiety, sleep, service utilization, embarrassment about memory problems, risky behaviors and unmet care needs of persons with dementia.

Of importance, 42 (86 %) studies reported a statistically significant difference between a treatment and control group condition for at least one outcome measure; although most studies also reported mixed results (e.g., a benefit in some domains but not others). Most studies examined immediate treatment effects. It is difficult to determine if treatment effects had long term benefits. We were able to identify only 3 (6 %) that assessed a long-term effect (e.g., follow-up occurred $\geq$ 12 months following termination of the intervention [34, 59, 60]. Delay in institutionalization, more days living at home and improved ability to keep persons with dementia at home were all found to be benefits in interventions that maintained contact with individuals beyond a year (e.g., [60, 65]).

Taken as a whole, there appears to be a strong corpus of research testing novel interventions directed at individuals with dementia living at home. Nevertheless, the use of different measures makes it virtually impossible to compare treatment effects and evaluate the merits of a single intervention relative to another or whether

Table 1 Summary of randomized clinical trials targeting outcomes for persons with dementia (n = 49)

Author/Date Country	Sample/Stage of disease	Intervention	# Sessions/Length/ Duration	Fidelity reported	Results related to PwD Intervention effects
Avila et al. [27] Brazil	N = 16 Mild to moderate	Neuropsychological rehabilitation—cognitive training, dementia education, coping strategies	22 sessions/40 min/22 weeks	NR	At 22 weeks, no changes in global function, cognitive function, ADL, QoL, or problem behaviors
Bass et al. [28] USA	N = 157 NR	Care consultation—dementia education, case management, care planning	12 sessions/NR/12 months	NR	At 12 months, ↓utilization of direct care community services & Kaiser case management visit ; no change in utilization of medical services (ER visits, hospital admissions, or physician visits)
Bass et al. [29] USA	N = 333 Mild to severe	"Partners in Dementia Care" intervention—care-coordinating program which addresses medical and non-medical concerns of persons with dementia and their caregivers	14 sessions[a]/NR/12 months	Yes (Biweekly refresher training and care reviews were completed)	At 6 months, ↓relationship strain, depression, unmet need, and embarrassment; no change in isolation
					At 12 months, ↓ unmet need and embarrassment; no change in relationship strain, isolation, and depression
Belle et al. [30] USA	N = 642 Moderate to severe	"REACH II" multicomponent intervention—dementia education, case management, counseling, behavioral management, problem solving skills training, telephone support	12 sessions/NR/6 months	NR	At 6 months, ↓ problem behaviors for Hispanic and White participants; no change in rates of institutionalization
Burgener et al. [31] USA	N = 54 Severe dementia	Educational and behavioral intervention—dementia education, behavioral management	1 session/90 min/1 month	NR	At 6 months, ↑ self-care ability; no change in problem behaviors
Burgio et al. [32] USA	N = 118 Moderate dementia	Psychosocial interventions ("REACH I")—dementia education, behavioral management, problem-solving, cognitive restructuring, environmental modification	8 sessions/1 h/6 months	Yes (Weekly case review meetings, audiotaped sessions)	At 6 months, ↓ problem behaviors for Black spouses

(continued)

Table 1 (continued)

Author/Date Country	Sample/Stage of disease	Intervention	# Sessions/Length/ Duration	Fidelity reported	Results related to PwD Intervention effects
Chang et al. [33] USA	N=65 Moderate dementia	Cognitive behavioral intervention—dementia education, behavioral management, coping strategies, case management	8 sessions/ 18.3 min[a]/8 weeks	NR	At 12 weeks, ↑behavioral disturbance; no change in ADL
Chien and Lee [34] Hong Kong	N=92 Mild to moderate dementia	Psychosocial intervention (family supportive group program)—dementia education, case management, behavioral management, discussion, psychological support, problem-solving	10 sessions/2 h/5 months	NR	At 12 months, ↓in rates of institutionalization At 18 months, ↓in rates of institutionalization and problem behaviors
Clare et al. [35] UK	N=113 Early stage of dementia	Cognitive rehabilitation—cognitive training (face-name learning, maintaining attention), coping strategies, relaxation therapy (for attention-placebo condition)	8 sessions/1 h/8 weeks	Yes	At 8 weeks (post treatment), ↑ goal performance and satisfaction At 6 months, ↑Memory performance subscale
Dias et al. [36] India	N=81 Mild to moderate dementia	Home care program—dementia education, case management, behavioral management, coping strategies, psychiatric assessment and treatment, support group meetings	12 sessions/ 45 min/6 months	NR	At 3 and 6 months, no changes in problem behaviors and ADL functioning)
Eloniemi-Sulkava et al. [37] Finland	N=100 Mild to severe dementia	Comprehensive support program—dementia education, case management, counseling, problem solving, support group meetings, coping strategies	Varies/NR/2 years	NR	At 1 year, ↓ rate of institutionalization At 2 years, no change in rate of institutionalization
Eloniemi-Sulkava et al. [38] Finland	N=125 Mild to severe dementia	Multicomponent support program—dementia education, case management, support group meetings, physical exercise, behavioral management, coping strategies, medical investigations and treatments	Varies/NR/2 years	Yes (Only CG group meetings were tape recorded)	At 6 and 12 months, no difference in rate of institutionalization At 18 months, ↓rate of institutionalization At 24 months, no change in rate of institutionalization
Fitzsimmons and Buettner [39] USA	N=30 NR	Therapeutic recreation intervention—activity engagement, sensory stimulation, coping strategies for persons with problem behaviors	6–10 sessions/ 1–2 h/2 weeks	NR	At 2 weeks,↓ in agitation and passivity

Gavrilova et al. [40] Russia	N=60 NR	"10/66 Dementia Research group" caregiver intervention—dementia education, behavioral management, problem-solving, coping strategies	5 sessions/30 min/5 weeks	NR	At 6 months, no change in problem behaviors or quality of life
Gerdner et al. [41] USA	N=237 Moderate to severe dementia	Psychoeducational intervention—dementia education, behavioral management, environmental modification, activity engagement	NR/NR/12 months	NR	At 12 months, ↓ in problem behaviors for non-spousal dyads; no change in functional status
Gitlin et al. [42] USA	N=171 NR	Home environmental intervention—dementia education, environmental modification, behavioral management	5 sessions/90 min/3 months	Yes (Formal case reviews, on-site observation of randomly selected visits, and follow-up interviews with CGs)	At 3 months, ↑ in IADL function, no change for self-care or problem behaviors
Gitlin et al. [43] USA	N=190 Moderate to severe dementia	"REACH I" home environmental skill-building program (now called Skills$_2$Care^{Tm}—dementia education, case management, environmental modification, behavioral management, coping strategies, problem solving, adaptive equipment	6 sessions/90 min/6 months	Yes (Case reviews and checklist)	At 6 months, no differences in IADL and ADL function and problem behaviors
Gitlin et al. [44] USA	N=127	Same study as [43]	Same as [43]	Same as [43]	At 6 months,↓ problem behaviors which was sustained to 12 months
Gitlin et al. [45] USA	N=60 Mild to severe dementia	Tailored activity program—dementia education, behavioral management, problem solving, environmental modification, activity engagement, coping strategies	8 sessions/90 min/4 months	NR	At 4 months,↓ problem behaviors including agitation and argumentation
Gitlin et al. [75] USA	N=237 Mild to severe dementia	Biobehavioral environmental intervention ("COPE")—dementia education, case management, environmental modification, activity engagement, caregiver training in home safety, coping strategies	10 sessions/60 min/4 months	Yes (audiotapes reviewed)	At 4 months, ↑ functional status (and specifically for IADLs), activity engagement. Trend in ↑ quality of life; no change in agitated behaviors At 9 months, ↑ in ability of caregivers to keep person at home; no change for function or problem behaviors

(continued)

Table 1 (continued)

Author/Date Country	Sample/Stage of disease	Intervention	# Sessions/Length/ Duration	Fidelity reported	Results related to PwD Intervention effects
Gitlin et al. [80] USA	N = 272 Mild to severe dementia	Advancing caregiver training ("ACT") — dementia education, case management, medical behavior management, medical screening, problem-solving, environmental modification, activity engagement, coping strategies	11 sessions/ 85 min[a]/4 months	Yes (Audiotapes were reviewed)	At 16 weeks,↓ in targeted problem behaviors
Gormley et al. [46] UK	N = 62 Moderate to severe dementia	Behavior management program — dementia education, behavior management, environmental modification	4 sessions/NR/8 weeks	NR	At 8 weeks, : Aggressive behavior (RAGE) (↓, p = .071), RAGE scores over time (↓), BEHAVE-AD (No difference)
Graff et al. [47] Netherlands	N = 135 Mild to moderate dementia	Occupational therapy — dementia education, behavior management, environmental modification, activity engagement, coping strategies	10 sessions/1 h/5 weeks	NR	At 6 and 12 weeks, ↑ quality of life and health status; ↓depression
Guerra et al. [48] Peru	N = 58 Mild to severe dementia	"10/66 Caregiver Intervention" — dementia education, behavior management	5 sessions/30 min/5 weeks	NR	At 6 months, no change in problem behaviors and quality of life
Horvath et al. [49] USA	N = 108 Mild to severe dementia	Home Safety Toolkit (HST) — self-directed, self-paced intervention, which consists of a booklet and sample items	1 session/NR/3 months	Yes (Simulated home visits and regular review meetings)	At 3 months: ↓ risky behaviors and accidents
Huang et al. [50] Taiwan	N = 48 Mild to severe dementia	Caregiver training program — dementia education, behavior management, environmental modification	2 sessions/2–3 h/2 weeks	NR	At 3 weeks and 3 months,↓ problem behaviors (except for "physically aggressive behavior" subscale)
Huang et al. [51] Taiwan	N = 129 Mild to severe dementia	Caregiver-training program with telephone consultation — dementia education, case management, behavior management, environmental modification, coping strategies	2 sessions/NR/3 weeks	Yes (Research nurses and three experts met monthly for case conferences)	At 3 months, ↓ in physically aggressive behaviors
Jansen et al. [52] Netherlands	N = 99 Early symptoms of dementia	Case management — dementia education, behavior management, coping strategies	2 sessions/10.8 h/ year[a]/12 months	Yes (Audiotaped interviews)	At 6 and 12 months, no changes in cognitive functioning, daily living functioning, neuropsychiatric symptoms, and quality of life

Kiosses et al. [53] USA	N = 30 Mild dementia	Problem adaptation therapy ("PATH")—dementia education, environmental modification, behavior management, activity engagement	12 sessions/NR/12 weeks	Yes (Weekly supervision of therapist)	Over 12 weeks, ↓ in depression and disability
Lam et al. [54] Hong Kong	N = 102 Mild dementia	Case management—dementia education, medical treatment, cognitive training, behavior management, environmental modification, activity engagement, coping strategies	4 sessions/NR/4 months	NR	At 4 months, ↓ neuropsychiatric symptoms and depression; no change in quality of life and cognitive state
					At 8 months, ↓ cognitive state; no change in neuropsychiatric symptoms, depression, and quality of life
					None of the changes at 4 and 12 months showed significant group difference.
Livingston et al. [55] UK	N = 173	Manual based coping strategy program ("START")—case management, behavior management	8 sessions/NR/8–14 weeks	Yes (94 % of randomly selected audio-recorded sessions were rated)	At 4 and 8 months, no change in quality of life
Marriott et al. [56] UK	N = 44 Moderate to severe dementia	Cognitive-behavioral family intervention—dementia education, behavior management, coping strategies	14 sessions/NR/7 months	NR	At 9 months, ↓ problem behaviors; no change in ADL function, depression, psychotic symptoms, cognitive function, dementia severity
					At 12 months, ↑ ADL function; no change in problem behaviors and other outcomes
McCurry et al. [57] USA	N = 36 Mild to severe dementia	Sleep education program ("NITE-AD")—sleep hygiene education, physical exercise, light exposure, environmental modification, activity engagement	6 sessions/1 h/2 months	Yes (Tape-recorded sessions)	At 2 and 6 months, ↓ time awake at night and depression, ↑exercise days

(continued)

Table 1 (continued)

Author/Date Country	Sample/Stage of disease	Intervention	# Sessions/Length/Duration	Fidelity reported	Results related to PwD Intervention effects
McCurry et al. [58] USA	N = 132 Mild to moderate dementia	Walking, light exposure, and a combination intervention ("NITE-AD")—sleep hygiene education, physical exercise, behavior management	6 sessions/1 h/8 weeks	Yes (Audiotapes reviewed)	At 8 weeks, ↓ total wake time; no change in subjective sleep quality, sleep percentage, number of awakenings, and total sleep time
					At 6 months, no change in total wake time, subjective sleep quality, sleep percentage, number of awakenings, and total sleep time.
Mittelman et al. [59] USA	N = 206 Mild to severe dementia	Comprehensive support and counseling intervention—dementia education, problem solving, behavior management, emotional support, coping strategies	6 sessions/1.5 h/4 months	NR	At every 6 months up to 8 years, ↓ rate of institutionalization
Mittelman et al. [60] USA	N = 406 Mild to severe dementia	Counseling and support intervention—dementia education, individual and family counseling, ad hoc telephone counseling, support group participation, case management, coping strategies	6 sessions/NR/NR	NR	At every 6 months until 11 years, ↓ rate of institutionalization
Moniz-Cook et al. [61] UK	N = 113 NR	Psychosocial intervention—dementia education, case management, clinical supervision, behavior management, coping strategies	4 sessions/NR/18 months	Yes but poor (Only 2 interventionists sustained the ongoing clinical supervision requirement)	Over 18 months, ↑ Cognitive level, ↓ problem behaviors
Nobili et al. [62] Italy	N = 69 Moderate to severe dementia	Structured educational intervention—dementia education, behavior management, environmental modification, coping strategies	2 sessions/60 or 90 min/NR	NR	At 12 months, ↓ problem behaviors, no change in rate of institutionalization
Pitkala et al. [63] Finland	N = 210 Mild to severe dementia	Exercise trial—dementia education, behavior management, physical exercise	104 sessions/1 h training, twice a week/12 months	NR	At 6 and 12 months, ↑ physical function (motor function, cognitive function); no change on mobility function
Quayhagen et al. [64] USA	N = 78 NR	Cognitive remediation—dementia education, cognitive stimulation, problem-solving, behavior management	12 sessions/NR/12 weeks	NR	At 3 and 9 months, ↑cognitive and behavioral functioning

Samus et al. [65] USA	N = 303 Mild to severe dementia	Care coordination intervention ("MIND")—dementia education, case management, problem-solving, behavior management, activity engagement, coping strategies	2 sessions/NR/18 months	Yes (Observation, meetings, tracking software)	At 18 months, ↑ number of days living at home, quality of life; no change in unmet care needs, proxy-rated quality of life, problem behaviors and depression
Stanley et al. [66] USA	N = 32 Mild to moderate dementia	Cognitive-behavioral therapy ("Peaceful Mind")—dementia education, cognitive training, behavior management, coping strategies	20 sessions/47 min[a]/6 months	Yes (Audiotape reviewed)	At 3 months, ↓ anxiety on one measure but not another; ↑ quality of life; At 6 months, no change in anxiety
Steinberg et al. [67] USA	N = 27 Mild to moderate dementia	Exercise program ("MIND" study)— dementia education, physical exercise (aerobic fitness, strength training, balance and flexibility training)	3 sessions/2 h/12 weeks	NR	At 12 weeks, ↑ hand function task, no change in functional performance, timed 8 foot walk, chair sit to stand
Suttanon et al. [68] Australia	N = 40 Mild to moderate dementia	Balance, strengthening, and walking exercise program—dementia education, physical exercise	6 sessions/15 min/6 months	NR	At 6 months, ↓ fall risk; ↑ functional reach; no change in falls rate, step test, timed chair stand, timed up and go, balance, limits of stability, walking, step quick turn, sit to stand, quality of life
Tappen et al. [69] USA	N = 68 Early stage of dementia	Cognitive training—spaced retrieval, functional task training, compensatory strategies, behavior management	24 sessions/1 h/12 weeks	NR	At 3 months, ↑cognitive and functional performance, no change in functional dependence
Tchalla et al. [70] France	N = 96 Mild to moderate dementia	Home-based technologies coupled with teleassistance service (HBTec-TS)— nightlight path, remote intercom, electronic bracelet, central hot line, etc.	NA/NA/12 months	NR	Over 12 months, ↓falls at home
Teri et al. [71] USA	N = 72 NR	Pleasant events and caregiver problem solving—dementia education, behavior management, activity engagement, coping strategies	9 sessions/1 h/9 weeks	Yes (Meetings)	At 9 weeks and 6 months, ↓ depression; no change in cognition, functional status

(continued)

Table 1 (continued)

Author/Date Country	Sample/Stage of disease	Intervention	# Sessions/Length/ Duration	Fidelity reported	Results related to PwD Intervention effects
Teri et al. [72] USA	N = 153 Moderate to severe dementia	Exercise plus behavioral management—dementia education, physical exercise, behavior management, activity engagement	12 sessions/1 h/3 months	Yes (Videotaped and reviewed)	At 3 months, ↑ physical role function, # of persons who exercised; ↓ depression, # of restricted activity days; no change in mobility
					At 12 months, ↑ physical role function; no change in other outcomes
Teri et al. [73] USA	N = 95 Moderate dementia	Home-based counseling with family caregivers ("STAR-Caregiver")—dementia education, problem-solving, behavior management, activity engagement, coping strategies	8 sessions/1 h/8 weeks	Yes (Audiotapes and paperwork; 95 % adherence rate)	At 2 and 6 months, ↑ quality of life, ↓ problem behaviors
Vreugdenhil et al. [74] USA	N = 40 Mild to moderate dementia	Home exercise program—daily exercises and walking	NR/>30 min walking/4 months	NR	At 4 months, ↑ cognitive function, physical and ADL function

NA not applicable, *NR* not reported

↑ = improvement in the outcome, ↓ = decrease in the outcome

[a]Average duration or number of completed sessions

Table 2 Type and frequency of intervention strategies tested

Intervention strategies	Example	# of studies (%)
Education about dementia	Education session, written material, videotape	49 (100 %)
Behavioral management	ABC approach, problem solving, caregiver communication techniques	41 (84 %)
Coping strategy	Stress management technique, emotional/psychological support, relaxation technique, counseling	29 (59 %)
Case management	Arranging services, making referral, addressing financial & legal issues	20 (41 %)
Environmental modification	Modification of home conditions, use of assistive devices or tools, home safety, home-based technologies for fall prevention	18 (37 %)
Activity engagement	Meaningful activities for person with dementia, pleasant events	13 (27 %)
Psychological, emotional and social support for caregiver	Developing social support network, sharing of the emotional impact of caregiving, improving interpersonal relationships between family members, support group participation	12 (24 %)
Cognitive training	Cognitive rehabilitation, cognitive stimulation, face-name association learning	8 (16 %)
Physical exercise	Daily walking, tailored home-based exercise including endurance, balance, and strength training	8 (16 %)
Sleep education	Exercise, light exposure	2 (4 %)

targeting one entity (person with dementia only, caregiver, or dyad) versus another is more beneficial to the person with dementia with respect to a particular outcome measure.

Interventions

A wide range of behavioral intervention strategies were tested. Although there is not an agreed upon approach to classifying non-pharmacologic strategies, those reviewed here can be grouped, for efficiency purposes, into ten broad types: education, behavioral management, psychosocial coping, case management, environmental modification/home safety/fall, activity engagement, support group, cognitive training, physical exercise, and sleep education.

Most studies tested a combination of strategies. For example, the provision of education about dementia to family caregivers was included in every intervention, instructing caregivers in behavioral management techniques were present in 41 (84 %) studies, helping caregivers learn effective coping strategies (e.g., stress management, relaxation techniques) in 29 (59 %) studies, case management (e.g., arranging services, addressing legal and financial issues) in 20 (41 %) studies, and

environmental modification (e.g., modification of physical environments, simplifying communications and tasks, using assistive devices) in 18 (37 %) studies (Table 2). While many interventions directly targeted the caregiver and their well-being, they appear to have direct benefit to and address the unmet needs of persons with dementia. Also, caregivers serve in the capacity of a therapeutic agent in the delivery, oversight and management of many of these strategies.

Interventions were highly variable in dose, intensity and duration ranging from a single visit to 104 sessions over 12 months, although contacts averaged approximately 1 h in length. No studies tested the dose response relationship and therefore it is not possible to conclude whether more is better and for which types of outcomes. However, from this review it appears that more exposure does seem to be a requisite for certain outcomes such as prevention of relocation.

Glass Half Full

From a historical perspective, targeting persons with dementia themselves for intervention has been a focus of inquiry only in recent years. This may reflect in part the long-standing societal view that as a progressively disabling and incurable illness, there is nothing that can be done to improve the well-being of this population.

Nevertheless, our search revealed a growing, active and increasingly robust body of research that is testing interventions that target a wide range of needs of individuals with dementia. We found evidence that some intervention components affected certain outcomes (e.g. exercise improved functional outcomes, behavior management improved quality of life, and case management delayed time to institutionalization); some interventions appeared to be suitable for persons with dementia across all disease stages; and some interventions appeared to be more appropriate for individuals at a specific disease stage (e.g. cognitive training for early stage dementia). Despite mixed findings across the pooled studies, positive outcomes were reported for every area of concern including for example reductions in functional dependence [42, 75], behavioral symptoms [16], and institutionalization [60]. Noteworthy is that the positive outcomes reported in these studies reviewed here have not been achieved with current pharmacologic agents. Thus, this review provides further and substantial evidence of the important role of non-pharmacologic approaches in the treatment and care of individuals with dementia. It suggests as others have that with the right mix of services and support, persons with dementia can stay at home with life quality [76].

Effective interventions were theory based, appeared to conduct pilot testing before implementation, emphasized skill building, attended to fidelity, and tailored strategies to persons and their physical and social environments. Interventions that impacted distal outcomes (e.g. time to institutionalization) appeared to achieve desired benefits by affecting intermediate factors such as reductions in behaviors or increasing caregiver support [77]. Additionally, no adverse events were reported in these studies; thus they appear to be of low to no risk, highly feasible to implement and acceptable to persons with dementia and their families. As such, these interventions present a menu of options from which the clinician can choose from depending upon resources, time, identified or targeted problem area or unmet need, and desired outcomes.

Glass Half Empty

Despite the strength of this growing body of evidence for interventions that support persons with dementia at home, there are significant limitations that the next generation of intervention studies must address.

First, as shown by Fig. 1, the needs of persons with dementia change with disease progression. As such, a comprehensive, integrated, long-term and multi-faceted dementia care model of service delivery would be necessary that integrates key proven interventions along the disease trajectory. Furthermore, although home dwelling persons with dementia share common characteristics, each person differs in terms of his or her individual strengths and needs, as well as response to specific intervention methods or techniques. Thus, there is no one specific intervention approach that will be effective for all persons, families and their living environments.

It was unclear from this review whether certain persons achieved better outcomes following specific home-based interventions than others. Benefits may vary by demographic subgroup, disease type or stage, caregiver characteristics or other factors. Future research is warranted to examine moderating effects of effective interventions to evaluate generalizability and enhance targeting of interventions. Also, as caregivers serve in many of these studies as the therapeutic agent, it is unclear whether certain interventions are easier than others for families to implement or whether some caregivers do better with some approaches than others. In addition, studies in this review did not address the optimal timing for delivering interventions to achieve the highest benefit for persons with dementia.

Another set of limitations concerns the delivery characteristics of interventions. Interventions were not always clearly characterized making their replication, dissemination, translation and wide-spread implementation and uptake challenging. For example, few if any interventions discuss how much exposure would be necessary in order to achieve a desired effect. There are no guidelines for when to start or stop a particular intervention protocol, how long or how many sessions would be required for benefits to be derived, and how long benefits endure. Moreover, as many of these interventions are necessarily dependent upon family caregivers to provide and continue to use the intervention, greater attention to their characteristics, capabilities and role in intervention delivery is warranted. Some interventions may require too much effort or time for families. Treatment failures may be the result of the intervention protocol or the inability of families to adhere to required actions. Distinguishing between these reasons would help to refine treatment development. These are all critical clinically-oriented questions that would be important to evaluate in future efforts to maximize the relevance and 'real-world' dissemination potential of interventions.

A related point is that many interventions are complex and multi-component. While that makes them more relevant and beneficial to persons with dementia, it may in turn limit their scalability and raise issues as to the necessary readiness and preparation of the workforce to provide these interventions. Future multi-component intervention trials would benefit from theory-based modeling of individual components and rigorous process evaluation of treatment delivery [78, 79]. These analytic strategies would allow for the systematic tailoring of interventions to individual settings or healthcare systems and help to identify core components of an intervention from which to establish a minimum dose necessary to achieve meaningful improvements.

Limitations also concern measurement. The wide variation in outcome measures prohibits cross-study comparisons. Additionally, most outcome measures rely on proxy report, typically a family member, that are subject to bias by latent variables such as caregiver depression or perceived poor quality of life. Traditional psychometric methods provide limited information about a measure's reliability and validity for a specific use. A high global reliability coefficient does not indicate that there will be high measurement precision for different ranges of caregiver burden, for example. Techniques associated with item response theory can provide greater precision of measurement properties to identify these

problems and assist with future measurement construction.

The measures used in most of these 49 intervention studies do not provide an understanding of "clinically meaningful" changes. For example, it is difficult to discern if small changes in the mean score of a functional measure constitutes a clinically meaningful change for the person with dementia or their caregiver or a qualitative improvement in daily life. Future trials need to consider the clinical significance of observed statistically significant changes.

Yet another limitation is the lack of understanding concerning the mechanisms by which these interventions are effective. With few exceptions studies have not examined mediation and moderation effects [42, 77, 80]. At a more fundamental level, the field needs to further develop, test, and apply bio-measures to further characterize mediators of treatment efficacy and clarify the mechanism underlying the effect of interventions [81]. It would be helpful to identify those individuals most likely to benefit from an effective treatment. As such, bio-measures could be used to provide selection criteria or information on differential treatment responses. In addition, bio-measures could be used to clarify the clinically meaningful nature of intervention effects on various outcomes. If it could be shown that changes from these interventions are clinically meaningful in the short and long term, that information would help refine intervention approaches, advance their clinical relevance and galvanize the field.

Future Directions for Intervention Research

Each person with a dementia, whether living alone or with others, has a different family situation and environmental context. Therefore, it is important to assess the strengths and needs of persons with dementia vis a vis their support structure and home environment. As home life is embedded in a cultural context, it is essential to consider the family's culture, primary language and resources when providing home interventions. The role of the household context and culture in designing and implementing the interventions reviewed here were not discussed but should be a concern for future research.

Also needed is the development and testing of a basic package or set of intervention components that could be adjusted based on need and disease stage. For example, as per Fig. 1, we know that persons with dementia and their caregivers need education, problem solving skills and specific strategies across the spectrum of the disease; however, content may vary by disease stage and the constellation of unique challenges encountered.

When considering home-based interventions, it is also important to evaluate their cost and reimbursement potential in order to determine long term sustainability. Many payment sources fail to cover the cost of home-based interventions and will only reimburse for direct patient care only leaving caregiver training or coordination of services an important but unfunded need of families. Other variables to consider are the staff that will be providing the service. If more than one clinician is providing treatment, it is important to consider close collaboration between these professionals as to preserve the fidelity of the intervention. Health information technology may facilitate this process. For example, Bass et al. [29] and Samus et al. [65] each used an electronic care coordination information system for care coordinators in different organizations to share case information and plan together intervention delivery as well as to monitor treatment fidelity.

As we have discussed, future studies should address a host of questions that will enhance the clinical relevance and hence implementation potential of efficacious interventions. The next generation of interventions need to better link the purpose of the intervention to disease stage and etiology, caregiver and care receiver characteristics and unmet needs, examine both objective and subjective measures of desired outcomes, consider if certain groups benefit more than others, identify optimal dosing and if and when booster sessions are needed, and the underlying mechanisms by which interventions work.

Finally, this review was purposely limited to outcomes related to the person with dementia. Nevertheless, of equal concern is the well-being of the over 15 million families who provide care for and assistance to individuals with dementia. It is unclear whether interventions that target the person with dementia have a positive impact on the family caregiver. While there is increasing evidence that the reverse is true, this should be the focus as well for future research.

Conclusions

Collectively, the past 15 years has yielded important interventions that improve different facets of the well-being of individuals with dementia. While this review of available research did not allow us to definitively quantify the impact of dementia interventions, we are able to suggest approaches that seem more likely to have a modest impact in the short run than others. Of the ten categories of interventions identified, evidence of moderate improvements for home dwelling persons with dementia appear strongest for multi-component interventions that include caregiver education about dementia, behavior management, activity engagement and case management. Thus, inclusion of attention to the needs of caregivers may bolster treatment effects for persons with dementia.

Unfortunately, the literature provided no definitive guidance on the specific components of the multi-factor interventions or on whether the benefits of such interventions justify costs of these interventions in terms of maintaining long term clinically, meaningful improvements for caregivers. Effective interventions in the reviewed studies often combined outcome measures of health and well-being and diverse, non-specified intervention strategies and were not designed in a way to determine which specific components of a multi-component intervention would be most effective.

As dementia is a prolonged disease (upwards to 20 years), individuals have a wide range of needs that endure and change over time. As we have shown, a vast array of interventions can be employed now by the field, although more refinements and continual development of novel interventions are also warranted. Current interventions form a menu from which clinicians and service settings can choose from for implementation. In the future, these and the next generation of interventions must be integrated into a broader, more comprehensive overarching framework of dementia care in which improving quality of life at home is an essential ingredient to managing the disease over time. Of note is that inclusion of the caregiver in the delivery of interventions represents a significant paradigm shift in our current health care system in which the focus continues to be on treating the "patient" as a single entity. As this review as well as others concerning caregiver interventions suggest, in the case of dementia, the family serves as the "therapeutic agent" [14] and therefore, must be part of treatment approaches.

Acknowledgements Dr. Gitlin has been supported for research reported in this article in part by funds from the National Institute on Aging and the National Institute on Nursing (Research Grant # RO1 AG22254), the National Institute on Aging (R01 AG041781-01A1), and Alzheimer's Grant NPSASA-10-174265).

Dr. Hodgson has been supported for research reported in this article in part by funds from the National Institute on Aging and National Institute on Nursing Research (Grant K23 NR012017).

References

1. Callahan CM, Arling G, Tu W, Rosenman MB, Counsell SR, Stump TE, et al. Transitions in care for older adults with and without dementia. J Am Geriatr Soc. 2012;60(5):813–20.
2. Alzheimer's Association. 2013 Alzheimer's disease facts and figures. Alzheimers Dement J Alzheimers Assoc. 2013;9(2):208–45. doi:10.1016/j.jalz.2013.02.003.
3. World Health Organization. Dementia caregiving and caregivers. Dementia: a public health priority. Geneva: WHO Press; 2014. p. 67–80.
4. Rabins PV, Lyketsos CG, Steele CD. Practical dementia care. New York, NY: Oxford University Press; 2006.
5. Black BS, Johnston D, Rabins PV, Morrison A, Lyketsos C, Samus QM. Unmet needs of community-residing persons with dementia and their informal caregivers: findings from the maximizing independence at home study. J Am Geriatr Soc. 2013;61(12):2087–95.
6. Gitlin LN, Hodgson N, Piersol CV, Hess E, Hauck WW. Correlates of quality of life for individuals with dementia living at home: the role of home environment, caregiver, and patient-related characteristics. Am J Geriatr Psychiatry. 2014;22(6):587–97. doi:10.1016/j.jagp.2012.11.005.
7. Hodgson N, Gitlin LN, Winter L, Hauck WW. Caregiver's perceptions of the relationship of pain to behavioral and psychiatric symptoms in older community-residing adults with dementia. Clin J Pain. 2014;30(5):421–7. doi:10.1097/AJP.0000000000000018.
8. Ice HG. Daily life in a nursing home: has it changed in 25 years? J Aging Stud. 2002;16(4):345–59.
9. von Kutzleben M, Schmid W, Halek M, Holle B, Bartholomeyczik S. Community-dwelling persons with dementia: what do they need? What do they demand? What do they do? A systematic review on the subjective experiences of persons with dementia. Aging Ment Health. 2012;16(3):378–90.
10. Miranda-Castillo C, Woods B, Orrell M. The needs of people with dementia living at home from user, caregiver and professional perspectives: a cross-sectional survey. BMC Health Serv Res. 2013;13:43-6963-13-43. doi:10.1186/1472-6963-13-43[doi].
11. Samus QM, Rosenblatt A, Steele C, Baker A, Harper M, Brandt J, et al. The association of neuropsychiatric symptoms and environment with quality of life in assisted living residents with dementia. Gerontologist. 2005;45 suppl 1:19–26.
12. Scherder EJ, Bogen T, Eggermont LH, Hamers JP, Swaab DF. The more physical inactivity, the more agitation in dementia. Int Psychogeriatr. 2010;22(08):1203–8.
13. Riley RJ, Burgener S, Buckwalter KC. Anxiety and stigma in dementia: a threat to aging in place. Nurs Clin North Am. 2014;49(2):213–31.
14. Gitlin LN, Hodgson N. Caregivers as therapeutic agents in dementia care: the evidence-base for interventions supporting their role. In: Gaugler JE, Kane RL, editors. Family caregiving in the new normal. Amsterdam: Elsevier. 2015; 305–353.
15. Maslow K. Translating innovation to impact: evidence-based interventions to support people with Alzheimer's disease and their caregivers at home and in the community. A white paper; 2012.
16. Brodaty H, Arasaratnam C. Meta-analysis of non-pharmacological interventions for neuropsychiatric symptoms of dementia. Am J Psychiatry. 2012;169(9):946–53. doi:10.1176/appi.ajp.2012.11101529.
17. Gitlin LN. Good news for dementia care: caregiver interventions reduce behavioral symptoms in people with dementia and family distress. Am J Psychiatry. 2012;169(9):894–7. doi:10.1176/appi.ajp.2012.12060774.
18. Gitlin LN, Kales HC, Lyketsos CG. Nonpharmacologic management of behavioral symptoms in dementia. J Am Med Assoc. 2012;308(19):2020–9. doi:10.1001/jama.2012.36918.

19. O'Neil ME, Freeman M, Christensen V, Telerant R, Addleman A, Kansagara D. Non-pharmacological interventions for behavioral symptoms of dementia: a systematic review of the evidence; 2011. doi:NBK54971 [bookaccession].

20. Olazaran J, Reisberg B, Clare L, Cruz I, Pena-Casanova J, Del Ser T, et al. Nonpharmacological therapies in Alzheimer's disease: a systematic review of efficacy. Dement Geriatr Cogn Disord. 2010;30(2):161–78. doi:10.1159/000316119.

21. Cohen-Mansfield J. Nonpharmacologic interventions for inappropriate behaviors in dementia: a review, summary, and critique. Am J Geriatr Psychiatry. 2001;9(4):361–81.

22. McLaren AN, LaMantia MA, Callahan CM. Systematic review of non-pharmacologic interventions to delay functional decline in community-dwelling patients with dementia. Aging Ment Health. 2013;17(6):655–66.

23. Hodgson NA, Black BS, Johnston D, Lyketsos C, Samus QM. Comparison of unmet care needs across the dementia trajectory: findings from the maximizing independence at home study. J Geriatr Palliat Care. 2014;2(2):5.

24. Trahan MA, Kuo J, Carlson MC, Gitlin LN. A systematic review of strategies to foster activity engagement in persons with dementia. Health Educ Behav. 2014;41(1 Suppl):70S–83S. doi:10.1177/1090198114531782.

25. Dias A, Samuel R, Patel V, Prince M, Parameshwaran R, Krishnamoorthy E. The impact associated with caring for a person with dementia: a report from the 10/66 dementia research group's Indian network. Int J Geriatr Psychiatry. 2004;19(2):182–4.

26. Harker J, Kleijnen J. What is a rapid review? A methodological exploration of rapid reviews in health technology assessments. Int J Evid Based Healthc. 2012;10(4):397–410.

27. Avila R, Carvalho IAM, Bottino CMC, Miotto EC. Neuropsychological rehabilitation in mild and moderate Alzheimer's disease patients. Behav Neurol. 2007;18(4):225–33.

28. Bass DM, Clark PA, Looman WJ, McCarthy CA, Eckert S. The Cleveland Alzheimer's managed care demonstration: outcomes after 12 months of implementation. Gerontologist. 2003;43(1):73–85.

29. Bass DM, Judge KS, Snow AL, Wilson NL, Morgan RO, Maslow K, et al. A controlled trial of partners in dementia care: veteran outcomes after six and twelve months. Alzheimers Res Ther. 2014;6(1):9. doi:10.1186/alzrt242 [doi].

30. Belle SH, Burgio L, Burns R, Coon D, Czaja SJ, Gallagher-Thompson D, et al. Enhancing the quality of life of dementia caregivers from different ethnic or racial groups: a randomized, controlled trial. Ann Intern Med. 2006;145(10):727–38. doi:145/10/727 [pii].

31. Burgener SC, Bakas T, Murray C, Dunahee J, Tossey S. Effective caregiving approaches for patients with Alzheimer's disease. Geriatr Nurs. 1998;19(3):121–6. doi:S0197-4572(98)90055-6 [pii].

32. Burgio L, Stevens A, Guy D, Roth DL, Haley WE. Impact of two psychosocial interventions on White and African American family caregivers of individuals with dementia. Gerontologist. 2003;43(4):568–79.

33. Chang BL. Cognitive-behavioral intervention for homebound caregivers of persons with dementia. Nurs Res. 1999;48(3):173–82.

34. Chien WT, Lee IYM. Randomized controlled trial of a dementia care programme for families of home-resided older people with dementia. J Adv Nurs. 2011;67(4):774–87.

35. Clare L, Linden DE, Woods RT, Whitaker R, Evans SJ, Parkinson CH, et al. Goal-oriented cognitive rehabilitation for people with early-stage Alzheimer disease: a single-blind randomized controlled trial of clinical efficacy. Am J Geriatr Psychiatry. 2010;18(10):928–39. doi:10.1097/JGP.0b013e3181d5792a.

36. Dias A, Dewey ME, D'Souza J, Dhume R, Motghare DD, Shaji KS, et al. The effectiveness of a home care program for supporting caregivers of persons with dementia in developing countries: a randomised controlled trial from Goa, India. PloS One. 2008;3(6), e2333. doi:10.1371/journal.pone.0002333.

37. Eloniemi-Sulkava U, Notkola IL, Hentinen M, Kivela SL, Sivenius J, Sulkava R. Effects of supporting community-living demented patients and their caregivers: a randomized trial. J Am Geriatr Soc. 2001;49(10):1282–7. doi:49255 [pii].

38. Eloniemi-Sulkava U, Saarenheimo M, Laakkonen ML, Pietila M, Savikko N, Kautiainen H, et al. Family care as collaboration: effectiveness of a multicomponent support program for elderly couples with dementia. Randomized controlled intervention study. J Am Geriatr Soc. 2009;57(12):2200–8. doi:10.1111/j.1532-5415.2009.02564.x.

39. Fitzsimmons S, Buettner LL. Therapeutic recreation interventions for need-driven dementia-compromised behaviors in community-dwelling elders. Am J Alzheimers Dis Other Demen. 2002;17(6):367–81.

40. Gavrilova SI, Ferri CP, Mikhaylova N, Sokolova O, Banerjee S, Prince M. Helping carers to care—the 10/66 dementia research group's randomized control trial of a caregiver intervention in Russia. Int J Geriatr Psychiatry. 2009;24(4):347–54. doi: 10.1002/gps.2126.

41. Gerdner LA, Buckwalter KC, Reed D. Impact of a psychoeducational intervention on caregiver response to behavioral problems. Nurs Res. 2002;51(6):363–74.

42. Gitlin LN, Corcoran M, Winter L, Boyce A, Hauck WW. A randomized, controlled trial of a home environmental intervention effect on efficacy and upset in caregivers and on daily function of persons with dementia. Gerontologist. 2001;41(1):4–14.

43. Gitlin LN, Winter L, Corcoran M, Dennis MP, Schinfeld S, Hauck WW. Effects of the home environmental skill-building program on the caregiver-care recipient dyad: 6-month outcomes from the Philadelphia REACH initiative. Gerontologist. 2003; 43(4):532–46.

44. Gitlin LN, Hauck WW, Dennis MP, Winter L. Maintenance of effects of the home environmental skill-building program for family caregivers and individuals with Alzheimer's disease and related disorders. J Gerontol A Biol Sci Med Sci. 2005; 60(3):368–74. doi:60/3/368 [pii].

45. Gitlin LN, Winter L, Burke J, Chernett N, Dennis MP, Hauck WW. Tailored activities to manage neuropsychiatric behaviors in persons with dementia and reduce caregiver burden: a randomized pilot study. Am J Geriatr Psychiatry. 2008;16(3):229–39.

46. Gormley N, Lyons D, Howard R. Behavioural management of aggression in dementia: a randomized controlled trial. Age Ageing. 2001;30(2):141–5.

47. Graff MJ, Vernooij-Dassen MJ, Thijssen M, Dekker J, Hoefnagels WH, Olderikkert MG. Effects of community occupational therapy on quality of life, mood, and health status in dementia patients and their caregivers: a randomized controlled trial. J Gerontol A Biol Sci Med Sci. 2007;62(9):1002–9. doi:62/9/1002 [pii].

48. Guerra M, Ferri CP, Fonseca M, Banerjee S, Prince M. Helping carers to care: the 10/66 dementia research Group's randomized control trial of a caregiver intervention in Peru. Revista Brasileira De Psiquiatria. 2011;33(1):47–54.

49. Horvath KJ, Trudeau SA, Rudolph JL, Trudeau PA, Duffy ME, Berlowitz D. Clinical trial of a home safety toolkit for Alzheimer's disease. Int J Alzheimers Dis. 2013;2013:913606.

50. Huang HL, Shyu YI, Chen MC, Chen ST, Lin LC. A pilot study on a home-based caregiver training program for improving caregiver self-efficacy and decreasing the behavioral problems of elders with dementia in Taiwan. Int J Geriatr Psychiatry. 2003;18(4):337–45. doi:10.1002/gps.835.

51. Huang HL, Kuo LM, Chen YS, Liang J, Huang HL, Chiu YC, et al. A home-based training program improves caregivers' skills and dementia patients' aggressive behaviors: a randomized controlled trial. Am J Geriatr Psychiatry. 2013;21(11):1060–70. doi:10.1016/j.jagp.2012.09.009.

52. Jansen APD, van Hout HPJ, Nijpels G, Rijmen F, Dröes RM, Pot AM, et al. Effectiveness of case management among older adults with early symptoms of dementia and their primary informal caregivers: a randomized clinical trial. Int J Nurs Stud. 2011;48(8):933–43. doi:10.1016/j.ijnurstu.2011.02.004.

53. Kiosses DN, Arean PA, Teri L, Alexopoulos GS. Home-delivered problem adaptation therapy (PATH) for depressed, cognitively impaired, disabled elders: a preliminary study. Am J Geriatr Psychiatry. 2010;18(11):988–98. doi:10.1097/JGP.0b013e3181d6947d.

54. Lam LC, Lee JS, Chung JC, Lau A, Woo J, Kwok TC. A randomized controlled trial to examine the effectiveness of case management model for community dwelling older persons with mild dementia in Hong Kong. Int J Geriatr Psychiatry. 2010;25(4):395–402. doi:10.1002/gps.2352.

55. Livingston G, Barber J, Rapaport P, Knapp M, Griffin M, King D, et al. Clinical effectiveness of a manual based coping strategy programme (START, STrAtegies for RelaTives) in promoting the mental health of carers of family members with dementia: pragmatic randomised controlled trial. Br Med J. 2013;347:f6276.

56. Marriott A, Donaldson C, Tarrier N, Burns A. Effectiveness of cognitive-behavioural family intervention in reducing the burden of care in carers of patients with Alzheimer's disease. Br J Psychiatry. 2000;176:557–62.

57. McCurry SM, Gibbons LE, Logsdon RG, Vitiello MV, Teri L. Nighttime insomnia treatment and education for Alzheimer's disease: a randomized, controlled trial. J Am Geriatr Soc. 2005;53(5):793–802.

58. McCurry SM, Pike KC, Vitiello MV, Logsdon RG, Larson EB, Teri L. Increasing walking and bright light exposure to improve sleep in community-dwelling persons with Alzheimer's disease: results of a randomized, controlled trial. J Am Geriatr Soc. 2011;59(8):1393–402. doi:10.1111/j.1532-5415.2011.03519.x.

59. Mittelman MS, Ferris SH, Shulman E, Steinberg G, Levin B. A family intervention to delay nursing home placement of patients with Alzheimer disease: a randomized controlled trial. J Am Med Assoc. 1996;276(21):1725–31.

60. Mittelman MS, Haley WE, Clay OJ, Roth DL. Improving caregiver well-being delays nursing home placement of patients with Alzheimer disease. Neurology. 2006;67(9):1592–9. doi:10.1186/1472-6963-13-43 [pii].

61. Moniz-Cook E, Elston C, Gardiner E, Agar S, Silver M, Win T, et al. Can training community mental health nurses to support family carers reduce behavioural problems in dementia? An exploratory pragmatic randomised controlled trial. Int J Geriatr Psychiatry. 2008;23(2):185–91. doi:10.1002/gps.1860.

62. Nobili A, Riva E, Tettamanti M, Lucca U, Liscio M, Petrucci B, et al. The effect of a structured intervention on caregivers of patients with dementia and problem behaviors: a randomized controlled pilot study. Alzheimer Dis Assoc Disord. 2004;18(2):75–82.

63. Pitkala KH, Poysti MM, Laakkonen ML, Tilvis RS, Savikko N, Kautiainen H, et al. Effects of the Finnish Alzheimer's disease exercise trial (FINALEX): a randomized controlled trial. JAMA Int Med. 2013;173(10):894–901. doi:10.1001/jamainternmed.2013.359.

64. Quayhagen MP, Quayhagen M, Corbeil RR, Roth PA, Rodgers JA. A dyadic remediation program for care recipients with dementia. Nurs Res. 1995;44(3):153–9.

65. Samus QM, Johnston D, Black BS, Hess E, Lyman C, Vavilikolanu A, et al. A multidimensional home-based care coordination intervention for elders with memory disorders: the maximizing independence at home (MIND) pilot randomized trial. Am J Geriatr Psychiatry. 2014;22(4):398–414.

66. Stanley MA, Calleo J, Bush AL, Wilson N, Snow AL, Kraus-Schuman C, et al. The peaceful mind program: a pilot test of a cognitive-behavioral therapy-based intervention for anxious patients with dementia. Am J Geriatr Psychiatry. 2013;21(7):696–708.

67. Steinberg M, Leoutsakos JM, Podewils LJ, Lyketsos CG. Evaluation of a home-based exercise program in the treatment of Alzheimer's disease: the Maximizing Independence in Dementia (MIND) study. Int J Geriatr Psychiatry. 2009;24(7):680–5. doi:10.1002/gps.2175.

68. Suttanon P, Hill KD, Said CM, Williams SB, Byrne KN, LoGiudice D, et al. Feasibility, safety and preliminary evidence of the effectiveness of a home-based exercise programme for older people with Alzheimer's disease: a pilot randomized controlled trial. Clin Rehabil. 2013;27(5):427–38. doi:10.1177/0269215512460877.

69. Tappen RM, Hain D. The effect of in-home cognitive training on functional performance of individuals with mild cognitive impairment and early-stage Alzheimer's disease. Res Gerontol Nurs. 2014;7(1):14–24. doi:10.3928/19404921-20131009-01.

70. Tchalla AE, Lachal F, Cardinaud N, Saulnier I, Rialle V, Preux PM, et al. Preventing and managing indoor falls with home-based technologies in mild and moderate Alzheimer's disease patients: pilot study in a community dwelling. Dement Geriatr Cogn Disord. 2013;36(3-4):251–61. doi:10.1159/000351863.

71. Teri L, Logsdon RG, Uomoto J, McCurry SM. Behavioral treatment of depression in dementia patients: a controlled clinical trial. J Gerontol B Psychol Sci Soc Sci. 1997;52(4):159–66.

72. Teri L, Gibbons LE, McCurry SM, Logsdon RG, Buchner DM, Barlow WE, et al. Exercise plus behavioral management in patients with Alzheimer's disease: a randomized controlled trial. J Am Med Assoc. 2003;290(15):2015–22. doi:10.1001/jama.290.15.2015.

73. Teri L, McCurry SM, Logsdon R, Gibbons LE. Training community consultants to help family members improve dementia care: a randomized controlled

trial. Gerontologist. 2005;45(6):802–11. doi:45/6/802 [pii].

74. Vreugdenhil A, Cannell J, Davies A, Razay G. A community-based exercise programme to improve functional ability in people with Alzheimer's disease: a randomized controlled trial. Scand J Caring Sci. 2012;26(1):12–9. doi:10.1111/j.1471-6712.2011.00895.x.

75. Gitlin LN, Winter L, Dennis MP, Hodgson N, Hauck WW. A biobehavioral home-based intervention and the well-being of patients with dementia and their caregivers: the COPE randomized trial. JAMA. 2010;304(9):983–91. doi:10.1001/jama.2010.1253.

76. Gould E, Basta P. Home is where the heart Is—for people in all stages of dementia. Generations. 2013;37(3):74–8.

77. Roth DL, Mittelman MS, Clay OJ, Madan A, Haley WE. Changes in social support as mediators of the impact of a psychosocial intervention for spouse caregivers of persons with Alzheimer's disease. Psychol Aging. 2005;20(4):634.

78. Craig P, Dieppe P, Macintyre S, Michie S, Nazareth I, Petticrew M, et al. Developing and evaluating complex interventions: the new medical research council guidance. BMJ (Clin Res Ed). 2008;337:a1655. doi:10.1136/bmj.a1655.

79. Möhler R, Bartoszek G, Köpke S, Meyer G. Proposed criteria for reporting the development and evaluation of complex interventions in healthcare (CReDECI): guideline development. Int J Nurs Stud. 2012;49(1):40–6.

80. Gitlin LN, Winter L, Dennis MP, Hodgson N, Hauck WW. Targeting and managing behavioral symptoms in individuals with dementia: a randomized trial of a nonpharmacological intervention. J Am Geriatr Soc. 2010;58(8):1465–74. doi:10.1111/j.1532-5415.2010.02971.x.

81. Hodgson NA, Granger DA. Collecting saliva and measuring salivary cortisol and alpha-amylase in frail community residing older adults via family caregivers. JoVE (J Vis Exp);(82):e50815–e50815.

Experiences and Perspectives of Family Caregivers of the Person with Dementia

Jan McGillick and Maggie Murphy-White

Learning Objectives

After reading this chapter readers will be able to:

1. Identify the influence of gender, gender identity, relationship status, ethnicity, the stage of dementia and the use of health care settings upon the caregiving experience.
2. Examine factors that contribute to adverse and positive experiences of providing care for a person with dementia over time.
3. Cite evidence for the scope, societal value and costs of family care for those with dementia.

Who Are Today's Dementia Family Caregivers?

Millions of people worldwide are family caregivers supporting persons with Alzheimer's disease and related dementias such as Lewy Bodies that cause attendant changes in memory, judgment, behavior, thinking and function. These same caregivers are fighting daily to assure a person-centered approach: i.e., care that upholds the dignity, life story, personhood, humanity, well-being, comfort and core identity of those affected [1]. In this chapter, caregiving refers to attending to another individual's health needs without pay to include assistance with one or more activities of daily living (ADLs; such as bathing and dressing) as well as, extensive help with Instrumental Activities of Daily Living (IADL) such as money management, shopping, home maintenance [2]. The term care partners refers to family members or members of intentional kinship networks such as friends, members of faith communities and extended social or work related relationships. In the early stages of the disease, caregiving may lend itself to more mutual cooperation and shared responsibility; thus, creating partners in care, or care partners. Later in the disease, carers take on more of the surrogate decision-making and hands on, physical care roles.

Caregiving Facts and Figures

In 2013, 15.5 million American caregivers provided an estimated 17.7 billion hours of unpaid care for people with Alzheimer's disease and other dementias, valued at more than $220 billion. Eighty-five percent of help provided to all older adults in the United States is from family members [3]. Additionally, caregivers of people with dementia spend more hours per week

J. McGillick (✉)
Dolan Memory Care Homes, P.O. Box 4082,
Chesterfield, MO 63006, USA
e-mail: jmcgillick@dolancare.com

M. Murphy-White
339 Swan Lake Dr, Dardenne Prairie,
MO 63368, USA
e-mail: mmurphywhite@gmail.com

providing care than non-dementia caregivers. Additionally, they report greater employment complications, caregiver strain, mental and physical health problems, family time and less time for leisure [4]. The unique characteristics of those caring for people with dementia and their challenges are explored in this chapter.

Complex Composition of Caregivers

Caregivers come from many ethnic backgrounds, socioeconomic strata, communities, environments and family situations. There are many diversity factors to consider when profiling the caregiving population. Some less referred to in the literature include: sexual orientation or identity, employment status, distance carers, new Americans, those in military service, caring for a developmentally disabled elder or members of religious communities such as Catholic Sisters and Brothers. Those caring for more than one loved one with dementia is also expanding [5]. Data that summarizes some of these groups and caregiving relationships with the person with dementia is explored below.

Women as Caregivers

There are 2.5 times more women than men providing intensive "on-duty" care 24 h a day for someone with Alzheimer's. More than 60 % of Alzheimer's and dementia caregivers from the above categories are women. In 2009–2010 caregiving data was collected in eight states and the District of Columbia from the Behavioral Risk Factor Surveillance System (BRFSS) surveys. It indicates 65 % of caregivers of people with Alzheimer's disease and other dementias were women; 21 % were 65 years old and older; 64 % were currently employed, a student or a homemaker; and 71 % were married or in a long-term relationship [6]. Women's roles in caregiving are a significant focus for new research and resources. While many provide care for a family member, according to the Alzheimer's Association, women are still at the epicenter of the growing Alzheimer's epidemic [7]. As indicated in Table 1, the burdens of female caregivers are heightened by the amount of time they spend with the person with dementia.

Table 1 Comparisons of caregiver strains

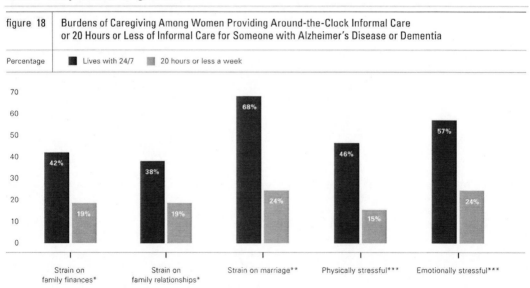

| figure 18 | Burdens of Caregiving Among Women Providing Around-the-Clock Informal Care or 20 Hours or Less of Informal Care for Someone with Alzheimer's Disease or Dementia |

Percentage   ■ Lives with 24/7   ▓ 20 hours or less a week

Created from data from the 2014 Alzheimer's Association Women and Alzheimer's Poll.[A17]

* A "great deal" or "good amount" of strain reported.

** Responded "Yes" when questioned whether caregiving was causing marital strain.

*** Responded 5 (very stressful) when asked to rate stress on a scale of 1-5.

Source: Alzheimer's Association 2014 Alzheimer's Disease Facts and Figures.

The typical family caregiver is a 49-year-old woman caring for her widowed 69-year-old mother who does not live with her. She is married and employed. Approximately 66 % of family caregivers are women. More than 37 % have children or grandchildren under 18 years old living with them [8]. National averages predict that women will spend an average of 27 combined years caring for children and parents over the course of their lifetime. As availability of earlier diagnosis and treatments that may work to plateau symptoms of Alzheimer's disease (AD) in some, become the norm, female carers could spend closer to 40 years in these roles either sequentially or simultaneously [9].

Men as Caregivers

Approximately 14.5 million caregivers are men. Male caregivers are less likely to provide personal care, but 24 % helped a loved one get dressed compared to 28 % of female caregivers; 16 % of male caregivers help with bathing versus 30 % of females. 40 % of male caregivers use paid assistance for a loved one's personal care (The National Alliance for Caregiving and AARP 2012). A national study of male caregivers revealed that the average male caregiver was a white, protestant, middle class, moderately well-educated, retired man who was 68 years old. Most caregivers were husbands taking care of their wives [10]. This may account for the lack of information regarding other male caregivers, such as sons.

Additional research regarding male caregiving is needed. In particular, research fully linking men's caregiving, to men's health issues as a means to articulate strategies to sustain the health and well-being of male caregivers. This seems especially relevant in light of the closing gender gap in life expectancy, which will ultimately see many men providing direct care to their partners [11].

Results of the 2014 Alzheimer's Association Women and Alzheimers Poll indicate that male caregivers are more likely to share the caregiver burden [2]. Participants of Male Caregiver Groups sponsored around the country by Alzheimer's Association chapters and other organizations, report perceptions of lowered stress and isolation and greater access to useful information than peers that do not participate in such groups.

A Male Caregiver's Perspective

MJ, an 80 year old spouse, cared for his wife Lisa, both at home and in a skilled nursing community for over 10 years. During the last four years of her life, he also helped start 2 support groups for male caregivers, attended collectively by about 30 men. He reports, "New guys are coming all the time. We have older men, but younger guys too. One story, that of a successful architect in the height of his career, really got to me. His wife was diagnosed at 52, and he just lost her at age 59. He quit his job to care for her. This group really helped him through all this and now he helps other guys.

MJ goes on to say... The big thing both the older and younger men share is guilt. And I let them know, you will never entirely get over that you just learn to live with it or keep it at bay. Another thing I notice again and again in our meetings is that us boys like specific answers. So the guys ask 'When will I know it is time to give up entire control over care, i.e.place my loved one in a care setting?' And there is no specific answer for that. You can't set your clock. But what often comes out in our discussions, is that we just want our loved one near us for as long as possible...sometimes even when it is no longer safe for either of us. We guys try to stretch our patience beyond our own strength without realizing it. They want a sign or a message about exactly the right time to make "the decision". That is just not the way life rolls out. One man, whose wife has Lewy body dementia keeps asking me 'when did you know?'. I asked him if he felt safe taking care of his wife and he responded "are you kidding? I never turn my back on her... last time I did she came after me."

Spouses as Caregivers

Caregiving for a spouse with dementia brings specific relational challenges. Many spouses experience denial which may be a beneficial coping mechanism as they become educated about the anticipated anguish and reality of what Alzheimer's will mean to their relationship. The spousal relationship will change throughout the course of the disease. Roles, responsibilities and intimacy will all begin to look different as the disease progresses [12]. Subtle adaptations may turn into major lifestyle and relational changes. Social transitions will occur as couples try to maintain friendships and networks. Spouses are the most likely caregivers to live 24/7 with the person with dementia. They may feel uniquely overburdened because they find it difficult to get away from the home, to take a break and to care for themselves. All caregivers struggle with the balance of caring for the person with dementia and caring for themselves. This struggle may have dramatic consequences. The *Journal of American Medical Association* reports that if you are a spousal caregiver between the ages of 66 and 96, and are experiencing ongoing mental or emotional strain as a result of your caregiving duties, there's a 63 % increased risk of dying over those people in the same age group who are not caring for a spouse. This indicates the urgent need for caregiving spouses to find resources and support [13].

Children and Others as Caregivers

Society well recognizes the role spouses often play as providers of care for persons with dementia, but providers in the field similarly observe, children, stepchildren, former spouses, grandchildren, nieces, nephews, siblings, friends, intentional family members, partners and even parents involved in some aspects of the caregiving role. The Aging, Demographics, and Memory Study (ADAMS), based on a nationally representative subsample of older adults from the Health and Retirement Survey, indicates over half of primary caregivers (55 %) of people with dementia took care of parents [14]. They may be assisted by a variety of "adjuncts" such as care managers, trust officers and legal guardians as well as a host of paid caregivers. Many children report the benefits of caring for their parent, including bringing the family closer and feeling good about taking care of someone. However, complications of caring for parents can include, struggling with role reversal, unresolved familial issues and resentment. Because adult children are the largest group of carers for people with dementia, there are many support groups, blogs and resources to provide support.

First Fear by Adult Daughter

In the very early times, before we even had a handle on what was going on with mom, I thought I was losing my ability to relate well with her or interpret what she was communicating to me. One minute she would be saying the most logical thing and another minute her thoughts seemed so confusing to me. It just did not make sense and I thought my own brain was playing tricks on me. Mom was living in Florida at the time. I would visit her and then my sister would and we would try to compare notes. But I think the most helpful thing we did together as siblings, was to decide to visit mom together so we could both experience in real time together what each of us had been noticing but doubting ourselves about. During this trip we witnessed together the early, but undeniable symptoms mom was experiencing and we were able to validate each others feelings and develop a game plan over time. I have moved mom here, close to me. And I do provide the care planning, the visits to her in her memory care assisted living and the financial oversight. But, I am so lucky, my sister and brother in law are incredible and available by phone. I call them almost daily to vent, report on mom's well being and bounce around ideas and decisions.

Club Sandwich Generation Caregivers

The "sandwich generation caregiver" is a nomenclature that has described a mid-life person who simultaneously cares for dependent minor children and aging parents. But the phenomenon of sandwich generation is now becoming more nuanced and multi-generational. A 65 year old may have a 90 year old parent, and also may have responsibilities for multiple elders in their family such as care of in-laws, middle aged children, grandchildren and even great-grandchildren. An 80 year old may have a 100 year old parent and a 60 year old adult child and all three generations suffer with a variety of comorbid, age related conditions. Data from recent years suggest that demographic changes (such as parents of dependent minors being older than in the past and the aging in general of the U.S. population) have led to increases in the number of what these authors call "Club Sandwich Families"; family members involved in three or more layers of familial caregiving. This is not unique to dementia care, but given that prevalence is on a dramatic rise, one can expect to see club sandwich generation caregivers growing as well. It is known that 30 % of Alzheimer's disease and dementia caregivers had children under 18 years old living with them [8, 15]. About one-third of elderly care recipients have Alzheimer's disease or another dementia [8]. Studies have found that sandwich generation caregivers are present in 8–13 % of households in the United States [16]. Studies concur that sandwich generation caregivers experience unique challenges related to the demands of providing care for both aging parents and dependent children. Such challenges include limited time, energy and financial resources [17, 18]. This leads to conjecture that "club sandwich caregivers" may be at exceptional risk for anxiety, depression and lower well-being due to the unique challenges these individuals experience [19].

> **RM's Perspective as A Sandwiched Caregiver**
>
> *RM is a 57 year old daughter who over the last four years from a distance has shared caring for her 80 year old dad with Lewy Bodies disease with her mom, the primary caregiver. She makes the trip to Virginia from her midwest city about every other month. After growing concerns about her mom, RM accompanied her to a neurologist who assessed her mother and diagnosed her with Alzheimer's disease. RM's 97 year old grandmother, who she tries to visit, lives in yet another town. Grandma is currently well cared for by a live in companion, but remains a concern. RM's son is preparing for his freshmen year out of town in college. In the midst of all this, she is struggling to get her parents to agree to sell their beloved home and relocate close to her. She is working to find a "memory care" assisted living community. Her goal is to find somewhere that can meet her mom's early stage needs and her dads later stage needs. The financial impact of all the involved travel, time off work and cost of care is staggering.*

Parents as Caregivers: When Your Child Has Dementia

As persons have access to more timely and accurate diagnosis, leading to earlier identification of dementia, parents of early onset individuals are also seen providing or coordinating care. Evidence-based information on this growing trend is lacking in the literature. It is a very difficult scenario as this may take place at a time of diminished health and financial resources for that parent. If other children, or spouses are available, they may find themselves sharing the care and supporting the grieving parent as a co-caregiver, adding to the collective familial stress.

A Mother's Story: My Daughter has early onset Alzheimer's Disease

I am 97 and experiencing some dementia myself, but I remember some of my earliest perceptions about my daughter's illness. I had a sister who suffered from Alzheimer's, but it was never openly acknowledged in our family. I can remember visiting her with my daughter, HM in the Veteran's home in which my sibling resided. Ironically, my sis had a very odd symptom at this stage of repeating poetry like phrases all in rhyme. They made no sense, but were amazing to listen to. So my daughter knew about AD at an early age.. I was in denial for a long time when it was my daughter HM's turn. What mother can admit that her adult, middle aged child, who still looked so young, had this disease? I took it personally and felt guilty. Like it was my fault she had gotten this. That was almost 14 years ago. Helen is my youngest and only female child. She always felt I favored her brothers and perhaps I did. I used to call her Suzie in those days. Now my daughter has been in a nursing home for 8 years. It is strange, but it is easier for me now that she seems more like a child. Her brother, my son, John brings me to visit and until 2 years ago she recognized me. I am calling her Suzie again.

Evidence is just emerging on the relatively newly recognized phenomenon of parents of individuals with Down syndrome (DS), who are at especially high risk of developing Alzheimer's disease. These parents in their 60s–80s may find themselves caring for a developmentally disabled adult with Alzheimer's disease. They may be particularly ill prepared for this possibility due to the lack of good medical care or cognitive screenings for persons aging with Down syndrome. Plus, information and education about the DS Alzheimer's risk factor is only recently being disseminated more widely by groups such as the National Association on Down Syndrome, the National Down Syndrome Society and the National Alzheimer's Association. Special care environments for these individuals are virtually lacking. Estimates show that Alzheimer's disease affects about 30 % of people with Down syndrome in their 50s. By their 60s, this number comes closer to 50 % [20]. Only 25 % of persons with DS live more than 60 years, and most of those have AD. Individuals with Down syndrome develop AD symptoms identical to those described in individuals without DS. Given the early age of onset (40s–50s) of AD in individuals with DS, their parents in their 70s and 80s may be navigating the difficult waters of getting accurate diagnosis for their adult child in a health care system not prepared for this presentation [21]. These caregivers fight a battle of poor awareness,

few appropriate medical services or knowledgeable professionals available to guide them. They also deal with the highly possible reality of outliving their child with AD [22].

Employed Caregivers

Another important aspect of caregiving to examine is employment status. Interestingly, working and non-working adult children are almost equally as likely to be caregivers. Eighty-one percent of Alzheimer's caregivers under the age of 65 are employed. Thirty-five percent of those over age 65 were employed while caregiving [8]. As the baby boomers postpone their retirement, the number of caregivers working into later years from 66 to 70+, will likely increase. Caregiving in any age group often means adjustments to work schedules are necessary, which may lead to job insecurity and elevated stress for caregivers. Table 2 indicates some of the consequences of juggling work and caregiving. Early retirement rates or breaks in employment to provide care, are also more prevalent in carers of people with dementia. It is reasonable to consider that these demands will affect the caregiver's economic status for years to come. The total estimated lost wages, pension and social security benefits of these caregivers are nearly $3 trillion. The estimated impact on lost Social Security benefits for the average caregiver is $303,000 [23].

Table 2 Impacts of family caregiving for a person with dementia on employment

figure 19	Consequences of Caregiving on Aspects of Employment Among Female and Male Caregivers
Percentage	▨ Women ■ Men

Created from data from the 2014 Alzheimer's Association Women and Alzheimer's Poll.[A17]

Source: Alzheimer's Association 2014 Alzheimer's Disease Facts and Figures.

While working and non-working adult children are almost equally as likely to provide care, adult children 50 and over who work, are more likely to have poor health than those who are not caregivers [23].

Long Distance Caregivers

Long distance caregiving can add unique and complicated challenges to an already stressful and emotional situation. Studies have defined a long distance caregiver in different ways. Some suggest the term apply to caregiving from 100 miles or more away from the person with dementia. Others indicate that the most important factor to define, is the amount of time it takes to travel to the person requiring care. Those studies propose that living an hour or more away constitutes a long distance caregiver.

Clearly long distance caregivers enlist the aid of others to provide the daily care of the person with dementia. Often, the long distance caregiver is not the primary caregiver, but plays the role of a counselor, helper or source of respite. Long distance caregivers who are the primary caregivers, 5 %, depend more heavily on paid caregivers. It has been estimated that

long distance caregiving costs twice as much as for those more proximate [24]. Additionally, these caregivers may spend more time away from other family, friends, work and home life as they travel frequently to see their loved one.

Families with special needs for caregiving support include those who may be deployed in or out of country due to military service, those who work overseas for non-governmental entities or work in a foreign country for international firms. As our world shrinks and becomes more interdependent, this group of long distance caregivers, coupled with the boomers anticipated needs for dementia care, raises both ethical and logistical questions. With the number of long distance caregivers increasing, it is important to explore resources and accessible support to these individuals. There may be some offset for these caregivers by other members of the family such as adult children moving back in with a demented parent for both economic and caregiving reasons as alluded to earlier in this chapter. Technology also holds promise for the possibility of closer communication between geographically dispersed caregivers and their loved one with AD. The availability of safety tracking systems, visual viewing, cueing and monitoring devices may become more affordable and routine for popular use.

Korean Granddaughter - Long Distance Caregiving

I am 31 and in the US working towards my PhD. But my heart is in Korea. I came to America to pursue a PhD in geriatric social work. My first intention was to study public policy, but after my grandmother was diagnosed with dementia, I quickly switched my interest to geriatric social work. I went home this summer and stayed longer than I intended to care for my grandmother. We have a very special relationship and I know I cheer her up. And yet her depression grows. She just suffered a second stroke and will probably have to go live in a nursing home soon after the hospital. The good news is my Aunt works there. The bad news is that I needed to return to America to complete my studies. Goodbye Grandma.

Ethnic Diversity Factors

Diversity among caregivers is an important factor to consider. African-Americans, are **two times more likely** to develop late-onset alzheimer's disease than whites and less likely to have a diagnosis of their condition, resulting in less time for treatment and planning. Clearly, this will impact the African-American caregivers stress and access to resources and support. A 2006 analysis [25] on caregivers of African-Americans with dementia, found that African-American primary caregivers are more likely to be adult children, extended family or friends rather than spouses who constitute the primary caregiver norm for white counterparts. She summarizes various studies on the explanatory models and strong cultural expectations around care of African-Americans with dementia. Lower use of formal care supports or long term care settings in this population has been well documented. Other recent research, about perceptions of African-American carers, regarding role strain versus positive aspects of caregiving report contrasting results. Some indicators propose that African-Americans find caregiving more rewarding than whites, while other studies demonstrate a wide range of psychological burden especially among higher educated female caregivers [26]. Among caregivers of people with Alzheimer's disease and other dementias, the National Alliance for Caregiving (NAC) and AARP found the following [14].

- Fifty-four percent of white caregivers assist a parent, compared with 38 % of individuals from other racial/ethnic groups.
- On average, Hispanic and African-American caregivers spend more time caregiving (approximately 30 h/week) than non-Hispanic white caregivers (20 h/week) and Asian-American caregivers (16 h/week).
- Hispanic (45 %) and African-American (57 %) caregivers are more likely to experience high burden from caregiving than whites (33 %) and Asian-Americans (30 %).

Data collection around many other groups of caregivers such as, Asian-American, new immigrant populations and among non-English speaking populations is scarce, but emerging.

Caregiving for and by LGBT Community

Often lesbian, gay, bisexual or transgender (LGBT) individuals have experienced challenges with family, friends, employers and service providers. This experience may create unique challenges for these caregivers. For example, LGBT individuals may seek medical care less regularly due to fear of inadequate treatment or discrimination. Regardless, a recent survey indicated respondents who were lesbian, gay, bi-sexual or transgendered were more likely than other respondents to have cared for an elderly family member in the last 6 months [27].

In a MetLife study, both men and women are likely to be caregivers in near equal proportions: 20 % men vs. 22 % women in the LGBT group, and 17 % men vs. 18 % women in the general population sample. Male caregivers report providing more hours of care than female caregivers: the average weekly hours of care provided by women from both the LGBT and general population samples is similar—26 vs. 28 h—but LGBT men provide far more hours of care than men from the comparison sample: 41 vs. 29 h. This reflects that about 14 % of the gay men indicate that they are full-time caregivers, spending over 150 h/week in this capacity, compared to 3 % of the lesbian and 2 % of the bisexual respondents [28].

As we explore diversity and relationships among caregivers there are a vast number of "invisible" or less visible sub-groups. There are many diverse groups not discussed in detail here; such as, vowed religious, military personnel, divorced spouses, former in-laws, and non-related caregivers. The key is recognizing that caregivers are extremely heterogeneous and each category bring their unique relationships, values, perspectives, history and beliefs to their caregiving experience.

Likely Course of the Caregiving Experience: A Family Disease Perspective—The First Fear to Last Tear Phases

Due to the slow, insidious progression of Alzheimer's and some other dementias, the duration of caregiving for these persons, averages 4–8 years after a diagnosis of Alzheimer's disease. As care improves and other wellness tactics are deployed it is not rare for otherwise healthy individuals to live as long as 15 or more years with dementia [29]. Table 3 illustrates the variations in the caregiving experience as the person with dementia moves through the disease process.

Physical Care

Though the care provided by family members of people with Alzheimer's disease and other dementias is somewhat similar to the help provided by caregivers of people with other conditions, dementia caregivers tend to provide more extensive assistance. Family members of people with dementia are more likely than caregivers of other older people to assist with any activities of daily living (ADL). Physical care demands can be wide-ranging and in some instances all-encompassing. Table 4 summarizes some of the most common types of dementia care provided. More than half of dementia caregivers report routinely helping loved one's getting in and out of bed, and about one-third provide help to their family member with dementia to locate and use the toilet, bathing, managing incontinence and assist with eating [8].

In the earliest phases of dementia, affected persons may not need physical care, but caregivers may notice worrisome signs of self-neglect or changes in personal grooming in their loved one. As caregivers notice things, like mom periodically sleeping in her street clothes at night or dad wearing the same stained slacks, they may become more physically involved with helping their loved one dress. Long distance caregivers may not have access to these clues to functional changes and most adult children are reluctant to comment or interfere with things as personal as grooming, dressing and bathing until absolutely necessary. Male spouses may be more sensitive to these subtle changes and assume a compensatory role in laying out clothing, helping with makeup and clothes shopping etc. In moderate stages, physical care demands become more difficult to ignore. The person with dementia may ask for needed help, but may also deny help, leading to stressful situations. As illness progresses physical care needs increase and are often provided in part by formal caregivers, like in home aides. Ideally this helps families "share the care" or provides respite. But in some circumstances the person with dementia will only accept care from their familiar loved one. Paid staff are

Table 3 Phases of the family experience

Stressful dimensions of the family experience	First suspicion to formal diagnosis	Minimal assistance to total care	Home to long-term care community (LTC)	Living in LTC	Persons death and beyond
Physical demands	Minimal: patient takes longer with ADL's	Demands significantly increase	Physical exhaustion as excessive physical demands precipitate move to LTC	Physical demands decrease but routine of visiting LTC can be tiring	Considerable relief of physical demands
Lifestyle disruptions	Minimal: concern is growing. There is less spontaneity and less enjoyment	Increases in proportion to practical and physical responsibilities. Need for respite	Total disruption; severe curtailment of leisure and freedom	Diminish, but visiting schedule continues to play a role	General return to normalization once adjustments are made
Psychological/emotional impact	Fears start early: of the unknown, of the future. Guilt may start here. Anticipatory grief begins. Hopelessness may begin with understanding of prognosis	Fear grows and proliferates. Guilt builds as needs are harder to meet. Grief builds as a result of loss of relationship. Hopelessness is intense and formal support is needed. Loneliness begins to intensify here	Fear related to LTC costs, and transition. Anger can be intense. Guilt very severe. Ambivalence about continued life. Grief very intense about care transfer. Hopeless remains intense. Loneliness is overwhelming	Some fears diminish. Anger continues. Guilt most severe. Grief and hopelessness may lessen as family resigns to LTC decision. Loneliness continues until family begins reintegration	Genetic fears may linger. Anger related to wasted years, martyrdom. Guilt not yet resolved. Grief will continue to resurface. Hopelessness lingers . Loneliness continues as family tries to reintegrate
Relationship strains	Pre-illness issues continue. Person with dementias forgetfulness, depression and personality changes	Conflicts intensify because of paranoia, emotional outbursts and frustration	Severe strain regarding opinions about care issues	Tensions may continue over care issues	Diminished however unresolved feelings may remain
Practical problems	Minimal at first, but rapidly increasing	Increase with need for financial, legal and community resource support	Increasing costs, complexity and frustration	Often severe due to depletion of financial resources	Often minimal resources are available to rebuild
Ethical	Ethical tension can be significant. They can be burdensome depending upon religious and moral values. Strain may be related to limiting independence, facing mortality, end of life issues, broken promises, objective evaluations and uncertain future				

Adapted from Alzheimer's Association Train the Trainer Manual. Author, Carl Bretscher, MSW

Table 4 Comparisons of those caring for demented or non-demented persons

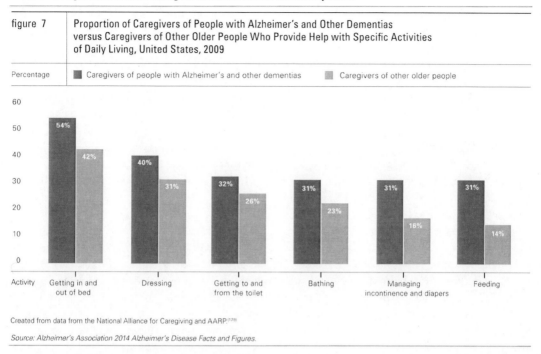

figure 7 | Proportion of Caregivers of People with Alzheimer's and Other Dementias versus Caregivers of Other Older People Who Provide Help with Specific Activities of Daily Living, United States, 2009

Created from data from the National Alliance for Caregiving and AARP.[178]

Source: Alzheimer's Association 2014 Alzheimer's Disease Facts and Figures.

often not available for care at night. Scheduling and oversight of paid, in-home workers could add a level of stress for the primary caregiver. During this phase, families learn to simplify many physical tasks, adapt the environment for both caregiver and person with dementia and limit choices to acceptable options. There is a great deal of information available through caregiving groups. However, little of this information provides specific breakdown of how to accomplish specific tasks, such as bathing, oral care, body mechanics and changing a bed with someone in it. Others learn to adapt and respond to physical care demands by trial and error. Few in home teaching resources for caregivers are available due in part to reimbursement and insurance funding mechanisms. Caregivers may actually find pride in the hands on care they provide, as they seek to retain their loved ones former appearance and preferences. However, if caregivers experience resistance or aggression from the person with dementia during personal care, the demands become both a source of physical and emotional drain for the care provider.

Physical decline is a risk for carers of people with dementia. Caregivers self-report a decline in their own health condition while caregiving.

Their emergency room visits and use of hospital services increase 25 % while caregiving [30].

Families using supportive information learn to "choose their battles", adapt expectations, simplify tasks and perform them in short spurts at the best time of day for the person with dementia. These techniques and others may mitigate the strain of providing physical care.

In the later stages of AD/related dementias caregivers have experienced the worst impacts of declining health. Often times family members provide care for their declining loved one beyond what is safe. Caregivers must assess their own physical ability to manage complete incontinence, poor ambulation, total dependent care so that the person with dementia and the carer remain safe. Many in the dementia care field have witnessed the not uncommon circumstance of the caregiver dying before the person with dementia. Roughly 30 % of caregivers die before their loved one [31]. This may leave a person with dementia without a caregiver or may require other family members to quickly assume this duty.

Advocacy roles may grow, but the physical care demands may be met in a way that now allows family caregivers to resume a more predictable work or social life, sleep better at night or take long-withheld vacations. Other families who are aware of, qualify and use hospice care for their loved one, may find relief at this stage from some of the physical care demands as they also receive emotional and spiritual support.

Lifestyle Changes

The psychological strains of caregiving have been measured in many ways [32]. Major disruptions in lifestyle, such as a caregiver relocating to be near the person with dementia or giving up employment to provide care are easily measured. The impact of more subtle changes in caregiver roles and activities are more difficult to gauge. In the first stages, caregivers may feel confused as their loved one seems to choose to engage in fewer shared activities or conversations. A caregiver may notice and grieve a change in spontaneity or enjoyment in the person with dementia. As care demands grow, caregivers may have to give up poker nights, bowling leagues, church or synagogue activities for fear of leaving the affected person alone, which can lead to social isolation, depression, and even resentment. A shift in who pays the bills or does the cooking, may feel uncomfortable or unfamiliar to the care partner taking on these tasks. The need to accompany the person with dementia to all medical appointments becomes time-consuming. Caregivers may then begin to neglect their own medical needs. Employed caregivers may experience lower work performance or work satisfaction and a more limited social life as weekends become absorbed with parent care responsibilities. Seeking to coordinate a patchwork of services for the person living with Alzheimer's such as having them attend day programs or hiring in home help may be quite helpful, but can also change the rhythm and privacy in the caregiver's life. The most commonly cited disruption in the mid-stage of illness is the impact on driving cessation. This can have major lifestyle repercussions for caregivers especially for those living in rural communities or in those families in which the person with dementia was the sole driver [33]. It is highly beneficial

for families to seek advice, counsel, information and referral from groups such as AARP, Alzheimer's Disease Research Centers and the Alzheimer's Association to support them early on in the disease around matters such as driving, curtailment of leisure, locus of control issues and exhaustion from these disruptions. The families using these supports report high levels of satisfaction and relief when they are able to find social networks that foster positive changes in lifestyle, despite the disease [34].

In later stages of illness, especially when the person with dementia may have been moved to a care setting. Spouses or those living with the person with dementia, absorb the impact of lifestyle changes. But, these are not all negative. In some instances this can be a time to re-invest in neglected work life. Spouses that visit their loved ones often in "the Home" may become friendly with other frequent visitors, residents and staff. Support groups for those with family members in long term care may provide a therapeutic and social outlet. Remaining lifestyle stressors, may be affected by comorbid conditions that can result in numerous moves, rehabilitation stays or hospitalizations secondary to the primary dementia. Throughout the disease progression caregivers are called upon to frequently adapt their lifestyle based on the needs of the person with dementia.

Emotional Care

The emotional aspect of the journey with Alzheimer's begins for family members in the "first fear stage." Self-doubt about whether to seek assessment for a loved one is emotional. Some families have to contemplate and devise elaborate plans to even get a parent to see a physician. Many carers report that the diagnosis was communicated abruptly and without regard or support for the feelings of the person with dementia or their family. Anger, denial and confusion are common responses that can linger. Disease awareness and the normative experience of being a boomer generation caregiver has led to greater sense of empowerment of the caregiver. Caregivers are more likely now, than their counterparts 20 years ago, to understand Alzheimer's and other dementias as a brain disorder rather than a preventable malady or mental illness. Unfortunately, 24 % of Americans still believe that Alzheimer's disease is part of normal aging and that the disease is NOT fatal. But that number is decreasing as education and resources become more available [2]. Emotional support from peers who have already cared for an elder may be more available. As person centered care models and a culture shift in long term care environments has occurred, persons needing formal care may have more individualized, homelike and attractive environments in which to receive care. But many families still feel overwhelmed and guilt ridden when exploring care options. Early intervention such as receiving counseling for oneself as well as accessing expert and appropriate neurological care for the person with dementia can also diminish anxiety or guilt. Families provide care in the context of pre-existing relationships. The frustration and fear around just getting an accurate diagnosis may start a chain of feelings like "why didn't I notice this sooner" or "… perhaps if I'd spent more time with mom"…etc. As difficult behaviors appear, caregivers may have a range of feelings from anger, ambivalence, hopelessness, loss of control about the disease and the changes the person with dementia is experiencing. Finally, any unresolved conflicts within family members are often visible as the need to communicate and coordinate care of the affected person places more emotional demands on the family network. Feelings may submerge and re-emerge during difficult decisions like moving to long term care or end of life decisions.

Grief can be anticipatory and extensive as the carer tries to respond emotionally to their loved ones diminished capacity and changes in appearance, personality and health status. Falls, accidents and hospitalizations all become mini-crisis that evoke feelings. Fear and lack of control are often reported by family caregivers, as well as regret that unresolved issues can never be addressed with the person losing their memory [2].

Behavioral changes requiring interventions are evidenced in 80–90 % of elders living with a dementia at some time during the course of the disease [35]. Caregivers may feel many emotions including embarrassment for behavioral symptoms.

One of the most painful experiences families report is watching a loved one display behavior the carer never would have thought possible, such as cursing or disrobing. It is particularly challenging when caring for persons with a frontotemporal dementia which has a more behavioral symptomatic presentation [36]. Carers may blame themselves for these challenging behaviors. Many families find ways to modify or better accommodate behaviors by creating a more "forgiving or failure free" environment or adapting the way they communicate with their loved one with dementia. Others may seek emotional support through counseling, or pastoral guidance, which may make a substantial difference in stress and perception of burden.

At the later stage, families may be more knowledgeable about disease progression, may have received some formal counseling, and may have begun to utilize services that support the caregivers emotional healing. At the end of life, depending on the situation, families may still report loneliness and some fear of the unknown, but also feelings of relief, pride, reflection and closure.

Relational Dynamics

Caregiving for a loved one is accompanied by the interpersonal relationship that existed prior to dementia and caregiving. Certainly this complicates the relationship between care partners. If a relationship was without much strain before caregiving began, it is likely that the caregiving relationship can develop without intense issues. Conversely, when caregiving happens in an already strained relationship the challenges can quickly multiply [37].

In the early stages of the disease, caregivers may feel concerned about crossing an unspoken boundary. Their loved one is an adult and it can be stressful deciding when to begin assisting with decision making and caregiving. This stage can create strain if the person with dementia feels disrespected or undervalued. Decreasing decision making skills on the part of the person with dementia adds tension as the caregivers concerns over safety rise. As the person with dementia experiences cognitive decrements, the role of the caregiver as decision maker, becomes clearer and can lessen the relationship burden. Behavior issues are common and add tension to the relationship as caregivers try to understand and prevent challenging behaviors [38]. In the last stages of Alzheimer's disease, relationship strain decreases as caregivers have some resolve

with their role and relationship shifts. Yet, strain that existed prior to caregiving may remain unresolved and unlikely to be settled for the caregiver. This may add to their grief and loss [39]. Support through family/friends, grief counseling and hospice services can help to ease this unresolved pain.

A person with dementia reflects on relationships

I was diagnosed a few months ago and it feels pretty ironic since my mother also had this illness. It's also ironic because I spent years volunteering for the Alzheimer's Association. Now I'm backing away, I don't want to drive myself there anymore. It's getting harder and harder to stay involved. I'm glad I have some insight into what is happening to me. My husband, seems to be holding up pretty well. It's interesting once I tell people my diagnosis, they ask how I'm coping. Then they ask about my 3 kids and how are they are handling it. I am proud of them. They have come in from out of town,, visiting more often and went to the Alzheimer's Association for a care consultation to help my husband and I get all our affairs in order. All in all, I think my kids are coping pretty well. Maybe it is a blessing we have been through this before.

Practical Matters

Families step in to help the person with dementia with many essential affairs such as banking and finances, legal planning, accessing community resources, making end of life plans and adjusting living arrangements. Almost two-thirds of caregivers of people with Alzheimer's and other dementias advocate for their care recipient with government agencies and service providers (64 %), and nearly half arrange and supervise paid caregivers from community agencies (46 %) [8]. The task of managing practical matters may be a shared responsibility across several generations or may be managed by one key family member. Power of Attorney, health directives and other legal affairs need to be organized as early in the disease process as possible to assure the person with dementia has a voice, but this is not always possible. Many times adult children may be unaware of their parents' financial and legal affairs or feel awkward bringing this topic up. Confusion, suspicion or family discord can add

to the stress surrounding practical matters. There may be feelings of anger, disappointment and fear once caregivers determine the financial reality of caring for someone with an illness that lasts many years. Family members can be embarrassed or overwhelmed by their loved ones' need to apply for public benefits. Often families are uninformed about eligibility and what Medicaid, Medicare, veterans benefits and long term care insurance covers.

Abuse is an important concern. One in nine seniors report being abused, neglected or exploited in the past 12 months; the rate of financial exploitation is extremely high, with 1 in 20 older adults indicating some form of perceived financial mistreatment in the recent past (National Adult Protective Services Association Internet). Consequently, some family members may also be concerned about others in or outside the family financially exploiting their loved one.

Some carers may place themselves in financial risk in an effort to help pay for the person with dementia's care. Education and resources can assist with these complex practical concerns. Families may be so busy providing essential physical care that they have limited time and resources to investigate and plan around legal and financial matters or their parents may be reluctant to share needed documents and information. Early planning for these practical matters can reduce strain, cost and frustration for family caregivers.

Ethical Dilemmas

The last domain in this construct of Phases of Family Experience is ethical decision making. Family members may assist the person who has dementia with numerous decisions involving autonomy, self-determination, safety and risk throughout the disease process. Examples include: choosing medical practitioners, sharing the diagnosis, balancing risk with autonomy, determining capacity and competency and advocating for ethical care. The progressive nature of the disease makes decision-making a moving target. Particularly in situations involving early onset dementias, families have not typically had the crucial conversations that outline preferences for treatment, care and good death scenarios. Families generally want their loved one involved in decision making as long as possible. Degrees of capacity fluctuate for persons with dementia so a decision specific strategy is often engaged. Some tools caregivers use are advance directives, living wills, power of attorney for both financial and health related decisions, guardianship, conservatorship, Do Not Resuscitate orders and POLST guidelines (Physician Orders for Life Sustaining Treatment.) The legal nuances among these choices may vary from state to state impacting long distance caregivers and members of the LGBT community particularly. Few families will have formal training in medical ethics concepts such as surrogacy or best interest standards, but can generally discern concepts of consent, assent and dissent in practical caregiving situations. **Viki Kind's** book, *Caregiver's Path to Compassionate Decision Making: Making Choices for Those Who Can't* [40] and the Group Principles outlined in the work of Beauchamp

and Childress [41] may be consumer friendly resources for caring families.

Another issue caregivers' may confront is lack of access to ethicists at crucial times such as during a hospital stay or a critical change in condition. Families planning ahead can educate and prepare themselves to engage with the person with dementia around those difficult decision such as when to stop driving, sell a home, apply for Medicaid or hospice care and when to end life sustaining treatments. Knowing what the person with dementia perceives as a good death while they are still able to express their opinion relieves doubt and provides comfort to families [42]. Caregivers may turn to advance counseling with pastoral care, care managers, social workers, elder law attorneys, Alzheimer's Association Helplines and websites to prepare to make these ethical choices.

Family Perspectives Across the Care Continuum: Evidence Based Best Practices

Medical Care: Getting the Diagnosis

Awareness of Alzheimer's disease is low, but growing. Persons that have a history in their family may be more aware of disease risks. Since Alzheimer's disease occurrence is sporadic many caregivers are not prepared to seek diagnosis for their loved one. Despite concerns and episodes of memory loss, forgetfulness and accidents, most families report feeling guilty suggesting that a person seeks assessment. Additionally, it is often very difficult to convince a person with memory loss to seek diagnosis. Diagnosis may involve a trusted primary care physician or may be performed at a large and unfamiliar academic institution. Other challenges may include living in a community with few diagnostic resources, or physicians not familiar with diagnosing dementia. The best practices for diagnosis are outlined in the Alzheimer's Association's, Principles for a Dignified Diagnosis [43].

Some families experience conflict during diagnosis. For example, they may feel the diagnosis should be hidden from the affected person or its importance or significance downplayed by the practitioner. Some of the questions families have at this time of pre-post diagnosis are: *Who should we to go to? Can I trust this doctor? Can I trust this diagnosis?* Carers may not understand the steps in the diagnostic process or the purpose behind various tests leading to confusion about the results. They report the way the diagnosis was communicated was insensitive or hurried. While some families have a "can do" attitude and remain positive, doubts such as, *I can't do this alone, no one else understands what I am going through, or I'm sick too*, arise. Adult children, especially those in the "club sandwich" generation report feeling overwhelmed. Families express frustration that no one has explained what to do next, what comes

next or what the action steps are they are supposed to take now. They often have questions about the length and projection of the illness, which can be down played by some practitioners. They may be confused about the efficacy cost or side effects of medications and treatment. After the appointment where diagnosis is given, caregivers may leave, not understanding that they are dealing with a long term, terminal illness. Unfortunately, families may not find out about resources such as the Alzheimer's Association until they have already experienced these situations. Hopefully, with advice from friends, clergy or health care providers, families reach out for the education and support that they will now need.

Judy's Story

Unlike the previously discussed experiences, Judy found the diagnosis process very helpful. She had realized that her father, who lives alone had forgotten to pay some bills. She also noticed him repeating a few recent conversations. Judy had some concerns, but her dad denied any issue and became argumentative when she brought it up. Judy asked to attend her Dad's upcoming annual exam with his primary care physician. Judy had called ahead to the doctors office and let them know about her concerns. The doctor offered to do a brief assessment during the visit. The assessment took only a few minutes, but indicated that something may be going on with Dad's memory. Dad was not thrilled but agreed to do what the doctor said. The doctor explained that there are many things that can cause memory problems so it is best to get a thorough exam. Judy and her father were then referred to a diagnostic center. There, several tests were conducted. Judy was interviewed separately from her father so that she could report on changes that she had noticed. It was a long day, but in the end it was confirmed that Dad had Alzheimer's Disease. They met with a social worker who informed them about resources and first steps to take. Judy reports that it was a very emotional time for both of them. But after a short time, they got busy planning and learning what they needed to know about the disease.

Using Community Education and Support Resources

Caregivers differ in their approach to accessing community education and support resources. They also differ in the relative value that they place on utilization. Some families may choose to "handle it on our own". Others want to take full advantage of everything that is available [44]. One challenge for careers is the enormous amount of ever changing information about both the disease as well as treatment protocols. For example, information for families dealing

with stroke, Parkinsons disease and AD related dementias may have to select among a vast array of information and education opportunities. Other caregivers such as those dealing with more rare dementias such as supranuclear palsy, Lewy body, Down syndrome associated dementia or frontal temporal lobe dementias may lack access to resources specific to their needs. Family members of younger onset individuals, affected by any type of dementia often feel that the information is skewed to an older population. Other real or perceived barriers may be living in a rural community, or technology limitations since many resources are now accessed or delivered online. Although some services for caregivers like support groups have been around for years, families may perceive attendance as one more task on their "to do" list. They may also have difficulty having someone stay with their loved one while they are out to attend education programs or they cannot use respite because their loved one is unaccepting of anyone else in the home. There is insufficient research about receiving information alone i.e., online, versus at an in person education or support group. Some families may perceive that they already know everything because of a previous caregiving experience thus missing out on newer services or technology supports.

Caring at Home-Community Care Services

When asked, most elders as well as their family members state they (the elder) prefers to remain at home or in the home of a family member. According to the Pew Research Center [45], 22 % of older women and 16 % of older men reside in multigenerational households. Families become increasingly aware that their loved ones' decreased insight and judgment, poses many challenges for living totally alone. Home health care is more readily available to families, but vary in quality. More expensive private home care companies are innovating to provide more ala carte services such as pet care, transportation and hair care services. But the growing expense to families of providing in home oversight, to a live alone elder with cognitive impairment, is either unaffordable or does not provide the total piece of mind caregivers need.

According to Mollica [46], families often select home care first in hopes of avoiding moving to long term care and to lower costs. Caregivers of persons with dementia are often advised to avoid changes, maintain a familiar environment to retain a sense of lifestyle continuity. Services in the home may fit these criteria for varying periods of time. A family member residing with the memory impaired person, may decide that home care can no longer address increasing "nocturnal wandering", severe incontinence and other symptom related behaviors such as aggressivity. In addition to financial and safety concerns the person with dementia may eventually lack of recognition and trust of the caregiver (family and/or paid). Families then ask: *Where should my loved one with AD/dementia live? Is my loved one's home or my home still appropriate? What is the practicality or financial impact of assuring in-home care is a safe, accessible environment for later stages of disease? Are family and other resources sufficient and proximate enough to sustain living at home? Should I relocate my loved one to a care center for more support?* Asking these difficult but necessary questions, can cause stress for families or create conflict and divisions difficult to repair. This is when other options of care can be considered.

Care Management

Care management services broker and coordinate needed supports for family members caring for persons with dementia. While this is a growing resource, many families do not know about care management or cannot afford it. Care management may be delivered to carers from public, private non-profit, private for-profit or hospital, social services or home care affiliated organizations. Since care management is referred to by a number of names such as case coordination, case management or transitional care services, it may be confusing for some family members to identify. Long distance caregivers may be more likely to use this type of assistance to coordinate care and decisions about their loved one with dementia. Since awareness of case management resources is low among family members, they may feel guilty or inadequate if they have not discovered this resource earlier in the disease process. Use of care management represents another affordability decision at a time of scarce resources. Geriatric care managers provide initial assessments and assistance with care of a loved one including crisis management, interviewing in-home helpers, or assisting with placement in a long term care community. The evidence base for the efficacy of care management services is being established. Some family members may feel they do not need this outside assistance or should be providing all the care coordination themselves. Older spouses may not be comfortable using this relatively "new" service to support them in their caregiving role. This may change as medical homes and transitional care services are becoming a more entrenched standard of care.

Adult Day Care

Adult Day Service (ADS) centers offer a wide range of services for the person with dementia who lives in a private home. Typically ADS is sought by caregivers who are concerned about leaving their loved one at home alone. Or, it is often a great resource for improved social interaction or respite for the caregiver. For the caregiver of a person with dementia, running errands, spending social time with friends, or even personal hygiene can suffer because of the need for 24/7 supervision of their loved one. ADS can provide a break so that the caregiver can tend to needs that might otherwise not be possible. Family caregivers show an increase in the beneficial stress hormone DHEA-S on days when they use an adult day care service for their relatives with dementia, according to researchers at Penn State and the University of Texas at Austin (2014). While many families may have guilt about their loved ones it can be an essential piece to caring for the caregiver.

The Adult Day Centers also benefit the person with dementia. The increased social interaction, physical activity, and cognitive stimulation can improve the general welfare of the person with dementia. In contrast, ADS participants are more likely to experience behavior problems and poor sleep on days when they remained at home [47]. ADS programs are expanding and improving their models of care to meet the needs of people with dementia. They should be considered as a promising resource.

Assisted Living

Family caregivers may perceive the need for assisted living during the mid to later course of their family members' illness. It is difficult to tell whether a parent, another family member or loved one needs more help. The following warning signs in the following figure have been suggested as indicators that additional formal support such as assisted living may be appropriate for an adult with cognitive impairment.

Indicators of need for a protective living setting:

- The refrigerator is empty or filled with spoiled food. The person with dementia is losing weight. Shopping, cooking or remembering to eat is becoming difficlt.

- Frequent bruises may be a sign of falling, or mobility and balance problems.

- The person with dementia wears the same clothes repeatedly or neglects personal hygiene. This can indicate that doing laundry and bathing is physically challenging.

- The house and yard isn't clean and tidy as it used to be.

- Loved one forgets important things, including doctor's appointments and when to take medication.

- Loved one has lost interest in relationships and outings, appears depressed and isolated.

- Family notices strange or inappropriate behavior.

In the U.S., each state has its own definition or specific licensing requirements for assisted living. Families may be uncertain about the services provided for a loved one in any level of care.

For example other common names for assisted living include:

• Residential care
• Board and care
• Congregate care
• Adult care home
• Adult group home
• Alternative care facility
• Sheltered housing

One of the challenges families confront when making a relocation decision on behalf of a relative with dementia is understanding the differences among a general assisted living community, a memory care assisted living and a nursing home. Assisted living models of all kinds have been on sharp rise in the last two decades a while the once phenomenal growth in nursing home beds has decreased by 7 %. Often their perception is more favorable towards assisted living as they may believe it is a more intimate, cost effective and homelike environment. Choosing the "correct" level of care may be difficult due to a number of factors. First, families may be in denial about their loved ones progressive care needs. Some assisted living is all inclusive in terms of fees and supports an aging in place model. Families, however can be surprised if there has not been full disclosure about the extent to which a residential care setting will go, to care for a demented person's behaviors and physical care needs. Caregivers can experience disruption of multiple moves. They may believe a general assisted living facility (ALF) will be the final transition to be made by their loved one. Later, they may be informed that mom or dad needs a memory support program located elsewhere [48]. Then finally, at the last stage of the Alzheimer's journey, when a loved one is at their frailest or most confused, families are confronted with yet another move to a skilled setting. Zimmerman and Fletcher [49] have documented that the emotional factors for families using a skilled or ALF alternative are more alike than different. Family guilt may be heightened, as well as exhaustion and financial duress increased, when multiple moves are required due to lack of initial awareness of levels of care. ALF families may spend more time in dialogue with physicians, monitoring finances and taking their loved one out socially. Caregivers using skilled settings for their loved ones spend an equal amount of caregiver energy monitoring changes in physical status and communicating with multiple levels of staff involved in their loved ones care. In both assisted living or skilled nursing settings, caregivers report using their time to advocate for quality of life and providing activity focused visits. Carers express feelings of relief related to decreased demands for physical care interventions with their loved ones. New roles become available. As some families who are frequent visitors network with other families; take an interest in those other families' loved ones, and form meaningful relationships and alliances. More often however, families visit at their convenience, focus on their loved ones needs, interface only with their loved one and perhaps with staff and remain somewhat isolated in their roles. Guilt, grief, loneliness, relief and ambiguous mourning are often the sentiments expressed by family members who move the person with dementia to any level of care.

Discrete memory care settings have emerged since the late 1990s. Families using these settings may experience more understanding and feelings of assurance from staff specifically trained in dementia care. They may also have had preexisting relationships with other families through support groups or Alzheimer's Association programs and may be better educated about the disease process leading them to seek out these specialized care settings. Once the immediate physical care needs are addressed through placement, families may have attended to the legal, financial and end of life decisions. If not, placement will prompt these discussions. Some settings stress the availability and desirability of hospice as the next option in the Alzheimer's course. But many families who are exhausted by decisions and transitions still may not be as prepared as desirable for the last set of decisions they may have to make for their loved one [50].

Moving to a Nursing Home

When Dell went into the nursing home it was a strange relief to me. For the last 2 years she had needed someone with her continually, because she kept getting lost while she was out walking the dog. Then she began feeling unsafe at home and was inconsolable. Dell, herself, stated she needed and wanted to go to a nursing home. That is unusual isn't it? She thought it was the safest place, but the family was not ready. We did go ahead and add her to the waiting list at a local long term care community. She became more and more frantic and insistent about not being at home. One night, at the suggestion of a Helpline, we took her outside and tried to get her back in the house by telling her it was the nursing home. That did not work and her son ended up driving her around for hours. When he took his mom to his home to rest she would not get out of the truck. She kept saying she wanted to go to a nursing home. So we agreed to do it and begged the home to take her abruptly. It has been a big adjustment for us all. This illness is an ongoing balancing act. It is not easy to go where the person with dementia leads you. I still miss her . I wish her sons visited her more. But I have heard guys have a harder time with all this.

Hospitalization

> *They fall asleep in a world they know and wake up in a world of pink coats and green coats, bright lights and unfamiliar faces*

Hospitalization can be a frightening time for both the person with dementia and their caregiver. Often it is not the Alzheimer's symptoms that bring a person with dementia to the hospital. People with dementia can have many comorbid conditions that often result in hospitalization [51]. It has been documented that hospital staff in general are not educated about the special needs of people with dementia during hospitalization. Table 5 shows results of a small but recent study examining the preparedness of hospital staff to meet the special needs of the patient with dementia. As indicated in the table, even though the staff report that more than 32 % of their patients have dementia, the majority of staff have had no specific education about how to meet these special needs. As caregivers, it can be challenging to understand the complex and often chaotic world of the hospital. Staff may not recognize the

persons' dementia and then may not initiate contact to update information and communicate appropriately with caregivers in addition to the primary "patient". This leaves families feeling uniformed and helpless.

> *There was no one around. I couldn't even leave mom long enough to go to the bathroom.*

Families may expect hospital staff to be knowledgeable about dementia and appropriate approaches toward care. The discrepancy between the perceptions of the family caregiver and the reality of hospital staff skills is clear. Consequently, hospitalization for the person with dementia, and their care partners is extremely stressful. While staff education is essential to shifting this paradigm, families can engage as advocates for their loved ones. Caregivers want to understand their role at the hospital. Most are the primary caregivers and feel responsible 24/7. So, now that their loved one is in the hospital: What is their role? There are many questions inherent to hospitalization. Families often wonder about when they are allowed to be present, about restraints, medication

Table 5 Hospital staff education

Participants (540)	Mean
Age	45.7
Years of practice	17.6
% of Patients >65 years	66.9
% of Patients with Dementia	32.4
Staff reported amount of Dementia-related care education	
None	176
<3 h	136
>3 h	58

Adapted from Alzheimer Dis Assoc Disord. 2010 Oct–Dec; 24(4): 372–379. doi: 10.1097/WAD.0b013e3181e9f829

changes and about changes in the patients' level of independence. They may not feel empowered to address questions or concerns with health care providers such as hospitalists or know ways to make hospitalization more successful. Caregivers are so focused on trying to get current medical information that they may be slow to ask questions about what kind of care of care they need to provide or coordinate when their loved one leaves the hospital [51]. Returning home can be an area of concern and stress on a family caregiver dependent upon the changes that the person with dementia experienced during hospitalization. Carers may question and worry about whether the hospitalization has moved them closer to needing nursing home care for their loved one. Hospitalization ideally may be an opportunity for families to gain greater insight onto their loved ones needs, current medical information and support for making short term and long term arrangements for care. as hospitals place greater emphasis on transitional care planning.

Family Participation in Dying Process

The demands of caregiving may intensify as people with dementia approach the end of life. In the year before the person's death, 59 % of caregivers felt that they were "on duty" 24 h a day, and many felt that caregiving during this time was extremely stressful. One study of end of life care found that 72 % of family caregivers said that they experienced relief when the person with dementia died [52]. Consequently, preparing for this stage of the disease is essential. In a caregiving journey that can last 8–12 years, most carers are depleted in many realms by this stage of the disease. Preparing for death of a person with dementia is variable amongst caregiving families. Family members may be dealing with a loved one who has given consideration or made explicit plans about their end of life wishes. According to www.conversationproject.org, 60 % of people say that making sure that their family is not burdened by tough decisions is "extremely important". Yet, 56 % have not communicated their end of life wishes [53]. Care partners of someone in the very early stages of Alzheimer's disease ideally make it a priority to have that difficult conversation while the person is still able to express their wishes. As the person declines, it can be a great comfort to the person with dementia and their care partners to know that their wishes regarding end of life care are clear and will be respected. Advance directives are the legal document that once signed and witnessed, express the details of what a person wants at the end of life. While forms can be free and are easily accessible online, families should have them reviewed by an elder law attorney. Unfortunately, many people miss the opportunity to know or understand the wishes of their loved one with dementia. There are still ways to prepare for end of life decisions. Caregivers can consider the things they know from the past about the person with dementia. How have they handled other illness? What have they said, possibly to or about others, during conversations about death or dying? It is important for the caregiver to find support, both personal and professional, during this stage of the disease.

Hospice

Hospice can be a positive option not only for the person with dementia, but also their caregivers. There are many cultural norms and beliefs surrounding the use of hospice care by dementia caregivers. Some families believe hospice equates to "giving up on" the person with dementia or hastening their death. Some may even equate the use of hospice as a death wish [54]. Other families believe, that because hospice is

typically reserved for those with 6 months or less to live, it is not a viable option for their loved one with Alzheimer's disease. It is important for caregivers to talk with healthcare providers about hospice even before the need becomes evident. Families engaged in a hospice program report many perceived advantages to the program [55]. Other families reflect that waiting until too near death may be a missed opportunity for the person with AD/related dementias to experience a dignified death. The hospice focus on palliative care can be a great relief for caregivers as they see their loved one more comfortable. Hospice also offers caregivers significant support through death preparedness and grief counseling. Many hospice programs offer unique services such as chaplaincy, music therapy, aromatherapy and pet therapy to aid in celebrating the dignity of the dying person with dementia.

Caring for someone on Hospice

Terry is on hospice now for the second time. The first time it was such a comfort and we appreciated all the extra help. With her doctor, we were able to take her off all her medications, but one. Her appetite, especially for the milk shakes I bring each visit, remained strong. She did not lose weight and was discharged from hospice. But this time she is not eating or drinking and when I saw her like this I just came apart. We can still listen to our favorite music from Les Miserables. She loves "I Dreamed a Dream". It is so hard, but volunteering with the Alzheimer's Association has helped me turn this all into a positive.

Family as Advocates

Merriam-Webster defines an advocate as, one that supports or promotes the interest of another. Caregivers of a person with dementia are thrust into the role of advocate in so many ways during the entire course of the illness. At some stage people with dementia are no longer able to express their wishes. Caregivers, become the advocates to meet this need.

Advocacy on medical issues may start for the caregiver even before diagnosis. Caregivers are often helping the person with memory concerns manage existing chronic conditions and obtain an accurate diagnosis. This may require multiple

long office visits and being persistent to get the attention of medical personnel. As the needs of the person with dementia change, caregivers will advocate for appropriate medications, living arrangements and services. Possibly the most important medical advocacy comes at the end of life when a caregiver needs to make sure that the person's wishes are upheld and respected.

Socially, caregivers play a big role helping the person with dementia maintain relationships and navigate the outside world. Social isolation is a common report of caregivers. Friends and other family members may withdraw from contact due to a lack of understanding or discomfort [56]. Yet, social interaction can be very good for a person with dementia and so caregivers may have to advocate by educating and making friends feel more comfortable around the person with dementia. Additionally, it may not be apparent that a person has dementia simply by their appearance. Consequently, service staff at restaurants or grocery stores may not understand the behavior or social limitations of the person with dementia.

Social Challenges

A care partner once shared with her support group, that she and her husband were no longer allowed to "walk" in the mall together because the mall staff were concerned about the behavior of her husband. The caregiver contacted the Alzheimer's Association for support and spent a lot of time working with mall staff. Her goal as an advocate was to maintain the ritual of morning walks at the mall, which calmed and promoted health for her loved one with dementia.

Political advocacy is essential to educating the regulators and policy makers about dementia and the needs of those with the disease [57]. Many organizations work at the local and federal levels to meet with politicians to gain financial support for research and services. Caregivers have a personal story to share with these law makers that can impact future care and finding a cure.

Reflections on Burden Versus Privilege of Caregiving

Caregivers of persons with dementia vary in their perceptions of burden versus privilege based on the many factors mentioned in this chapter. This includes long held views on reciprocity, ethnically influenced values, culturally accepted practices and the pre/post disease relationship to the affected individual. The ability to resolve, compartmentalize, integrate, and respond to, what may be a 20 year journey with a confusing disease process, may differ based on social, financial and spiritual resources available to caregivers. Many studies have shown that Alzheimer's disease and related disorders' caregivers, suffer from depression and other adverse physical and psychological repercussions. There have been encouraging studies on the effects of comprehensive support programs on depression in caregivers. A myriad of psychosocial and educational intervention programs (as will be explored in subsequent chapters), can support the primary caregiver and family members over the entire course of the disease in ways that ameliorate the potential negative effects of caregiving. Models include individual and family counseling available 24/7, enrollment and participation in research trials, socialization programs and support group participation. Programs pioneered by Alzheimer's Associations and Alzheimer's Disease Research Centers across the United States, for affected individuals and their family members, have been shown to positively impact the excess burden associated with caregiving. Studies have shown that caregivers engaged in these interventions were significantly less depressed than those in the not so engaged in similar services,. These results suggest that enhancing long-term social support can have a significant impact on negative consequences of caregiving. Factors influencing caregiving experiences in the future include the availability of normalization and socialization opportunities for caregivers to share with their loved one, creative use of technology to support safety and societal acceptance of memory impaired persons. The social isolation and stigma experienced by caregivers even a decade ago, is being replaced with a more accepting attitude toward cognitive impairment. Normative experiences with neurological diseases are now shared among "Baby Boomers" and the availability of more person-centered and dignified care settings to care for the memory impaired, may remove some of the guilt associated with using long term care options.

It usually takes time and reflection for families, in the throes of physical caregiving, to integrate the emotional experience and accept the entirety of the caregiving experience as a privilege. When this acceptance occurs caregivers report positive feelings of re-engagement with a parent in a new and different way; a sense of fidelity toward a spouse or the ability to celebrate the newly found skills living in the moment with a memory impaired loved one. Families express gratitude for the strengths they were able to tap to take care of someone living with dementia and express pride in the lesson the situation served for future generations and younger members within the family. An indicator of this is the burgeoning literature written by caregivers about their experiences. The attitudes toward the caregiving experience are, as one would expect, largely influenced by pre-existing life views and life's stories as well as the need family member have to repay, reward or resolve their prior familial relationship with the person with dementia. Caregiving remains rich investigative territory for gerontologists, social and health care researchers in decades to come as the "Boomers" experience and engage in the "Age of Dementia" and await long anticipated cure.

Discussion Questions

1. Are family members better equipped to assume caregiving roles?
2. Is caring for a person with dementia any different than any other caregiving role?
3. What are some of the most promising resources caregivers can utilize to create an optimal quality of life caregiving experience?

References

1. Gillick MR. The critical role of caregivers in achieving patient-centered care. JAMA. 2013;310(6):575–6.
2. Alzheimer's Association. Late stage caregiving: your role as a caregiver. 2014.
3. Gitlin LN, Schultz R. Family caregiving of older adults. In: Prohaska RT, Anderson LA, Binstock RH, editors. Public health for aging society. Baltimore, MD: The Johns Hopkins University Press; 2014. p. 181–204.
4. Ory MG, Hoffmann RR, Yee JL, Tennstedt S, Schulz R. Prevalence and impact of caregiving: a detailed comparison between dementia and nondementia caregivers. Gerontologist. 1999;39(2):177–86.
5. Rava S. Swimming solo: a daughters memoir of her parets, his parents and Alzheimer's disease. Sewanee, TN: Plateau books; 2011.
6. Bouldin ED, Anderson E. Caregiving across the United States: caregivers of persons with Alzheimer's disease or dementia in 8 states and the District of Columbia. Data from 2009 and 2010 Behavioral Risk Factor Surveillance System [Internet]. 2010
7. Meuser TM, Berg-Weger M, Chibnall JT, Harmon AC, Stowe JN. Assessment of readiness for mobility transition (ARMT): a tool for mobility transition counseling with older adults. J Appl Gerontol. 2013;32(4):484–507. doi:10.1177/0733464811425914.
8. Caregiving NAf, AARP. Caregiving in the U.S. Unpublished data analyzed under contract for the Alzheimer's Association. 2009.
9. Fuller-Jonap F, Haley WE. Mental and physical health of male caregivers of a spouse with Alzheimer's disease. J Aging Health. 1995;7(1):99–118.
10. Ohio department of aging. Whom does caregiving affect? 2009. Available from: http://aging.ohio.gov/resources/publications/Caregiver_Fact_Sheet_1-866.pdf
11. Robinson CA, Bottorff JL, Besut B, Oliffe JL, Tomlinson J. The male face of caregiving: a scoping review of men caring for a person with dementia. Am J Mens Health. 2014;8(5):409–26.
12. National Institute on Aging. Alzheimer's disease and education center: intimacy sexuality and Alzheimer's disease: a resource list. 2008. Available from: http://www.nia.nih.gov/alzheimers/intimacy-sexuality-and-alzheimers-disease-resource-list
13. Bookwala J, Schulz R. A comparison of primary stressors, secondary stressors, and depressive symptoms between caregiving husbands and wives: The caregiver health effects study. Psychology and aging. 2000;15:607–616.
14. Fisher GG, Franks MM, Plassman BL, Brown SL, Potter GG, Llewellyn D, et al. Caring for individuals with dementia and cognitive impairment, not dementia: findings from the aging, demographics, and memory study. JAM Geriatr Soc. 2011;59(3):488–94.
15. Schumacher LAP, MacNeil R, Mobily K, Teague M, Butcher H. The leisure journey for sandwich generation caregivers. Ther Recreat J. 2012;46(1):42–60.
16. Hammer LB, Neal MB. Working sandwiched-generation caregivers: prevalence, characteristics, and outcomes. Psychol-Manag J. 2008;11(1):93–112.
17. Riley LD, Bowen CP. The sandwich generation: challenges and coping strategies of multigenerational families. Fam J. 2005;13(1):52–8.

18. Loomis LS, Booth A. Multigenerational caregiving and well-being. J Fam Issues. 1995;16(2):131–48.
19. Rubin R, White-Means S. Informal caregiving: dilemmas of sandwiched caregivers. J Fam Econ Iss. 2009;30(3):252–67.
20. National down syndrome society. 2014. Available at: http://www.ndss.org/
21. Chen H. Down syndrome: prognosis. Updated 8.2014. Medscape [Internet]. 2014.
22. Lancet Neurology (The). Strengthening connections between Down syndrome and AD. Lancet Neurol 2013;12(10):931.
23. Institute MMM. The Metlife study of caregiving costs to working caregivers: double jeopardy for baby boomers caring for their parents. 2011.
24. Alzheimer's Association. Alzheimer's disease facts and figures. 2014. pp. 30–58.
25. Hargrave R. Caregivers of African-American elderly with dementia: a review and analysis. Annals Long-term Care. 2006;14(10).
26. Haley WE, Gitlin LN, Wisniewwski SR, Mahoney DF, Coons DW, Winter L, et al. Well-being, appraisal, and coping in African-American and Caucasian dementia caregivers: findings from the REACH study. Aging Ment Health. 2004;8(4):316–29.
27. Institue MLMM. Still out, still aging: the MetLife study of lesbian, gay, bisexual and transgender baby boomers. 2010.
28. Achenbaum WA. How boomers turned conventional wisdom on its head a historian's view on how the future may judge a transitional generation. Metlife mature market institute. 2012.
29. Ganguli M, Dodge HH, Shen C, Panday RS, DeKosky ST. Alzheimer's disease and mortality: a—year epidemiological study. Arch Neurol. 2005;62(5):779–84.
30. Caregiving NAf, Schulz R, Cook T, Pittsburgh UCfSURDoPUo. Caregiving costs: declining health in the Alzheimer's caregiver as dementia increases in the care recipient. 2011.
31. AgingCare.com. Thirty percent of caregivers die. 2014. Available from: http://www.agingcare.com/Discussions/Thirty-Percent-of-Caregivers-Die-Before-The-People-They-Care-For-Do-97626.htm
32. Mavarid M, Paola M, Spazzaumo L, Mastriforti R, Rinaldi P, Polidori C, et al. The caregiver burden inventory in evaluating the burden of caregivers of elderly demented patients: results from a multicenter study. Aging Clin Exp Res. 2013;17(1):46–53.
33. Carr D, Duchek JM, Meuser TM, Morris JC. Older adult drivers with cognitive impairment. Am Fam Physician. 2006;73(6):680–7.
34. Carr DB, Ott BR. The older adult driver with cognitive impairment "it's a very frustrating life". JAMA. 2010; 303(16):1632–41.
35. Kohm R, Surti GM. Management of behavioral problems in dementia. J Med Health. 2008;91(11):335–8.
36. Levy ML, Miller BL, Cummings JL, Fairbanks LA, Craig A. Alzheimer disease and frontotemporal dementias behavioral distinctions. Arch Neurol. 1996; 53(7):687–90.
37. Lyons KS, Zarit SH, Sayer AG, Whitlatch CJ. Caregiving as a dyadic process: perspectives from caregiver and receiver. J Gerontol Psychol Sci. 2002;57B(3):195–204.
38. Morris SE, Cuthbert BN. Research domain criteria: cognitive systems, neural circuits, and dimensions of behavior. Dialogues Clin Neurosci. 2012;14(2): 29–37.
39. Boss P. Ambiguous loss: Harvard University Press. Cambridge, MA.
40. Kind V. The caregiver's path to compassionate decision making: making choices for those who can't (Home Nursing Caring). Austin, TX: Greenleaf book group; 2010.
41. Beauchamp TL, Childress JF. Principles of biomedical ethics. 5th ed. New York: Oxford University Press; 2001.
42. Kolcaba KY, Fisher EM. A holistic perspective on comfort care as an advance directive. Crit Care Nurs Q. 1996;18(4):66–76.
43. Alzheimer's Association. Alzheimer news: new statement to medical community demands a dignified diagnosis of dementia. 2009.
44. Robinson KM, Buchwalter KC, Reed D. Predictors of use of services among dementia caregivers. West J Nurs Res. 2005;27(2):126–40.
45. Pew Research Center. The return of the multigenerational family household. A social and demographic trends report. 2010.
46. Mollica RF. Coordinating services across the continuum of health, housing, and supportive services. J Aging Health. 2003;15:165–88.
47. Zarit SH, Kim K, Femia EE, Almeida DM, Savla J, Molenaar PCM. Effects of adult day care on daily stress of caregivers: a within-person approach. J Gerontol Ser B Psychologic Sci Soc Sci. 2011.
48. Kane RL, West JC. It shouldn't be this way—the failure of long term care. Nashville, TN: Press V; 2005.
49. Zimmerman S, Sloane PD, Fletcher S. The measurement and importance of quality in tomorrow's assisted living. In: Golant S, Hyde J, editors. The assisted living residence: a vision for the future. Baltimore: Johns Hopkins University Press; 2008.
50. Span P. The new old age: caring and coping. Avoiding the call to hospice. 2009.
51. Silverstein NM, Maslow K. Improving hospital care for persons with dementia. New York: Springer; 2006.
52. Schulz R, Mendelsohn AB, Haley WE, Mahoney D, Allen RS, Zhang S, et al. End-of-life care and the effects of bereavement on family caregivers of persons with dementia. N Engl J Med. 2003;349(20): 1936–42.
53. Conversationproject.org. 2014.
54. Wilder HM, Oliver DP, Demiris G, Washington K. Informal hospice caregiving: the toll on quality of life. J Soc Work End Life Palliat Care. 2008;4(4):312–32.
55. Raleigh H, Robinson ED, Hoey J, Marol K, Jamison TM. Family care perceptions of hospice support. J Hosp Palliat Care Nurs. 2006;8(1):25–33.

56. Robinson J, Fortinsky R, Kleppinger A, Shugrue N, Porter M. A broader view of family caregiving: effects of caregiving and caregiver conditions on depressive symptoms, health, work, and social isolation. J Gerontol: Soc Sci. 2009;64B(6):788–98.
57. Alzheimer's Association. Nearly 60 percent of people worldwide incorrectly believe that Alzheimer's disease is a typical part of aging. Alzheimer's News 2014 [Internet]. 2014.
58. SAGE. The issues—disability [cited 2014]. Available from: http://www.sageusa.org/issues/disability.cfm#sthash.veWCfUpO.dpufthere
59. Association NAPS. Policy and advocacy: elder financial exploitation.
60. Bookman A, Kimbrel D. Families and elder care in the twenty-first century. Future Child. 2011;21(2):117–40.
61. Bretcher C. Alzheimer's Association, Saint Louis Chapter. Train the trainer manual. 2013.
62. Brookmeyer R, Corrada MM, Curriero FC, Kawas C. Survival following a diagnosis of Alzheimer disease. Arch Neurol. 2005;59(11):1764–7.
63. Curry LA, Wetle T. Ethical considerations. In: Evashwick CJ, editor. The continuum of long term care. 3rd ed. Clinton Park, NY: Thomson Delmar Learning; 2005. p. 279–92.
64. Evashwick CJ. The continuum of long term care. Clifton Park, NY: Thomson Delmar Learning; 2005.
65. Gaugler JE, Mittelman MS, Hepburn K, Newcome R. Clinically significant changes in burden and depression among dementia caregivers following nursing home admission. BMC Med. 2010;8:85.
66. Gentry M. Challenges of elderly immigrants. Hum Serv Today. 2010;6(2):1–4.
67. Gorospe E. Elderly immigrants: emerging challenge for the U.S. healthcare system. Internet J Healthc Adm. 2005;4(1).
68. Greenlee K. Leaving the farm. Generations. 2013;37(3):6–7.
69. Morris LW, Mobily RG, Britton PG. The relationship between marital intimacy, perceived strain and depression in spouse caregivers of dementia sufferers. Br J Med Psychol. 1988;61(3):231–6.
70. Noelker LS, Whitlatch CJ. Informal caregiving. In: Evashwick CJ, editor. The continuum of long-term care. 3rd ed. Clifton Park, NY: Thomson Delmar Learning; 2005. p. 29–48.
71. Roth DL, Haley WE, Hovarter M, Perkins M, Wadley VG, Suzanne J. Family caregiving and all-cause mortality: findings from a population-based propensity-matched analysis. Am J Epidemiol. 2013;178(10):1571–8.
72. Schulz R. Research priorities in geriatric palliative care: informal caregiving. J Palliat Med. 2013;16(9):1008–12.
73. Services USDoHaH. Frontotemporal disorders: information for patients, families and caregivers: national institutes of health. 2014.
74. Tay L, Chua KC, Chan M, Lim WS, Ang YY, Koh E, et al. Differential perceptions of quality of life (QoL) in community-dwelling persons with mild-to-moderate dementia. Int Psychogeriatr. 2014;26(8):1273–82.

Interventions to Support Caregiver Well-Being

Meredeth A. Rowe, Jerrica Farias, and Marie Boltz

Introduction

The majority of persons with dementia (estimated to be 75 %) receive care and support provided by family caregivers [1]. Whether they are fulfilling the role of care providers (providing hands-on care) or care managers (arranging for others to provide care), they contribute care and services essential to the health and well- being of persons with dementia. Families of persons with dementia are often referred to as "invisible second patients" [2]. The purpose of this chapter is to describe the caregiver's physiological, emotional, and psychological changes that occur when providing care to a person with dementia, and to describe interventions designed to support caregiver well-being.

As described in Chapter "Experiences and Perspectives of the Family Caregiver of the Person with Dementia" (McGillick, Murphy-White), the effects of caregiving are often positive; however, the caregiving role appears to take

M.A. Rowe, PhD, RN, FAAN, FGSA (✉)
J. Farias, RN, MSN
University of South Florida College of Nursing,
12901 Bruce B. Downs Blvd., Tampa,
FL 33612, USA
e-mail: mrowe1@health.usf.edu

M. Boltz, PhD, RN, GNP-BC, FGSA, FAAN
William F. Connell School of Nursing, Boston
College, Mahoney Hall, 140 Commonwealth Avenue,
Chestnut Hill, MA 02467, USA
e-mail: boltzm@bc.edu

a toll upon physical and psychological, and financial well–being of family members. In an early investigation, stressed caregivers had earlier mortality and more morbidity than caregivers experiencing less stress [3]. In subsequent studies, researchers identified psychological morbidity of caregiving including high levels of perceived burden [4–8], depression [4, 5, 7–10], loneliness, decreased social support [10], and high levels of perceived stress [11].

A recent review on the physiologic consequences of caregiving details multiple studies that have examined the effect of the caregiving experience on physical consequences of caregiving [12]. The most conclusive findings were the impact of caregiving on both cognitive and immune function. In terms of cognitive function, being a dementia caregiver was associated with poorer function in specific domains of cognitive function (processing speed, attention and concentration) as well overall functioning. Furthermore, in one study, spousal dementia caregivers were found to be almost seven times more likely to get Alzheimer's disease themselves after being a caregiver [13]. Immune function in caregivers was worse particularly with the immune markers of TNF-α and C-reactive protein, both consistently elevated indicating immune dysfunction [12].

A series of articles have been published detailing the impact of caregiving on biomarkers of cardiovascular disease. Researchers have found evidence of two pathophysiologic mechanisms of

© Springer International Publishing Switzerland 2016
M. Boltz, J.E. Galvin (eds.), *Dementia Care*, DOI 10.1007/978-3-319-18377-0_13

coronary heart disease, vascular inflammation and altered clotting profiles [14–19]. When high levels of role overload or depression were present in the caregivers, the biomarkers profiles were more abnormal.

The mechanisms of caregiving-associated physiologic and psychological changes are currently being investigated and proposed mechanisms for the physiologic changes include emotional demands of caregiving, poor sleep, sustained vigilance, and interference with caregivers' health promoting behaviors [20–22]. The most prominent psychologic change is depression with a number of risk factors for higher levels of depression already identified. These include the caregiver having lower educational levels [23], lower income [24], being a spouse caregiver [25], being female [26], and being Caucasian (compared with being African American) [27]. Predictors of high levels of depressive symptomatology include poorer self-rated health [28], smaller social networks [29] and use of dysfunctional (emotion-focused) coping [30]. Caregiver stress (including role overload, captivity, or burden) both mediates [31] and contributes directly to depressive symptoms [32]. Additionally, sources of psychological strain are due to competing demands within the family and work setting, role changes within the family, insufficient information sharing and engagement in decision-making with health care providers [4]. Care recipient characteristics that are associated with caregiver depression include poorer cognitive function [33], higher dependence in activities of daily living (ADL) [25], and behavioral manifestations of distress in the patient [34].

Caregiver Well-Being Theoretical Models

Psychological Stress Models

In the Poulshock and Deimling model [35], dementia leads to caregiver burden which can manifest as strain in a number of ways that either could be exacerbated (e.g., by behavioral symptoms or health problems of the caregiver) or ameliorated (e.g., by support of others or competencies) by other factors. The model of caregiver stress offered by Pearlin and colleagues [36] describes four main areas that contribute to caregiver stress: the background context (including the influence of other life events and support systems), the primary stressors of the illness (such as amount of help required by the patient and behavioral symptoms), secondary role strains (such as family conflict and social life), and intrapsychic strains such as personality and competence [35, 37]. In a review of the Pearlin model, Campbell and colleagues reported that the strongest predictors of caregiver burden were sense of role captivity (feelings of being "trapped" in a role), caregiver fatigue and burnout, quality of relationship with the care receiver, and adverse life events outside of the caregiving role [37]. The Pearlin model obtained a satisfactory fit across race or ethnicity in subsequent research, despite significant racial differences in each of the latent constructs [38]. Results suggest that interventions must target different aspects of the stress process to provide optimal benefit for individuals of different cultural or ethnic backgrounds.

Physiologic Stress Models

Later models describe physiological responses to the caregiving role, particularly caregivers who perceive the role as stressful. Caregivers of persons with dementia demonstrate exaggerated cardiovascular responses to stressful conditions which put them at greater risk for the development of high blood pressure or heart disease [39–43]. Depression and anxiety in caregivers of persons with dementia have been associated with prolonged platelet activation [40, 42, 44], sympathetic activation and increased norepinephrine [40, 45–50]. The chronically stressed caregivers have been shown to have elevated cortisol levels [51–53], reduced lymphocyte sensitivity to glucocorticoids [54], impaired cellular immunity [54–58], increased cardiovascular disease biomarker activity [59–61].

Cross-sectional studies over the past two decades indicate that approximately two-thirds of dementia caregivers report they are having trouble sleeping with mixed findings on whether there are reductions in the quantity and quality of nightly sleep [62]. Predisposing and precipitating demographic (increasing age and female gender, dementia type) and medical risk factors (multiple co-morbidities, obstructive sleep apnea, restless leg syndrome) can be contributors to caregivers' poor sleep [63–65]. However, a growing body of literature suggests that the unique circumstances faced by dementia caregivers contribute to poor sleep, and this results in physiologic consequences that may contribute to their elevated risk of heart disease, for instance [17, 19, 39, 60, 66, 67].

Chronic caregiver stress has also been implicated as a contributor to cognitive decline in caregivers of persons with dementia [54, 68–70]. A theoretical model of chronic stress offered by Vitaliano and colleagues [69], as well as a longitudinal study of spousal caregivers [70] suggest a higher risk of cognitive impairment or dementia in caregiver. This is hypothesized to be effected by several mediators, including psychosocial (e.g., depression, loneliness, social isolation, sleep problems), behavioral (e.g., exercise, diet), and physiological (e.g., metabolic syndrome and inflammation) variables. This research has important implications because it considers modifiable risk factors for dementia that, if unchecked, may compromise the lives of caregivers and their ability to function.

Campbell, Rowe, and Marsiske expand the stress model with the supposition that stress in dementia caregiver produces consequences for both the caregiver (morbidity, mortality) and dyad (behavioral symptoms in the person with dementia and the caregiver's response) [71]. The caregiver's appraisal and adaptation to primary stressors (care recipient disability, problem behaviors, loss) and secondary stressors (family conflict, work difficulties) are manifest as behavioral and emotional responses which yield these consequences.

Moving Beyond Stress Models

Piercy and colleagues [34] offer a modified ecological contextual model developed by Williams [29] that includes five distinct contexts that influence caregiver mental health. The sociocultural context includes caregiver gender, marital status, education, and employment status. The situational context addresses the cognitive, functional, and behavioral status of the care recipient. The temporal context examines timing of the caregiver role by examining caregiver age and kin relationships to care recipients to determine whether or not caregiving is an "on" or "off" time experience. The interpersonal context examines formal and informal support received by the care dyad. Finally, the personal context includes psychosocial characteristics of caregivers or their personal situations that affect mental health.

The next step in this line of research is to untangle the concept of 'caregiver stress' as it relates to caregiver health. It will be critical to have a better understanding of the subcomponents that underlie a caregiver reporting high levels of stress. For instance the results of two qualitative studies illuminate the role poor sleep plays in changes in caregiver health [21, 72]. The effects of poor sleep were found to be quite pervasive with downstream consequences of loss of energy, mood changes including an increase in depressive symptoms, and social isolation. These changes resulted in a decreased desire to engage in health promoting activities. Once specific subcomponents of caregiver stress are uncovered more targeted interventions can be planned with the hope of reducing the effect of caregiving on health.

Interventions Focused on Improving Caregivers' Psychologic Health

Counseling

In the New York University Caregiver Intervention (NYUCI), Mittelman and colleagues showed that structured, individualized family counseling, supplemented with support groups and ad hoc (crisis or transitional) counseling, led to sustained benefits in reducing depressive symptoms in spouse caregivers of patients with Alzheimer's disease [73, 74]. The NYUCI was replicated in a multisite program in Minnesota

[75]. Consistent with the original randomized clinical trial, assessments of this program showed decreased depression and distress among caregivers [76]. Some of the challenges in the community setting included having caregivers complete the full six counseling sessions and acquiring complete outcome data. Given the challenges faced in the community setting, the researchers concluded that web-based training for providers may be a cost-effective way to realize the maximum benefits of the intervention on caregiver depression [76].

Problem solving therapy (PST) lessened depression symptoms, particularly among caregivers of persons with newly diagnosed early dementia [77]. PST also lowered caregivers' anxiety levels, and led to lessening of negative problem orientation.

Role-Related Educational Programs

Comprehensive educational program have demonstrated improvements in caregiver psychological wellbeing, self-efficacy, and preparedness [78]. Judge and colleagues combined educational skills (used with the caregivers) and cognitive rehabilitation skills training (used with the persons with dementia) into a single protocol for addressing the dyad's care issues and needs [79]. Key domains addressed by the intervention included: education about dementia and memory loss; effective communication; managing memory; staying active; and recognizing emotions and behaviors. Intervention caregivers compared to controls, had decreased symptoms of depression and anxiety, and less care-related strain as indicated by lower emotional health strain, dyadic relationship strain, role captivity, and higher caregiving mastery.

Using trained community consultants to provide a systematic, structured yet individualized approach to teach family caregivers resulted in reduced behavioral and psychiatric disturbances in people with Alzheimer's disease [80]. The focus of the intervention was teaching caregivers to monitor problems, identify possible events that trigger disturbances, and develop more effective

responses. It successfully improved caregivers' quality of life, and reduced subjective burden and reactive responses to dementia care recipients' problem behaviors.

Caregiver-focused interventions for persons affected by dementia have largely been described in developed countries [81]. One randomized controlled trial, carried out in communities based in two talukas (administrative blocks) in Goa, India, tested the effectiveness of home care advisors who were supervised by a counselor and a psychiatrist [82]. The caregivers in the intervention group received information on dementia, including support of patient mental well-being, supplemented with support groups. The intervention led to significant improvements in caregiver mental health and perceived burden; nonsignificant reductions were observed for behavior disturbances and functional ability in patients.

Cognitive Behavioral Therapy

Cognitive behavioral therapy (CBT), a structured, time-limited, problem-focused form of psychotherapy is an "action-oriented" approach which has improved the psychological wellbeing of dementia caregivers. For instance, cognitive reframing, a component of CBT, focuses on family carers' maladaptive, self-defeating or distressing cognitions about their relatives' behaviors and about their own performance in the caring role [83]. A Cochrane systematic review concluded that this intervention can reduce psychological morbidity and subjective stress but not perceptions of coping or burden [83]. CBT has been implemented in various cultures and languages [84–86] and has also demonstrated efficacy as a group intervention [87, 88].

Group Support Interventions

For almost 30 years, researchers have examined the impact of caregiver support groups on outcomes of both caregiver and care recipient [89, 90]. Across a number of studies including those recently published [91], caregivers report these groups as helpful and positive experiences, however there is little evidence that there are improvements in caregiver psychological health. The overall lack of effectiveness, at least in terms of caregiver health outcomes, is compounded by the fact that most caregivers do not participate in these groups that are generally widely available [92].

Meditation and Mindfulness

Dementia caregivers who practice mindfulness meditation have experienced decreases in levels of depression and burden [93–96]. Additionally, there is evidence that daily meditation practices [97], including yoga meditation [98] by family dementia caregivers can lead to improved mental and cognitive functioning along with lower levels of depressive symptoms, and anxiety, as well as improved self-efficacy. Clinical benefits have been accompanied by an increase in telomerase activity suggesting the intervention may reduce stress-induced cellular aging [98]. Similarly, in a randomized controlled trial, yogic meditation has shown to reverse the transcription of pro-inflammatory cytokines and decreased the transcription of innate antiviral response genes previously observed in healthy individuals confronting a significant life stressor [99].

Polarity therapy (PT) is another complementary therapy that has been tested to relieve dementia caregiver stress. In a randomized trial with American Indian and Alaskan Native family caregivers, PT was found to be feasible and culturally acceptable, and improved to reduce stress, depression and pain, and improve perception of vitality and general health [100].

Interventions Focused on Improving Caregivers' Physical Health

Psychoeducational Interventions

Unique psychoeducational interventions show early promise in reducing health risks in caregivers. The Pleasant Events Program (PEP), a 6-week Behavioral Activation intervention was designed to reduce cardiovascular disease (CVD) risk and depressive symptoms in caregivers [101]. CVD risk markers interleukig-6 (IL-6) The PEP program participants demonstrated less depression and reductions in IL-6 as compared to the control group. The researchers recommend that future research should examine the efficacy of PEP for improving other CVD biomarkers and seek to sustain the intervention's effects.

Interventions to Improve Caregiver Sleep

Sleep disturbance is a prevalent and complex issue within the family caregiver population. Caregivers have high amounts of unwanted wake time during the night, affecting the overall health of the caregivers themselves [102] including their cognitive status [103], as well as the well-being of care recipients [102]. Poor sleep has been associated with increased coagulation activity and endothelial dysfunction, plasma IL-6 and D-dimer levels [14, 17, 104]. This is one possible mechanism explaining how disturbed sleep secondary to the caregiving role might be associated downstream with cardiovascular disease, particularly in older people under chronic stress.

The effect of the short-term use of cranial electrical stimulation has been tested in caregivers and found not to improve sleep disturbances, depressive symptoms, or caregiving appraisal [105]. During periods wherein family members with dementia received institutional respite in community hospitals, caregivers who remained at home showed improvements in sleep disturbances. Nevertheless, for patients, respite care worsened already disturbed sleep patterns, demonstrating the need to target sleep management of patients during respite care [106]. In the home care setting, a pilot 5-week behavioral sleep intervention combining relaxation, stimulus control, and sleep hygiene with personal goal setting demonstrated trends toward improved sleep quality and less depression, warranting future investigation [107, 108].

When a nighttime monitoring system (NMS) was used, caregivers qualitatively reported improved "peace of mind" due to the reliable alerts signaling the whereabouts of the person with dementia [72]. Generally, caregivers reported improved quality of sleep, although some caregivers reported more awakenings due to the system alerts. However, neither quantitative measures of sleep nor sleep quality were improved by the NMS [109]. The researchers concluded that future research should investigate multimodal interventions using both technologies to improve safety of the care recipient [109] as well as therapies to improve chronic insomnia sleep patterns.

Exercise Interventions

Engaging in physical activity in general has been associated with positive health benefits including reduced risk of chronic illness, improved functional abilities, and improved mood and cognition [110, 111]. The benefits of exercise may be especially relevant to caregivers [112]. Regular exercise may increase the strength and endurance needed to perform the demanding physical tasks of the role; reduce stress, anxiety, and depression; intervene to prevent negative physiological responses to chronic stress (i.e., cardiovascular, immunologic, stress hormones, neurotransmitters); and promote self-efficacy and personal control. Studies show, however, that caregivers have less time and opportunity to exercise as their role-related responsibilities increase [113, 114] and the importance of pre-caregiving factors [115]. Home-based physical activity telephone interventions have yielded increases in total weekly physical activity levels, self-efficacy of caregivers, sleep quality, positive affective emotions, and cognitive ability [116–120]. However, involvement in vigorous physical activity is limited. Some of the barriers identified by Farran and colleagues include non-conducive weather conditions, heavy responsibilities in both caregiving and non-caregiving domains, and negative feelings such as anxiety and depressive symptoms [119].

Hirano and colleagues used pedometers to provide feedback to caregivers participating in home-based exercise program (three times per week for 12 weeks) of moderate intensity [120]. Participants reported less burden and improved sleep. The average number of steps taken, recorded by pedometers, was significantly higher in the intervention group as compared to the control group. Yu and Smartwood evaluated the subjective perceptions of the feasibility and impact of a 6-month, moderate-intensity aerobic exercise intervention by dyads of older adults with Alzheimer's disease and their family caregivers [121]. Both groups identified that participation was feasible and socially rewarding but did not believe that cognition was impacted by the exercise. The caregivers reported that the exercise reduced their stress and improved the attitude of the person with dementia.

Interventions That Use Technology

Recently, researchers have examined the effectiveness of of technology-based interventions including the use of telephones, videos, the internet, and monitoring devices.

Improved caregiver psychosocial well-being have been demonstrated to some extent with variety of technology-enhanced delivery methods including support groups conducted telephonically [88, 122], counseling via the telephone [123–128], combined in-home and counseling sessions [129, 130], video conferencing combined with telephone counseling [131], and a telephone-based exercise intervention [117].

The internet offers a feasible mechanism to assess caregiver status and needs and offers low-cost, convenient, individually tailored psychosocial programs [88, 132–134]. In a randomized controlled study conducted by Blom and colleagues, an internet course guided by a psychologist was associated with less caregiver depression [134]. Similarly, psychoeducational programs have demonstrated improvements in caregiver burden [135, 136] and depression in pre-post evaluation [136]. Support groups have been facilitated by using videoconferencing and internet forums with preliminary evidence of effect on caregiving outcomes [91, 135, 137–139].

Caregivers in a CBT skill training program delivered on a DVD reported that patient behaviors were appraised as less stressful and bothersome as compared to caregivers receiving a general educational program [140]. Preliminary work with in-home video monitoring uploaded via the Internet for interdisciplinary team review and feedback shows promise in reducing caregiving burden [141]. Professionals reported the value of video recordings for identifying antecedents and evaluating caregiver responses. The caregivers reported improved communication and behavior management, and ease of use.

Despite the statistically significant findings that occur in each of these studies individually, there are concerns whether the tested interventions have adequate evidence of clinically meaningful outcomes [142–145]. Problems of study design, recruitment of a generalizable sample, prevention of participant loss and the lack of replicated findings continue to be problematic in caregiver research.

Respite and Post Caregiving Interventions

Respite Services

Respite is commonly defined as short periods of personal private time and space away from the emotional, psychological, and physical demands of caregiving [146]. Respite interventions include companion and sitting services, home care provided around the clock, adult day care, and short term residential/in-patient care. Mavall and colleagues [8] explored the benefits of adult day care on caregiver experience and concluded that caregivers of persons with moderate to severe dementia would benefit from informal home support as a supplement to adult day care [147]. Zarit and others found that adult day care use lowered caregivers' exposure to stressors and improved behavior and sleep for people with dementia on days they had adult day care.

Although caregivers have described respite care as an important facilitator of coping, including supporting better sleep [148], a systematic review did not demonstrate any benefits or adverse effects from the use of respite care for people with dementia or their caregivers [149]. The authors of the review acknowledged the lack of high quality research in this area rather than an actual lack of benefit, and called for well-designed trials in this area.

Post-caregiving Interventions

Gaugler and colleagues examined the response of family caregivers during the transition of persons with dementia to nursing home care [74]. They found that institutionalization reduced caregiver burden and depressive symptoms, but enhanced counseling provided additional long-term benefits. The results offer some of the first clinical evidence of the benefits of enhanced counseling during the transition to institutionalization for caregivers of people with AD.

Responses to the death of relative with dementia are multifaceted. Bereavement after dementia caregiving can be associated with relief from the chronic strains of caregiving [150]. However, Schulz and colleagues found that approximately 25 % of caregivers remain depressed a year after the death, with depression while caregiving the strongest predictor of sustained depression after death [151]. Unfortunately, their increased grief reaction is too often overlooked by health professionals [139].

A multicomponent intervention, "Easing the Way," targeting grief symptoms in spouse caregivers of individuals with dementia was pilot tested [152]. The intervention is tailored to participants' grief, mental health, and learning needs, and includes supportive grief counseling, emotional support, education, skill building, and referral to community resources. Significant improvements were found from baseline to intervention completion for the measures of grief, depression, anxiety, positive states of mind, and self-efficacy in the intervention group. Another pilot study demonstrated the feasibility of a

12-week intervention that emphasizes knowledge, (2) skill in communication and conflict resolution, and (3) chronic grief management skill in family caregivers whose relative with Alzheimer's disease transitioned into a long-term care [153].

On a larger scale, the NYUCI research team examined the joint effects of bereavement and caregiver intervention on caregiver depressive symptoms in a randomized controlled trial [154]. The death of the care recipient led to reductions in depressive symptoms for both the intervention and the control groups. Enhanced support intervention led to lower depressive symptoms compared with controls both before and after bereavement. Post-bereavement group differences were stronger for caregivers of spouses who did not previously experience a nursing home placement. These caregivers maintained these differences for more than 1 year after bereavement.

Future Directions

Numerous types of interventions have been designed and tested with the goal of improving psychological health, and to a lesser extent physical health, of caregivers of persons with dementia. Despite the significant findings that occur in each of these studies individually, there are concerns whether the tested interventions have adequate evidence to be clinically meaningful [142–145] Problems of study design, recruitment of a generalizable sample, prevention of participant loss and the lack of replicated findings continue to be problematic in caregiver research. There is much opportunity to expand intervention with early evidence of effectiveness, create novel interventions particularly using technologic approaches, and personalize these interventions to meet the needs of individual caregivers. There are particularly significant gaps in terms of effective interventions that improve the physiologic health of caregivers.

There is a need to replicate interventional research in diverse ethnic groups, such as the randomized controlled trial of NYUCI with Hispanic caregivers who represent all types of family relatives (common law spouses, children, siblings, a nephew and nieces) [155]. Moore reported that gay caregivers experienced prejudice and insensitivity from health care providers, and experienced barriers to accessing health care benefits and employee leave to care for their partner with dementia [156]. Their distinct needs warrant attention both in clinical practice and program planning. Other underserved populations in the caregiver support arena include caregivers of persons with young-onset dementia [157] and intellectual disability [158], and families having relationship difficulty when caring for a member with dementia [159].

Cross-sectional data from the NINR—funded National Caregiver Training Project (data collected 1995–1997) indicated that the majority of caregivers did not attend support groups (73 %) or use respite services (79 %); nor did they participate in bereavement services [92, 160]. Among caregivers who did not use services, 78 % lived with the recipient and 77 % were spouses. The profile of non-users compared to users revealed that non-users were significantly older, more depressed, and received less social support. Thus, the utilization of caregiver interventions is a critical area for continued investigation in order to develop and sustain relevant and effective programs and services, including ones that meet the complex needs of the most vulnerable caregivers.

Factors associated with more successful interventions are: (1) the extent to which they are customized to the needs of the individual; (2) whether they offer long-term support; and (3) whether they involve interventions targeted to caregiver physical as well as psychological health. There is a critical need to move evidence-based interventions into practical, accessible, and cost-effective services for caregivers through translational research [75, 76, 106, 144, 161–163]. Caregivers provide the huge majority of care for persons with dementia and their care should be a major priority in the broader plan to care for persons with dementia.

References

1. Alzheimer's Association. 2014 Alzheimer's disease facts and figures. Alzheimers Dement. 2014;10(2): e47–92. PubMed PMID: 24818261.
2. Brodaty H, Donkin M. Family caregivers of people with dementia. Dialogues Clin Neurosci. 2009;11(2):217–28. PubMed PMID: 19585957. Pubmed Central PMCID: 3181916.
3. Zarit S, Zarit J. Families under stress: interventions for caregivers of senile dementia patients. Psychother Theor Res Pract. 1982;19:461–71.
4. Bjorkhem K, Olsson A, Hallberg IR, Norberg A. Caregivers' experience of providing care for demented persons living at home. Scand J Prim Health Care. 1992;10(1):53–9. PubMed PMID: 1589665. Epub 1992/03/01.
5. Drinka TJ, Smith JC, Drinka PJ. Correlates of depression and burden for informal caregivers of patients in a geriatrics referral clinic. J Am Geriatr Soc. 1987;35(6):522–5. PubMed PMID: 3553288. Epub 1987/06/01.
6. Farran CJ, Keane-Hagerty E, Tatarowicz L, Scorza E. Dementia care-receiver needs and their impact on caregivers. Clin Nurs Res. 1993;2(1):86–97. PubMed PMID: 8453391. Epub 1993/02/01.
7. Knight BG, Lutzky SM, Macofsky-Urban F. A meta-analytic review of interventions for caregiver distress: recommendations for future research. Gerontologist. 1993;33(2):240–8.
8. Pruchno RA, Resch NL. Husbands and wives as caregivers: antecedents of depression and burden. Gerontologist. 1989;29(2):159–65.
9. Evans-Bergman BF. Alzheimer's and related disorders: loneliness, depression, and social support of spousal caregivers. J Gerontol Nurs. 1994;March: 6–16.
10. Gallagher D, Rose J, Rivera P, Lovett S, Thompson LW. Prevalence of depression in family caregivers. Gerontologist. 1989;29(4):449–56.
11. Gallagher-Thompson D, Brooks J, Bliwise D, Leader J, Yesavage J. The relations among caregiver stress, "sundowning" symptoms, and cognitive decline in Alzheimer's disease. J Am Geriatr Soc. 1992;40:807–10.
12. Fonareva I, Oken BS. Physiological and functional consequences of caregiving for relatives with dementia. Int Psychogeriatr. 2014;26(5):725–47. PubMed PMID: 24507463. Pubmed Central PMCID: PMC3975665. Epub 2014/02/11.
13. Norton MC, Smith KR, Ostbye T, Tschanz JT, Corcoran C, Schwartz S, et al. Greater risk of dementia when spouse has dementia? The Cache County study. J Am Geriatr Soc. 2010;58(5): 895–900. PubMed PMID: 20722820. Pubmed Central PMCID: 2945313.
14. Mausbach BT, Ancoli-Israel S, von Kanel R, Patterson TL, Aschbacher K, Mills PJ, et al. Sleep disturbance, norepinephrine, and D-dimer are all related in elderly caregivers of people with Alzheimer disease. Sleep. 2006;29(10):1347–52. PubMed PMID: 17068989. Epub 2006/10/31.
15. Mausbach BT, Aschbacher K, Mills PJ, Roepke SK, von Kanel R, Patterson TL, et al. A 5-year longitudinal study of the relationships between stress, coping, and immune cell beta(2)-adrenergic receptor sensitivity. Psychiatry Res. 2008;160(3):247–55. PubMed PMID: 18708265. Pubmed Central PMCID: PMC2567282. Epub 2008/08/19.
16. Mausbach BT, Dimsdale JE, Ziegler MG, Mills PJ, Ancoli-Israel S, Patterson TL, et al. Depressive symptoms predict norepinephrine response to a psychological stress or task in Alzheimer's caregivers. Psychosom Med. 2005;67(4):638–42. PubMed PMID: 16046380. Epub 2005/07/28.
17. von Kanel R, Ancoli-Israel S, Dimsdale JE, Mills PJ, Mausbach BT, Ziegler MG, et al. Sleep and biomarkers of atherosclerosis in elderly Alzheimer caregivers and controls. Gerontology. 2010;56(1): 41–50. PubMed PMID: 19955705. Pubmed Central PMCID: PMC2844340. Epub 2009/12/04.
18. von Kanel R, Dimsdale JE, Mills PJ, Ancoli-Israel S, Patterson TL, Mausbach BT, et al. Effect of Alzheimer caregiving stress and age on frailty markers interleukin-6, C-reactive protein, and D-dimer. J Gerontol A Biol Sci Med Sci. 2006;61(9):963–9. PubMed PMID: 16960028. Epub 2006/09/09.
19. von Kanel R, Mausbach BT, Dimsdale JE, Mills PJ, Patterson TL, Ancoli-Israel S, et al. Cardiometabolic effects in caregivers of nursing home placement and death of their spouse with Alzheimer's disease. J Am Geriatr Soc. 2011;59(11):2037–44. PubMed PMID: 22091921. Pubmed Central PMCID: PMC3384995. Epub 2011/11/19.
20. Mahoney DF, Jones RN, Coon DW, Mendelsohn AB, Gitlin LN, Ory M. The Caregiver Vigilance Scale: application and validation in the Resources for Enhancing Alzheimer's Caregiver Health (REACH) project. Am J Alzheimers Dis Other Demen. 2003;18(1):39–48. PubMed PMID: 12613133. Epub 2003/03/05.
21. Simpson C, Carter P. Dementia caregivers' lived experience of sleep. Clin Nurse Spec. 2013;27(6):298–306. PubMed PMID: 24107753. Epub 2013/10/11.
22. Zanetti O, Frisoni GB, Bianchetti A, Tamanza G, Cigoli V, Trabucchi M. Depressive symptoms of Alzheimer caregivers are mainly due to personal rather than patient factors. Int J Geriatr Psychiatry. 1998;13(6):358–67.
23. Covinsky KE, Eng C, Lui LY, Sands LP, Sehgal AR, Walter LC, et al. Reduced employment in caregivers of frail elders: impact of ethnicity, patient clinical characteristics, and caregiver characteristics. J Gerontol A Biol Sci Med Sci. 2001;56(11):M707–13. PubMed PMID: 11682579. Epub 2001/10/30.

24. Schulz R, O'Brien AT, Bookwala J, Fleissner K. Psychiatric and physical morbidity effects of dementia caregiving: prevalence, correlates, and causes. Gerontologist. 1995;35(6):771–91. PubMed PMID: 8557205.

25. Pinquart M, Sorensen S. Helping caregivers of persons with dementia: which interventions work and how large are their effects? Int Psychogeriatr. 2006;18(4):577–95. PubMed PMID: 16686964. Epub 2006/05/12.

26. Alspaugh ME, Stephens MA, Townsend AL, Zarit SH, Greene R. Longitudinal patterns of risk for depression in dementia caregivers: objective and subjective primary stress as predictors. Psychol Aging. 1999;14(1):34–43. PubMed PMID: 10224630.

27. Haley WE, West CA, Wadley VG, Ford GR, White FA, Barrett JJ, et al. Psychological, social, and health impact of caregiving: a comparison of black and white dementia family caregivers and noncaregivers. Psychol Aging. 1995;10(4):540–52. PubMed PMID: 8749581.

28. Abdollahpour I, Nedjat S, Noroozian M, Salimi Y, Majdzadeh R. Caregiver burden: the strongest predictor of self-rated health in caregivers of patients with dementia. J Geriatr Psychiatry Neurol. 2014;27(3):172–80. PubMed PMID: 24614200. Epub 2014/03/13.

29. Williams IC. Emotional health of black and white dementia caregivers: a contextual examination. J Gerontol B Psychol Sci Soc Sci. 2005;60(6):P287–P95. PubMed PMID: 16260702.

30. Li R, Cooper C, Bradley J, Shulman A, Livingston G. Coping strategies and psychological morbidity in family carers of people with dementia: a systematic review and meta-analysis. J Affect Disord. 2012;139(1):1–11. PubMed PMID: 21723617.

31. Clyburn LD, Stones MJ, Hadjistavropoulos T, Tuokko H. Predicting caregiver burden and depression in Alzheimer's disease. J Gerontol B Psychol Sci Soc Sci. 2000;55(1):S2–13. PubMed PMID: 10728125.

32. Wright MJ, Battista MA, Pate DS, Hierholzer R, Mogelof J, Howsepian AA. Domain-specific associations between burden and mood state in dementia caregivers. Clin Gerontol. 2010;33:237–47.

33. Schoenmakers B, Buntinx F, Delepeleire J. What is the role of the general practitioner towards the family caregiver of a community-dwelling demented relative? A systematic literature review. Scand J Prim Health Care. 2009;27(1):31–40. PubMed PMID: 19040191. Epub 2008/12/02.

34. Piercy KW, Fauth EB, Norton MC, Pfister R, Corcoran CD, Rabins PV, et al. Predictors of dementia caregiver depressive symptoms in a population: the Cache County dementia progression study. J Gerontol B Psychol Sci Soc Sci. 2013;68(6):921–6. PubMed PMID: 23241850. Pubmed Central PMCID: PMC3894110. Epub 2012/12/18.

35. Poulshock SW, Deimling GT. Families caring for elders in residence: issues in the measurement of burden. J Gerontol. 1984;39(2):230–9. PubMed PMID: 6699382.

36. Pearlin LI, Mullan JT, Semple SJ, Skaff MM. Caregiving and the stress process: an overview of concepts and their measures. Gerontologist. 1990;30(5):583–94. PubMed PMID: 2276631. Epub 1990/10/01.

37. Campbell P, Wright J, Oyebode J, Job D, Crome P, Bentham P, et al. Determinants of burden in those who care for someone with dementia. Int J Geriatr Psychiatry. 2008;23(10):1078–85. PubMed PMID: 18613247.

38. Hilgeman MM, Durkin DW, Sun F, DeCoster J, Allen RS, Gallagher-Thompson D, et al. Testing a theoretical model of the stress process in Alzheimer's caregivers with race as a moderator. Gerontologist. 2009;49(2):248–61. PubMed PMID: 19363019. Pubmed Central PMCID: 2721662.

39. Vitaliano PP, Scanlan JM, Zhang J, Savage MV, Hirsch IB, Siegler IC. A path model of chronic stress, the metabolic syndrome, and coronary heart disease. Psychosom Med. 2002;64(3):418–35. PubMed PMID: 12021416. Epub 2002/05/22.

40. Aschbacher K, Mills PJ, von Kanel R, Hong S, Mausbach BT, Roepke SK, et al. Effects of depressive and anxious symptoms on norepinephrine and platelet P-selectin responses to acute psychological stress among elderly caregivers. Brain Behav Immun. 2008;22(4):493–502. PubMed PMID: 18054198. Pubmed Central PMCID: PMC2442159. Epub 2007/12/07.

41. Aschbacher K, von Kanel R, Dimsdale JE, Patterson TL, Mills PJ, Mausbach BT, et al. Dementia severity of the care receiver predicts procoagulant response in Alzheimer caregivers. Am J Geriatr Psychiatry. 2006;14(8):694–703. PubMed PMID: 16861374. Epub 2006/07/25.

42. Aschbacher K, von Kanel R, Mills PJ, Hong S, Roepke SK, Mausbach BT, et al. Combination of caregiving stress and hormone replacement therapy is associated with prolonged platelet activation to acute stress among postmenopausal women. Psychosom Med. 2007;69(9):910–7. PubMed PMID: 17991824. Epub 2007/11/10.

43. Chattillion EA, Ceglowski J, Roepke SK, von Kanel R, Losada A, Mills PJ, et al. Pleasant events, activity restriction, and blood pressure in dementia caregivers. Health Psychol. 2013;32(7):793–801. PubMed PMID: 22888824. Pubmed Central PMCID: PMC3572271. Epub 2012/08/15.

44. Aschbacher K, Roepke SK, von Kanel R, Mills PJ, Mausbach BT, Patterson TL, et al. Persistent versus transient depressive symptoms in relation to platelet hyperactivation: a longitudinal analysis of dementia caregivers. J Affect Disord. 2009;116 (1–2):80–7. PubMed PMID: 19131112. Pubmed Central PMCID: PMC2772124. Epub 2009/01/10.

45. Cacioppo JT, Burleson MH, Poehlmann KM, Malarkey WB, Kiecolt-Glaser JK, Berntson GG, et al. Autonomic and neuroendocrine responses to mild psychological stressors: effects of chronic stress on older women. Ann Behav Med. 2000;22(2):140–8. PubMed PMID: 10962707. Epub 2000/08/30.

46. Grant I, McKibbin CL, Taylor MJ, Mills P, Dimsdale J, Ziegler M, et al. In-home respite intervention reduces plasma epinephrine in stressed Alzheimer caregivers. Am J Geriatr Psychiatry. 2003;11(1): 62–72. PubMed PMID: 12527541. Epub 2003/01/16.

47. Irwin M, Brown M, Patterson T, Hauger R, Mascovich A, Grant I. Neuropeptide Y and natural killer cell activity: findings in depression and Alzheimer caregiver stress. FASEB J. 1991;5(15):3100–7. PubMed PMID: 1743441. Epub 1991/12/01.

48. Irwin M, Hauger R, Patterson TL, Semple S, Ziegler M, Grant I. Alzheimer caregiver stress: basal natural killer cell activity, pituitary-adrenal cortical function, and sympathetic tone. Ann Behav Med. 1997;19(2):83–90. PubMed PMID: 9603682. Epub 1997/04/01.

49. Mausbach BT, Chattillion E, Roepke SK, Ziegler MG, Milic M, von Kanel R, et al. A longitudinal analysis of the relations among stress, depressive symptoms, leisure satisfaction, and endothelial function in caregivers. Health Psychol. 2012;31(4):433–40. PubMed PMID: 22486550. Pubmed Central PMCID: PMC3393823. Epub 2012/04/11.

50. von Kanel R, Dimsdale JE, Patterson TL, Grant I. Association of negative life event stress with coagulation activity in elderly Alzheimer caregivers. Psychosom Med. 2003;65(1):145–50. PubMed PMID: 12554826. Epub 2003/01/30.

51. Gallagher-Thompson D, Shurgot GR, Rider K, Gray HL, McKibbin CL, Kraemer HC, et al. Ethnicity, stress, and cortisol function in Hispanic and non-Hispanic white women: a preliminary study of family dementia caregivers and noncaregivers. Am J Geriatr Psychiatry. 2006;14(4):334–42. PubMed PMID: 16582042. Epub 2006/04/04.

52. Clark MS, Bond MJ, Hecker JR. Environmental stress, psychological stress and allostatic load. Psychol Health Med. 2007;12(1):18–30. PubMed PMID: 17129930. Epub 2006/11/30.

53. Neri M, Bonati PA, Pinelli M, Borella P, Tolve I, Nigro N. Biological, psychological and clinical markers of caregiver's stress in impaired elderly with dementia and age-related disease. Arch Gerontol Geriatr. 2007;44 Suppl 1:289–94. PubMed PMID: 17317464. Epub 2007/02/24.

54. Oken BS, Fonareva I, Wahbeh H. Stress-related cognitive dysfunction in dementia caregivers. J Geriatr Psychiatry Neurol. 2011;24(4):191–8. PubMed PMID: 22228825. Pubmed Central PMCID: PMC3340013. Epub 2012/01/10.

55. Bauer ME, Vedhara K, Perks P, Wilcock GK, Lightman SL, Shanks N. Chronic stress in caregivers of dementia patients is associated with reduced lymphocyte sensitivity to glucocorticoids. J Neuroimmunol. 2000;103(1):84–92. PubMed PMID: 10674993. Epub 2000/02/16.

56. Bristow M, Cook R, Erzinclioglu S, Hodges J. Stress, distress and mucosal immunity in carers of a partner with fronto-temporal dementia. Aging Ment Health. 2008;12(5):595–604. PubMed PMID: 18855175. Epub 2008/10/16.

57. Redwine L, Mills PJ, Sada M, Dimsdale J, Patterson T, Grant I. Differential immune cell chemotaxis responses to acute psychological stress in Alzheimer caregivers compared to non-caregiver controls. Psychosom Med. 2004;66(5):770–5. PubMed PMID: 15385705. Epub 2004/09/24.

58. Thompson RL, Lewis SL, Murphy MR, Hale JM, Blackwell PH, Acton GJ, et al. Are there sex differences in emotional and biological responses in spousal caregivers of patients with Alzheimer's disease? Biol Res Nurs. 2004;5(4):319–30. PubMed PMID: 15068661. Epub 2004/04/08.

59. Mausbach BT, Patterson TL, Rabinowitz YG, Grant I, Schulz R. Depression and distress predict time to cardiovascular disease in dementia caregivers. Health Psychol. 2007;26(5):539–44. PubMed PMID: 17845105. Epub 2007/09/12.

60. Roepke SK, Allison M, Von Kanel R, Mausbach BT, Chattillion EA, Harmell AL, et al. Relationship between chronic stress and carotid intima-media thickness (IMT) in elderly Alzheimer's disease caregivers. Stress. 2012;15(2):121–9. PubMed PMID: 21790484. Pubmed Central PMCID: PMC3223262. Epub 2011/07/28.

61. Mausbach BT, Roepke SK, Ziegler MG, Milic M, von Kanel R, Dimsdale JE, et al. Association between chronic caregiving stress and impaired endothelial function in the elderly. J Am Coll Cardiol. 2010;55(23):2599–606. PubMed PMID: 20513601. Pubmed Central PMCID: PMC2892624. Epub 2010/06/02.

62. McCurry SM, Logsdon RG, Teri L, Vitiello MV. Sleep disturbances in caregivers of persons with dementia: contributing factors and treatment implications. Sleep Med Rev. 2007;11(2):143–53. PubMed PMID: 17287134.

63. McCurry SM, Vitiello MV, Gibbons LE, Logsdon RG, Teri L. Factors associated with caregiver reports of sleep disturbances in persons with dementia. Am J Geriatr Psychiatry. 2006;14(2):112–20. PubMed PMID: 16473975.

64. Creese J, Bedard M, Brazil K, Chambers L. Sleep disturbances in spousal caregivers of individuals with Alzheimer's disease. Int Psychogeriatr. 2008;20(1):149–61. PubMed PMID: 17466086.

65. Merrilees J, Hubbard E, Mastick J, Miller BL, Dowling GA. Sleep in persons with frontotemporal dementia and their family caregivers. Nurs Res. 2014;63(2):129–36. PubMed PMID: 24589648. Pubmed Central PMCID: PMC4151390. Epub 2014/03/05.

66. Mills PJ, Ancoli-Israel S, von Kanel R, Mausbach BT, Aschbacher K, Patterson TL, et al. Effects of gender and dementia severity on Alzheimer's disease caregivers' sleep and biomarkers of coagulation and inflammation. Brain Behav Immun. 2009;23(5):605–10. PubMed PMID: 18930805. Pubmed Central PMCID: PMC2757046. Epub 2008/10/22.

67. Moore RC, Harmell AL, Chattillion E, Ancoli-Israel S, Grant I, Mausbach BT. PEAR model and sleep outcomes in dementia caregivers: influence of activity restriction and pleasant events on sleep disturbances. Int Psychogeriatr. 2011;23(9):1462–9. PubMed PMID: 21429282. Pubmed Central PMCID: PMC3199377. Epub 2011/03/25.

68. Caswell LW, Vitaliano PP, Croyle KL, Scanlan JM, Zhang J, Daruwala A. Negative associations of chronic stress and cognitive performance in older adult spouse caregivers. Exp Aging Res. 2003;29(3):303–18. PubMed PMID: 12775440. Epub 2003/05/31.

69. Vitaliano PP, Murphy M, Young HM, Echeverria D, Borson S. Does caring for a spouse with dementia promote cognitive decline? A hypothesis and proposed mechanisms. J Am Geriatr Soc. 2011;59(5):900–8. PubMed PMID: 21568959. Epub 2011/05/17.

70. Norton MC, Piercy KW, Rabins PV, Green RC, Breitner JC, Ostbye T, et al. Caregiver-recipient closeness and symptom progression in Alzheimer disease. The Cache County Dementia Progression Study. J Gerontol B Psychol Sci Soc Sci. 2009;64(5):560–8. PubMed PMID: 19564210. Pubmed Central PMCID: 2728091. Epub 2009/07/01.

71. Campbell JL, Rowe MA, Marsiske M. Behavioral symptoms of dementia: a dyadic effect of caregivers' stress process? Res Gerontol Nurs. 2011;4(3):168–84. PubMed PMID: 20873693. Pubmed Central PMCID: PMC3140561. Epub 2010/09/30.

72. Spring HJ, Rowe MA, Kelly A. Improving caregivers' well-being by using technology to manage nighttime activity in persons with dementia. Res Gerontol Nurs. 2009;2(1):39–48. PubMed PMID: 20077992. Pubmed Central PMCID: PMC2946162. Epub 2010/01/19.

73. Mittelman MS, Roth DL, Coon DW, Haley WE. Sustained benefit of supportive intervention for depressive symptoms in caregivers of patients with Alzheimer's disease. Am J Psychiatry. 2004;161(5):850–6. PubMed PMID: 15121650. Epub 2004/05/04.

74. Gaugler JE, Roth DL, Haley WE, Mittelman MS. Can counseling and support reduce burden and depressive symptoms in caregivers of people with Alzheimer's disease during the transition to institutionalization? Results from the New York University caregiver intervention study. J Am Geriatr Soc. 2008;56(3):421–8. PubMed PMID: 18179495.

Pubmed Central PMCID: 2700042. Epub 2008/01/09.

75. Long KH, Moriarty JP, Mittelman MS, Foldes SS. Estimating the potential cost savings from the New York University Caregiver Intervention in Minnesota. Health Affairs (Millwood). 2014; 33(4):596–604. PubMed PMID: 24711320. Epub 2014/04/09.

76. Mittelman MS, Bartels SJ. Translating research into practice: case study of a community-based dementia caregiver intervention. Health Affairs (Millwood). 2014;33(4):587–95. PubMed PMID: 24711319. Epub 2014/04/09.

77. Garand L, Rinaldo DE, Alberth MM, Delany J, Beasock SL, Lopez OL, et al. Effects of problem solving therapy on mental health outcomes in family caregivers of persons with a new diagnosis of mild cognitive impairment or early dementia: a randomized controlled trial. Am J Geriatr Psychiatry. 2014;22(8):771–81. PubMed PMID: 24119856. Pubmed Central PMCID: PMC4021000. Epub 2013/10/15.

78. Kuzu N, Beser N, Zencir M, Sahiner T, Nesrin E, Ahmet E, et al. Effects of a comprehensive educational program on quality of life and emotional issues of dementia patient caregivers. Geriatr Nurs. 2005;26(6):378–86. PubMed PMID: 16373183. Epub 2005/12/24.

79. Judge KS, Yarry SJ, Looman WJ, Bass DM. Improved strain and psychosocial outcomes for caregivers of individuals with dementia: findings from Project ANSWERS. Gerontologist. 2013; 53(2):280–92. PubMed PMID: 22899427. Epub 2012/08/18.

80. Teri L, McCurry SM, Logsdon R, Gibbons LE. Training community consultants to help family members improve dementia care: a randomized controlled trial. Gerontologist. 2005;45(6):802–11. PubMed PMID: 16326662.

81. Brodaty H, Green A, Koschera A. Meta-analysis of psychosocial interventions for caregivers of people with dementia. J Am Geriatr Soc. 2003;51(5):657–64. PubMed PMID: 12752841.

82. Dias A, Dewey ME, D'Souza J, Dhume R, Motghare DD, Shaji KS, et al. The effectiveness of a home care program for supporting caregivers of persons with dementia in developing countries: a randomised controlled trial from Goa, India. PLoS One. 2008;3(6), e2333. PubMed PMID: 18523642. Pubmed Central PMCID: PMC2396286. Epub 2008/06/05.

83. Vernooij-Dassen M, Draskovic I, McCleery J, Downs M. Cognitive reframing for carers of people with dementia. Cochrane Database Syst Rev. 2011;(11):CD005318. PubMed PMID: 22071821. Epub 2011/11/11

84. Leone D, Carragher N, Santalucia Y, Draper B, Thompson LW, Shanley C, et al. A pilot of an intervention delivered to Chinese- and Spanish-speaking carers of people with dementia in Australia. Am J

Alzheimers Dis Other Demen. 2014;29(1):32–7. PubMed PMID: 24085251. Epub 2013/10/03.

85. Fialho PP, Koenig AM, Santos MD, Barbosa MT, Caramelli P. Positive effects of a cognitive-behavioral intervention program for family caregivers of demented elderly. Arq Neuropsiquiatr. 2012;70(10):786–92. PubMed PMID: 23060105. Epub 2012/10/13.

86. Losada A, Marquez-Gonzalez M, Romero-Moreno R. Mechanisms of action of a psychological intervention for dementia caregivers: effects of behavioral activation and modification of dysfunctional thoughts. Int J Geriatr Psychiatry. 2011;26(11):1119–27. PubMed PMID: 21061414. Epub 2010/11/10.

87. Marquez-Gonzalez M, Losada A, Izal M, Perez-Rojo G, Montorio I. Modification of dysfunctional thoughts about caregiving in dementia family caregivers: description and outcomes of an intervention programme. Aging Ment Health. 2007;11(6):616–25. PubMed PMID: 18074249. Epub 2007/12/13.

88. Kwok T, Au A, Wong B, Ip I, Mak V, Ho F. Effectiveness of online cognitive behavioral therapy on family caregivers of people with dementia. Clin Interv Aging. 2014;9:631–6. PubMed PMID: 24748781. Pubmed Central PMCID: PMC3990366. Epub 2014/04/22.

89. Haley WE, Brown SL, Levine EG. Experimental evaluation of the effectiveness of group intervention for dementia caregivers. Gerontologist. 1987;27(3):376–82.

90. Zarit SH, Anthony CR, Boutselis M. Interventions with care givers of dementia patients: comparison of two approaches. Psychol Aging. 1987;2(3):225–32. PubMed PMID: 3268213. Epub 1987/09/01.

91. McKechnie V, Barker C, Stott J. The effectiveness of an Internet support forum for carers of people with dementia: a pre-post cohort study. J Med Internet Res. 2014;16(e68). PubMed PMID: 24583789. Pubmed Central PMCID: PMC3961748. Epub 2014/03/04.

92. Robinson KM, Buckwalter K, Reed D. Differences between dementia caregivers who are users and non-users of community services. Public Health Nurs. 2013;30(6):501–10. PubMed PMID: 24579710. Epub 2014/03/04.

93. Hurley RV, Patterson TG, Cooley SJ. Meditation-based interventions for family caregivers of people with dementia: a review of the empirical literature. Aging Ment Health. 2014;18(3):281–8. PubMed PMID: 24093954. Epub 2013/10/08.

94. Khalsa DS. Mindfulness effects on caregiver stress: should we expect more? J Altern Complement Med. 2010;16(10):1025–6. PubMed PMID: 20954958. Epub 2010/10/20.

95. Mackenzie CS, Poulin PA. Living with the dying: using the wisdom of mindfulness to support caregivers of older adults with dementia. Int J Health Promot Educ. 2006;44(1):43–7.

96. Whitebird RR, Kreitzer M, Crain AL, Lewis BA, Hanson LR, Enstad CJ. Mindfulness-based stress reduction for family caregivers: a randomized controlled trial. Gerontologist. 2013;53(4):676–86. PubMed PMID: 23070934. Pubmed Central PMCID: PMC3709844. Epub 2012/10/17.

97. Waelde LC, Thompson L, Gallagher-Thompson D. A pilot study of a yoga and meditation intervention for dementia caregiver stress. J Clin Psychol. 2004;60(6):677–87. PubMed PMID: 15141399. Epub 2004/05/14. eng.

98. Lavretsky H, Epel ES, Siddarth P, Nazarian N, Cyr NS, Khalsa DS, et al. A pilot study of yogic meditation for family dementia caregivers with depressive symptoms: effects on mental health, cognition, and telomerase activity. Int J Geriatr Psychiatry. 2013;28(1):57–65. PubMed PMID: 22407663. Pubmed Central PMCID: PMC3423469. Epub 2012/03/13.

99. Black DS, Cole SW, Irwin MR, Breen E, St Cyr NM, Nazarian N, et al. Yogic meditation reverses NF-kappaB and IRF-related transcriptome dynamics in leukocytes of family dementia caregivers in a randomized controlled trial. Psychoneuroendocrinology. 2013;38(3):348–55. PubMed PMID: 22795617. Pubmed Central PMCID: PMC3494746. Epub 2012/07/17.

100. Korn L, Logsdon RG, Polissar NL, Gomez-Beloz A, Waters T, Ryser R. A randomized trial of a CAM therapy for stress reduction in American Indian and Alaskan Native family caregivers. Gerontologist. 2009;49(3):368–77. PubMed PMID: 19377083. Pubmed Central PMCID: PMC2682170. Epub 2009/04/21.

101. Moore RC, Chattillion EA, Ceglowski J, Ho J, von Kanel R, Mills PJ, et al. A randomized clinical trial of Behavioral Activation (BA) therapy for improving psychological and physical health in dementia caregivers: results of the Pleasant Events Program (PEP). Behav Res Ther. 2013;51(10):623–32. PubMed PMID: 23916631. Pubmed Central PMCID: PMC3774137. Epub 2013/08/07.

102. Kim H, Rose K. Sleep disturbances in family caregivers: an overview of the state of the science. Arch Psychiatr Nurs. 2011;25(6):456–68. PubMed PMID: 22114799.

103. Oken BS, Fonareva I, Haas M, Wahbeh H, Lane JB, Zajdel D, et al. Pilot controlled trial of mindfulness meditation and education for dementia caregivers. J Altern Complement Med. 2010;16(10):1031–8. PubMed PMID: 20929380. Pubmed Central PMCID: PMC3110802. Epub 2010/10/12.

104. von Kanel R, Dimsdale JE, Ancoli-Israel S, Mills PJ, Patterson TL, McKibbin CL, et al. Poor sleep is associated with higher plasma proinflammatory cytokine interleukin-6 and procoagulant marker fibrin D-dimer in older caregivers of people with Alzheimer's disease. J Am Geriatr Soc. 2006;54(3):431–7. PubMed PMID: 16551309. Epub 2006/03/23.

105. Rose KM, Taylor AG, Bourguignon C. Effects of cranial electrical stimulation on sleep disturbances,

depressive symptoms, and caregiving appraisal in spousal caregivers of persons with Alzheimer's disease. Appl Nurs Res. 2009;22(2):119–25. PubMed PMID: 19427574. Pubmed Central PMCID: PMC2713101. Epub 2009/05/12.

106. Widera E, Covinsky KE. Fulfilling our obligation to the caregiver: it's time for action: comment on "Translation of a dementia caregiver support program in a health care system–REACH VA". Arch Intern Med. 2011;171(4):359–60. PubMed PMID: 21357812. Epub 2011/03/02.

107. Simpson C, Carter PA. Pilot study of a brief behavioral sleep intervention for caregivers of individuals with dementia. Res Gerontol Nurs. 2010;3(1):19–29. PubMed PMID: 20128540. Epub 2010/02/05.

108. McCurry S, Logsdon R, Vitiello M, Teri L. Successful behavioral treatment for reported sleep problems in elderly caregivers of dementia patients: a controlled study. J Gerontol Psychol Sci. 1998; 53B(2):P122–9.

109. Rowe MA, Kairalla JA, McCrae CS. Sleep in dementia caregivers and the effect of a nighttime monitoring system. J Nurs Scholarsh. 2010;42(3):338–47. PubMed PMID: 20738745.

110. A new vision of aging: Helping older adults make healthier choices. Washington, DC: Center for the Advancement of Health, 2006 Contract No.: Issue Briefing No. 2.

111. The state of aging and health in America 2007. Whitehouse Station, NJ: Centers for Disease Control and Prevention and the Merck Company Foundation; 2007.

112. von Kanel R, Mausbach BT, Dimsdale JE, Mills PJ, Patterson TL, Ancoli-Israel S, et al. Regular physical activity moderates cardiometabolic risk in Alzheimer's caregivers. Med Sci Sports Exerc. 2011;43(1):181–9. PubMed PMID: 20473220. Pubmed Central PMCID: PMC3162319. Epub 2010/05/18.

113. Netz Y, Wu MJ, Becker BJ, Tenenbaum G. Physical activity and psychological well-being in advanced age: a meta-analysis of intervention studies. Psychol Aging. 2005;20(2):272–84. PubMed PMID: 16029091.

114. Lim K, Taylor L. Factors associated with physical activity among older people–a population-based study. Prev Med. 2005;40(1):33–40. PubMed PMID: 15530578.

115. Etkin CD, Prohaska TR, Connell CM, Edelman P, Hughes SL. Antecedents of physical activity among family caregivers. J Appl Gerontol. 2008;27(3):350–67. PubMed PMID: 25392600. Pubmed Central PMCID: 4226062.

116. Castro CM, King AC. Telephone-assisted counseling for physical activity. Exerc Sport Sci Rev. 2002;30(2):64–8. PubMed PMID: 11991539.

117. Connell CM, Janevic MR. Effects of a telephone-based exercise intervention for dementia caregiving wives: a randomized controlled trial. J Appl Gerontol. 2009;28(2):171–94. PubMed PMID:

21709757. Pubmed Central PMCID: PMC3121165. Epub 2009/04/01.

118. King AC, Baumann K, O'Sullivan P, Wilcox S, Castro C. Effects of moderate-intensity exercise on physiological, behavioral, and emotional responses to family caregiving: a randomized controlled trial. J Gerontol A Biol Sci Med Sci. 2002;57(1):M26–36. PubMed PMID: 11773209. Epub 2002/01/05.

119. Farran CJ, Staffileno BA, Gilley DW, McCann JJ, Yan L, Castro CM, et al. A lifestyle physical activity intervention for caregivers of persons with Alzheimer's disease. Am J Alzheimers Dis Other Demen. 2008;23(2):132–42. PubMed PMID: 18174315. Pubmed Central PMCID: PMC2758783. Epub 2008/01/05.

120. Hirano A, Suzuki Y, Kuzuya M, Onishi J, Ban N, Umegaki H. Influence of regular exercise on subjective sense of burden and physical symptoms in community-dwelling caregivers of dementia patients: a randomized controlled trial. Arch Gerontol Geriatr. 2011;53(2):e158–63. PubMed PMID: 20850878. Epub 2010/09/21.

121. Yu F, Swartwood RM. Feasibility and perception of the impact from aerobic exercise in older adults with Alzheimer's disease. Am J Alzheimers Dis Other Demen. 2012;27(6):397–405. PubMed PMID: 22871905. Epub 2012/08/09.

122. Bank AL, Arguelles S, Rubert M, Eisdorfer C, Czaja SJ. The value of telephone support groups among ethnically diverse caregivers of persons with dementia. Gerontologist. 2006;46(1):134–8. PubMed PMID: 16452294. Epub 2006/02/03.

123. Bormann J, Warren KA, Regalbuto L, Glaser D, Kelly A, Schnack J, et al. A spiritually based caregiver intervention with telephone delivery for family caregivers of veterans with dementia. Fam Community Health. 2009;32(4):345–53. PubMed PMID: 19752637. Epub 2009/09/16.

124. Tremont G, Davis JD, Bishop DS, Fortinsky RH. Telephone-delivered psychosocial intervention reduces burden in dementia caregivers. Dementia (London). 2008;7(4):503–20. PubMed PMID: 20228893. Pubmed Central PMCID: PMC2836858. Epub 2008/01/01.

125. van Mierlo LD, Meiland FJ, Droes RM. Dementelcoach: effect of telephone coaching on carers of community-dwelling people with dementia. Int Psychogeriatr. 2012;24(2):212–22. PubMed PMID: 21995966. Epub 2011/10/15.

126. Belle SH, Burgio L, Burns R, Coon D, Czaja SJ, Gallagher-Thompson D, et al. Enhancing the quality of life of dementia caregivers from different ethnic or racial groups: a randomized, controlled trial. Ann Intern Med. 2006;145(10):727–38. PubMed PMID: 17116917. Pubmed Central PMCID: PMC2585490. Epub 2006/11/23.

127. Glueckauf RL, Davis WS, Willis F, Sharma D, Gustafson DJ, Hayes J, et al. Telephone-based, cognitive-behavioral therapy for African American dementia caregivers with depression: initial findings.

Rehabil Psychol. 2012;57(2):124–39. PubMed PMID: 22686551. Epub 2012/06/13.

128. Martindale-Adams J, Nichols LO, Burns R, Graney MJ, Zuber J. A trial of dementia caregiver telephone support. Can J Nurs Res. 2013;45(4):30–48. PubMed PMID: 24617278. Epub 2014/03/13.

129. Burgio LD, Collins IB, Schmid B, Wharton T, McCallum D, Decoster J. Translating the REACH caregiver intervention for use by area agency on aging personnel: the REACH OUT program. Gerontologist. 2009;49(1):103–16. PubMed PMID: 19363008. Epub 2009/04/14.

130. Elliott AF, Burgio LD, Decoster J. Enhancing caregiver health: findings from the resources for enhancing Alzheimer's caregiver health II intervention. J Am Geriatr Soc. 2010;58(1):30–7. PubMed PMID: 20122038. Pubmed Central PMCID: PMC2819276. Epub 2010/02/04.

131. Gant JR, Steffen AM, Lauderdale SA. Comparative outcomes of two distance-based interventions for male caregivers of family members with dementia. Am J Alzheimers Dis Other Demen. 2007;22(2):120–8. PubMed PMID: 17545139. Epub 2007/06/05.

132. Gies C, Pierce L, Steiner V, van der Bijl J, Salvador D. Web-based psychosocial assessment for caregivers of persons with dementia: a feasibility study. Rehabil Nurs. 2014;39(2):102–9. PubMed PMID: 23703687. Epub 2013/05/25.

133. Hayden LJ, Glynn SM, Hahn TJ, Randall F, Randolph E. The use of Internet technology for psychoeducation and support with dementia caregivers. Psychol Serv. 2012;9(2):215–8. PubMed PMID: 22662739. Epub 2012/06/06.

134. Blom MM, Bosmans JE, Cuijpers P, Zarit SH, Pot AM. Effectiveness and cost-effectiveness of an internet intervention for family caregivers of people with dementia: design of a randomized controlled trial. BMC Psychiatry. 2013;13:17. PubMed PMID: 23305463. Pubmed Central PMCID: PMC3557221. Epub 2013/01/12.

135. Chiu T, Marziali E, Colantonio A, Carswell A, Gruneir M, Tang M, et al. Internet-based caregiver support for Chinese Canadians taking care of a family member with Alzheimer disease and related dementia. Can J Aging. 2009;28(4):323–36. PubMed PMID: 19925698. Epub 2009/11/21.

136. Finkel S, Czaja SJ, Schulz R, Martinovich Z, Harris C, Pezzuto D. E-care: a telecommunications technology intervention for family caregivers of dementia patients. Am J Geriatr Psychiatry. 2007;15(5):443–8. PubMed PMID: 17463195. Epub 2007/04/28.

137. Marziali E, Garcia LJ. Dementia caregivers' responses to 2 Internet-based intervention programs. Am J Alzheimers Dis Other Demen. 2011;26(1):36–43. PubMed PMID: 21282276. Epub 2011/02/02.

138. Beauchamp N, Irvine AB, Seeley J, Johnson B. Worksite-based internet multimedia program for family caregivers of persons with dementia.

Gerontologist. 2005;45(6):793–801. PubMed PMID: 16326661. Epub 2005/12/06.

139. Sanders S, Marwit SJ, Meuser TM, Harrington P. Caregiver grief in end-stage dementia: using the Marwit and Meuser Caregiver Grief Inventory for assessment and intervention in social work practice. Soc Work Health Care. 2007;46(1):47–65. PubMed PMID: 18032156. Epub 2007/11/23.

140. Gallagher-Thompson D, Wang PC, Liu W, Cheung V, Peng R, China D, et al. Effectiveness of a psycho-educational skill training DVD program to reduce stress in Chinese American dementia caregivers: results of a preliminary study. Aging Ment Health. 2010;14(3):263–73. PubMed PMID: 20425645. Epub 2010/04/29.

141. Williams K, Arthur A, Niedens M, Moushey L, Hutfles L. In-home monitoring support for dementia caregivers: a feasibility study. Clin Nurs Res. 2013;22(2):139–50. PubMed PMID: 22997349. Pubmed Central PMCID: PMC3633651. Epub 2012/09/22.

142. Boots LM, de Vugt ME, van Knippenberg RJ, Kempen GI, Verhey FR. A systematic review of Internet-based supportive interventions for caregivers of patients with dementia. Int J Geriatr Psychiatry. 2014;29(4):331–44. PubMed PMID: 23963684. Epub 2013/08/22.

143. Godwin KM, Mills WL, Anderson JA, Kunik ME. Technology-driven interventions for caregivers of persons with dementia: a systematic review. Am J Alzheimers Dis Other Demen. 2013;28(3):216–22. PubMed PMID: 23528881. Epub 2013/03/27.

144. Zarit SH, Femia EE. A future for family care and dementia intervention research? Challenges and strategies. Aging Ment Health. 2008;12(1):5–13. PubMed PMID: 18297475.

145. Samia LW, Hepburn K, Nichols L. "Flying by the seat of our pants": what dementia family caregivers want in an advanced caregiver training program. Res Nurs Health. 2012;35(6):598–609. PubMed PMID: 22911130. Epub 2012/08/23.

146. Upton N, Reed V. Caregiver coping in dementing illness–implications for short-term respite care. Int J Psychiatr Nurs Res. 2005;10(3):1180–96. PubMed PMID: 15960246. Epub 2005/06/18.

147. Mavall L, Thorslund M. Does day care also provide care for the caregiver? Arch Gerontol Geriatr. 2007;45(2):137–50. PubMed PMID: 17129621. Epub 2006/11/30.

148. Lee D, Morgan K, Lindesay J. Effect of institutional respite care on the sleep of people with dementia and their primary caregivers. J Am Geriatr Soc. 2007;55(2):252–8. PubMed PMID: 17302663. Epub 2007/02/17.

149. Maayan N, Soares-Weiser K, Lee H. Respite care for people with dementia and their carers. Cochrane Database Syst Rev [Internet]. 2014;(1). Available from: http://onlinelibrary.wiley.com/doi/10.1002/14651858.CD004396.pub3/abstract

150. Schulz R, Mendelsohn AB, Haley WE, Mahoney D, Allen RS, Zhang S, et al. End-of-life care and the effects of bereavement on family caregivers of persons with dementia. N Engl J Med. 2003; 349(20):1936–42. PubMed PMID: 14614169. Epub 2003/11/14.

151. Schulz R, Belle SH, Czaja SJ, McGinnis KA, Stevens A, Zhang S. Long-term care placement of dementia patients and caregiver health and well-being. JAMA. 2004;292(8):961–7. PubMed PMID: 15328328. Epub 2004/08/26.

152. Ott CH, Kelber ST, Blaylock M. "Easing the way" for spouse caregivers of individuals with dementia: a pilot feasibility study of a grief intervention. Res Gerontol Nurs. 2010;3(2):89–99. PubMed PMID: 20415358. Epub 2010/04/27.

153. Paun O, Farran CJ. Chronic grief management for dementia caregivers in transition: intervention development and implementation. J Gerontol Nurs. 2011;37(12):28–35. PubMed PMID: 22084962. Pubmed Central PMCID: PMC3708697. Epub 2011/11/17.

154. Haley WE, Bergman EJ, Roth DL, McVie T, Gaugler JE, Mittelman MS. Long-term effects of bereavement and caregiver intervention on dementia caregiver depressive symptoms. Gerontologist. 2008;48(6):732–40. PubMed PMID: 19139247. Pubmed Central PMCID: PMC2846300. Epub 2009/01/14.

155. Luchsinger J, Mittelman M, Mejia M, Silver S, Lucero RJ, Ramirez M, et al. The Northern Manhattan Caregiver Intervention Project: A randomised trial testing the effectiveness of a dementia caregiver intervention in Hispanics in New York City. BMJ Open. 2012;2(5). PubMed PMID: 22983877. Pubmed Central PMCID: PMC3467593. Epub 2012/09/18.

156. Moore W. Lesbian and gay elders: connecting care providers through a telephone support group. J Gay Lesbian Soc Serv. 2002;14:23–41.

157. Arai A, Matsumoto T, Ikeda M. Do family caregivers perceive more difficulty when they look after patients with early onset dementia compared to those with late onset dementia. Int J Geriatr Psychiatry. 2007;22:1255–61.

158. Jubb D, Pollard N, Chaston D. Developing services for younger people with dementia. Nurs Times. 2003;99(22):34–5. PubMed PMID: 12808749.

159. Peisah C, Brodaty H, Quadrio C. Family conflict in dementia: prodigal sons and black sheep. Int J Geriatr Psychiatry. 2006;21(5):485–92. PubMed PMID: 16676295.

160. Bergman EJ, Haley WE, Small BJ. Who uses bereavement services? An examination of service use by bereaved dementia caregivers. Aging Ment Health. 2011;15(4):531–40. PubMed PMID: 21500020. Epub 2011/04/19.

161. Stevens AB, Lancer K, Smith ER, Allen L, McGhee R. Engaging communities in evidence-based interventions for dementia caregivers. Fam Community Health. 2009;32(1 Suppl):S83–92. PubMed PMID: 19065098. Epub 2008/12/23.

162. Joling KJ, van Hout HP, Scheltens P, Vernooij-Dassen M, van den Berg B, Bosmans J, et al. (Cost)-effectiveness of family meetings on indicated prevention of anxiety and depressive symptoms and disorders of primary family caregivers of patients with dementia: design of a randomized controlled trial. BMC Geriatr. 2008;8:2. PubMed PMID: 18208607. Pubmed Central PMCID: PMC2259355. Epub 2008/01/23.

163. Zarit S, Femia E. Behavioral and psychosocial interventions for family caregivers. Am J Nurs. 2008;108(9 Suppl):47–53. quiz PubMed PMID: 18797226. Epub 2008/09/23.

Part IV

Dementia Continuing Care

Transitions in Care for the Person with Dementia

Marie Boltz

Introduction

Traditionally, transition in the gerontological and health services literature describes relocation from one health care setting to another [1, 2]. Thus, transitions of care refers to the actions involved in coordinating care for patients as they move through various components of the health care system [3]. The goal during a transition is to communicate the care that was provided, the patient's current status, and the need for follow-up care. The patient's and family's understanding of the clinical condition and treatments plan, as well as their preferences and perspectives should also be communicated [3, 4].

Older adults with dementia have greater nursing facility use, greater hospital and home health use, and more relocation transitions per person-year than those without dementia [5, 6]. During transitions in care, persons with dementia are typically experiencing significant changes in function and health, and family caregivers are experiencing increased stress and burden [7–13]. Consequently, negotiating transitions can be especially difficult for persons with dementia and their families [9, 13–15]. The heightened vulnerability of this population as well as the increased costs associated with transitions in care settings warrants close attention by the clinician and the health care administrator. This chapter describes best practices to improve the outcomes and experiences for transitions of the person with dementia within three care settings: primary care, the hospital, and long-term.

Primary Care: Considerations for Transitions

Timely detection of dementia (as described in Chapter "Detection of Dementia" by Galvin) is critical in order that supports can be put in place to help manage co-morbidities before they lead to acute problems and functional loss [16]. The point at which a person with dementia is formally diagnosed is when the family caregiver often assumes the role of caregiver [17]. Every effort should be made to include the patient in decision-making along with active engagement of the caregiver. Partnership with the caregiver is essential to detect changes in the patient's clinical and functional status, including signs of illness, as well identify the need for additional services and resources. Patients should be seen regularly, perhaps every 3–6 months, accompanied by their most consistent caregiver whenever possible. This allows the clinician to monitor the progression of cognitive and functional impairment, the response to medication, the signs of acute problems, the exacerbation of chronic disease, and

M. Boltz, PhD, RN, GNP-BC, FGSA, FAAN (✉)
William F. Connell School of Nursing, Boston
College, Mahoney Hall, 140 Commonwealth Avenue,
Chestnut Hill, MA 02467, USA
e-mail: boltzm@bc.edu

© Springer International Publishing Switzerland 2016
M. Boltz, J.E. Galvin (eds.), *Dementia Care*, DOI 10.1007/978-3-319-18377-0_14

caregiver coping [18]. The Healthy Aging Brain Care Monitor (HAB-C Monitor) is a clinically practical multidimensional tool to measure the patient's cognitive, functional, and behavioral/mood status, as well as caregiving stress. The HAB-C monitor utilizes caregiver report and has demonstrated good reliability and validity [19].

Counseling regarding physical activity, good nutrition, sleep hygiene, cognitive stimulation, and socialization is warranted to maximize function and health [20, 21]. Advance planning for both health care decisions and financial matters, is ideally addressed in the early stages of dementia when the patient is able to actively participate. Advanced care planning, the process of preparing and documenting preferences for future health decisions, is critical to guide treatment decisions across the care continuum [17]. However, advance directive completion rates in the United States continue to be low even among those with dementia. For example, a study of 127 patients without advance directives presenting for a cognitive evaluation found that 39 % still did not have directives after 5 years [22].

Evidence-Based Primary Care Models

Although not designed exclusively for patients with dementia, interdisciplinary models of care have demonstrated improvements in patient outcomes. The Collaborative Care Model, Guided Care Model, and GRACE Model offer the potential to promote aging in place and limit disruptions in care delivery.

The Collaborative Care Model (CCM) includes care provided by a team led by the primary care physician and a geriatric nurse practitioner who serves as the care manager [23]. Weekly meetings with a support team comprised of a geriatrician, geriatric psychiatrist, and a psychologist who review the care of new and active patients and monitor adherence to the standard protocols enhanced treatment planning and evaluation. Caregivers and patients receive education on communication skills; caregiver coping skills; legal and financial advice; patient exercise guidelines with a guidebook and videotape; and a caregiver guide provided by the local chapter of the Alzheimer's Association. Also the care manager is supported by a web-based longitudinal tracking system that manages the schedule for patient contacts, tracks the patient's progress and current treatments, and provides an instrument for communicating the patient's and caregiver's current clinical status to the entire care team. Patients participating in the CCM have shown significantly fewer behavioral and psychological symptoms of dementia and caregivers demonstrated less depression [23].

The Guided Care Model is a physician/nurse care coordination model, usually conducted for a long-term/indefinite amount of time [24]. The guided care nurse conducts a comprehensive home assessment, creates an evidence-based care guide and action plan for the patient; conducts monthly monitoring and self-management coaching; facilitates smooth transitions into and out of hospitals and other institutions; coordinate care by all providers; provides family caregiver education/support, and facilitates access to community based services. Guided Care [24, 25] as well as other nurse—coordinated programs [26], have positively influenced patient and physician satisfaction as well as caregiver burden, and demonstrated cost-savings.

Geriatric Resources for Assessment and Care of Elders (GRACE) is a practice-based care coordination model [27]. GRACE is conducted for a long-term/indefinite amount of time and requires a nurse practitioner and social worker who collaborate with the primary physician. The team offers in-home assessment and care management. Upon enrollment, the GRACE support team meets with the patient in the home to conduct an initial comprehensive geriatric assessment. The support team then meets with the larger GRACE interdisciplinary team (including a geriatrician, pharmacist, physical therapist, mental health social worker, and community-based services liaison) to develop an individualized care plan including activation of GRACE protocols for evaluating and managing common geriatric conditions. GRACE provides at least one in-home follow-up visit to review care plan, and one telephone or face-to-face contact per month, coordination of care, and collaboration with hospital discharge planners and a home visit after any hospitalization. The intervention was found to be cost-neutral for high-risk, low-income individuals aged 65 years or older in primary care due to reductions in hospital costs [27].

Hospitalization of the Person with Dementia

Older adults who have dementia are significantly more likely than those who do not to have an ED visit or be hospitalized [28, 29]. In a sample of 3,019 participants, age 65 years and older without dementia, of whom 494 developed dementia, Phelan and colleagues [30] compared rates of hospitalization among those who developed dementia with those who did not. After the onset of dementia, the average annual admission rate was more than twice the rate of years in persons without dementia, after adjustment for age, sex, nursing home residence, and other potential confounders. Moreover, the admission rate for "ambulatory care–sensitive conditions (ACSCs) for which proactive outpatient care might prevent the need for a hospital stay" was 78 % higher in persons with dementia, after full adjustment for covariates [30]. Bacterial pneumonia, congestive heart failure, urinary tract infection, dehydration, and duodenal ulcer were much more common in patients with dementia. Similarly, evidence suggests that the most common conditions precipitating hospital transfers in nursing home residents (e.g., pneumonia) can be treated with the same efficacy in the nursing home setting and therefore transfers are potentially avoidable [31–33].

As compared to older adults without cognitive impairment, hospitalized persons with dementia are more likely to experience delirium and behavioral manifestations of distress, as well as pressure ulcers, falls, nutritional problems, functional decline, hospital readmission, and increased morbidity/mortality [34–38]. Communication difficulties and persistent delirium can make post-acute rehabilitation difficult [38]. The additive stress of the hospitalization and the patient's increased functional dependency compound the

strain of the family caregiver [9] and increase the likelihood that the patient will be admitted to the nursing home for a long-term stay [39, 40]. The increased risks posed by hospitalization for both patient and family caregiver make it important to institute measures to: (1) prevent hospitalization when possible; (2) prepare patients and families for the possibility of hospitalization; and (3) when the patient is hospitalized, collaborate effectively with the post-acute setting to inform treatment plans, promote functional recovery, and prevent rehospitalization.

Efforts to Prevent Hospitalization

In order to prevent unnecessary hospitalization, access on a daily, 24 h-basis to an informed team member is critical. An acute care plan for potential emergencies should be accessible to on-call providers when there is an acute change in the patient's condition. Ideally this care plan reflects shared decision-making with the patient/caregiver and includes information on advance directives, medication use and history of problems, and caregiver wishes regarding choice of hospital and medical provider. Table 1 offers additional tips for the clinician on preventing and shortening hospitalization stays [18, 41].

Table 1 Approaches to prevent and shorten hospital stays

Keep immunizations up to date
Arrange or community resources to provide resource and respite
Encourage caregivers to utilize support services; monitor caregiver strain
Educate the caregiver to promptly report indications of illness including change in behavior, mentation, appetite, and sleep
Evaluate caregiver understanding of home safety and fall prevention and safe use of medications.
Whenever possible, arrange for diagnostics to be done on an outpatient as opposed to inpatient basis
Ensure prompt follow-up after the hospitalization
If possible arrange for diagnostic tests to be done before admission to shorten the hospital stay
Arrange for consultants to see the patient before he or she is admitted

Preparing Patients and Families for the Possibility of Hospitalization

The Alzheimer's Association [41] recommends that the caregiver prepare for an emergency room visit or unexpected hospital stay. Families can be advised to create an emergency kit in advance. Some items to include are: a list of current medications and food allergies, copies of advance directives, insurance information, name and phone number of medical provider, name and phone number of friends or family members who could stay with the person in the emergency room while the responsible party is filling out forms, a note explaining the person's dementia and particular needs, nonperishable snacks, a change of clothes, extra disposable briefs if they are usually worn, pen and paper to write down symptoms and doctor's or nurse's instructions or information. The Family Caregiver Report (Fig. 1) can be

---

Family Caregiver Report

Family Members, use this form to share information with staff about how your loved one is normally, When they are not sick or in crisis. Encourage patient involvement in the development of this information as much as possible. This information will help staff understand and provide for your loved one's needs.

Name: _____ What does he/she preferred to be called? _____

Where does he/she live? _____ Alone? Or with? _____

Does he/she become upset? Yes No How does he/she show this? _____

What triggers this? _____ What makes he/she feel comfortable? _____

In general, what helps he/she cope (for example, religion, music, certain people)? _____

What are fluids and simple foods does he/she enjoy? _____

Would he/she like chaplain to visit? Yes No What other religious/spritual activity would he/she desire? _____

What is his/her normal bedtime routine (for example, dentures in/out, call to family, a prayer, etc.)? _____

What kind of work did he/she do? _____

What are his/her interests or hobbies? _____

What else can you tell us that will help us care for him/her? Strengths/Challenges? _____

Does he/she normally need help...	Always	Sometimes	Never	Don't Know	Details
Understand where he/she is?					
Follow directions?					
Tell others what he/she needs?					
Tell others when he/she is in pain?					
Wear a hearing aid?					
Wear glasses?					
Have dentures?					
Using the bathroom?					
Walking?					
Getting out of bed?					
With bathing, brushing teeth, etc.?					
Dressing?					
Eating?					

Is there anything else you want the staff to know about him/her? _____

Name & relationship of person completing this form: _____

Fig. 1 (Permission by author: Maggie Murphy White). Source: This tool was created by Maggie Murphy -White, MA. Used with permission

used to orient staff to the needs and preferences of the person with dementia [42].

Family and friends play an important role motivating patients to be physically active as possible and providing cognitive stimulation [43]. Family should be counseled to let hospital staff who interacts with the person know that he or she has dementia, to report to the staff any increase in confusion, and provide information about his or her personal habits, diet or eating preferences, and medications that he or she is taking. Other important recommendations are to remain with the person as much as possible, or arrange coverage with family/friends to be present (especially upon awakening in the morning, when medications are given and procedures conducted, or when the physician visits or rounds are conducted). Notes at the bedside (if the person can read), telephone calls, and tape recording of familiar sounds and voices are ways of communicating and allaying anxiety when the family is unable to be present [41].

Hospital to Home

The traditional discharge record should include special transition considerations for the person with dementia. Emphasis should be placed on the patient's safety, functional recovery, need for follow-up care, and caregiver availability and capability [3, 9, 43]. See Table 2, Content of the Discharge Record.

The Transitional Care Model (TCM) provides comprehensive discharge planning and home follow-up by advanced practice nurses (APNs) to older adults at high risk for poor outcomes [44], including those with cognitive impairment [45]. The APN provides in-hospital assessment, home visits by the APN with available, ongoing telephone support, and continuity of medical care between hospital and primary care providers (facilitated by the APN accompanying patients to the first follow-up visit). The intervention is provided on average for 2 months post-discharge. The TCM resulted in fewer hospital readmissions for patients. Additionally, among those patients who are rehospitalized, the time between their

Table 2 The transitional record for the person with dementia: recommended items

Identified primary caregiver and contact information
Reason for hospitalization, treatment provided, response to treatment
Education provided to patient/caregiver and understanding demonstrated
Services and resources required (home care, local aging services, caregiver support)
Medications and treatments
Follow-up appointments
Baseline function, current function, and plan for functional recovery
Cognitive status, including presence of delirium
Plan to prevent/deal with behavioral manifestations of distress
Advance directives

discharge and readmission was longer and the number of days spent in the hospital was generally shorter than expected.

The Care Transitions Intervention (CTI) is a 4-week program facilitated by a Transitions Coach who works with patients with complex care needs and family caregivers to learn self-management skills to support transition from hospital to home [46]. The intervention includes one hospital visit, one home visit, and three follow up phone calls by the Transitions Coach. The transitions coach supports the patient and caregiver in developing and maintaining a personal health record for the patient, and provides coaching to make sure pertinent questions are asked and answered. Also, patients and their families are helped to develop self-care skills, including medication self-management and increased awareness of symptoms along with instructions on how to respond to them. CTI has demonstrated effectiveness in reducing hospital readmission rates [46].

Collaboration with the Post-acute Setting

The transfer of a person with dementia from the hospital to a nursing home, whether for short-term or long-term care, poses challenges [47]. Another new, unfamiliar environment can result in increased anxiety and decrements in cognition [13]. In general, communication between hospitals and nursing homes is fraught with problems creating potential for mistakes and adverse events [47–49]. Nurses have cited multiple inadequacies of hospital discharge information, including problems with medication orders, little psychosocial history, and inaccurate information regarding current health status. Other frequently under-reported yet critical clinical dimensions include cognitive history (including the presence of delirium) and physical function, specifically baseline function, and the potential to rehabilitate [49].

Given that behavioral manifestations of distress are common upon admission [50] an understanding of best ways to communicate potential stressors and coping mechanisms can promote comfort and function, and provide alternatives to psychoactive medication and the common negative sequelae [51]. Studies have shown, that contrary to common staff perception [52], family caregivers provide essential information to inform assessment, and can be instrumental to developing care plans that are tailored to the individual's need and are realistic and achievable [9, 42, 43]. The Family Caregiver Report (Fig. 1) can be utilized to provide information on the patient's function, preferences and needs.

End of Life Hospitalization

In general, advanced dementia patients with nutritional and severe functional impairment should be considered for palliative care evaluation. However, hospital transfers are common for those with dementia in the last 6 months of life [53, 54] despite poor outcomes and high mortality rates [31, 55, 56]. In the United States, approximately 16 % of those dying with dementia die in hospitals [57], despite widespread agreement that palliative care, rather than aggressive, life-sustaining care, should be provided to those with advanced dementia [17]. Often patients with anorexia, weight loss, and poor functional status will meet criteria for hospice admission with the diagnosis of failure to thrive even if they are unable to enroll with a dementia

diagnosis [58]. See Chapters "Dementia Palliative Care" by Brody and "Hospice Dementia Care" by Powers for discussion of palliative care and hospice, respectively.

Transition to Long-term Care

Although approximately 70 % of people with dementia are cared for at home by family, the duration and intensity of care needs cause many families to elect long-term care placement for care receivers as their needs increase [59]. The decision to seek institutional care is one of the most challenging transitions for family caregivers [17]. Smith and colleagues [60] identified predictors associated with time to nursing home placement. These included total number of years of education, age at onset of dementia, being single, living in a retirement or supervised apartment at onset, change in Charlson comorbidity score, and a change in the amount of daily assistance required.

A systematic review conducted by Gaugler and colleagues [61] found that the most consistent patient-related predictors of nursing home admissions in persons with dementia include the diagnosis of Alzheimer disease, severity of cognitive impairment, dependence in basic activities of daily living, behavioral symptoms, and depression. Caregiver-related characteristics that predicted nursing home placement included the severity of emotional stress, a desire to institutionalize the care recipient, and feelings of being "trapped" in care responsibilities [61].

Nursing home settings are federally licensed and regulated settings that provide room, board, 24 hour oversight, health monitoring, assistance with activities of daily living (ADLs), health services, recreational activities, and skilled nursing services [59]. Zimmerman and colleagues [62] report that the proportion of residents with dementia may be as high as 80 %. Further, the majority (90 %) of people with dementia utilize nursing home care at some point in their illness [63, 64], and 70 % of those with dementia receive end-of-life care in nursing homes [65].

Historically, nursing homes have been the primary long-term, institutional setting for persons with dementia [59]. Since the 1990's, however there has a surge in the number of residential care/assisted living (RC/AL) facilities, licensed by the states to provide non-medical, non-medical care, offering room, board, 24 h oversight, and assistance with activities of daily living. RC/AL are licensed by the States under various names, including sheltered housing, domiciliary care, intermediate care housing, personal care homes, adult foster care, assisted living, congregate care, and other names, and vary widely in size, structure, and services [59]. Recent estimates indicate that 45–67 % of RC/AL residents have dementia [62].

Alzheimer's (or dementia) special care units (SCUs) in RC/AL settings account for 5 % of all nursing home beds and approximately 11 % of RC/AL settings have a distinct dementia unit, wing, or floor [66]. Given the significant proportion of persons with dementia occupying both nursing homes and RC/AL, the majority of residents in both settings are clearly not in SCUs [6].

The Decision to Admit to Long-term Care

Several factors can influence the caregiver's selection of a nursing home for the person with dementia. They include the facility's geographic location, reputation, appearance, availability of services including medical care, financial factors (cost and/or coverage by insurance), and consumer ratings [59]. Family roles may influence the decision-making. A study conducted in Taiwan by Huang and colleagues [67] evaluated family members' decision-making factors regarding placement. The results showed that when making decisions about the placement of family members, spouses chose facilities according to their own life experiences, children considered medical treatment convenience, grandchildren preferred to collect relevant information on facilities, and other relatives preferred to decide based on introductions from government departments [67]. Results underscore the need for a mechanism of consultation that provides comprehensive

information to families and assistance with negotiating decisions, while including the prospective resident's needs and preferences.

Many consumer guides are available to assist the consumer to choose the long-term care setting that may be best for their family member. However, these guides do not appear to be derived from evidence and some have been developed by organizations with a financial interest in a certain long-term care product [59]. The website of the Centers for Medicare and Medicaid Services offers publicly available information to help families choose among nursing homes and includes quality of care ratings [68]. Additionally, the Alzheimer's Association CareFinder™, an interactive online guide proves education to consumers on how to recognize quality care, choose the best care options, and advocate for quality within a residence [69].

Person-Centered Care Approaches in Long-term Care

The admission and subsequent adjustment period can be a difficult time for people with dementia and their family caregivers. Admission has been linked to increased behavioral manifestations of distress, depression, decreasing cognition, frailty, and falls [70]. For caregivers, guilt, depression, feelings of failure, and continuing burden but also improvement in quality of life have been variously reported [70, 71]. Sury and colleagues [70] recommend ensuring that the person with dementia have input into decision to enter the long-term care setting, orientation procedures for the person with dementia and family member, and a "buddy" system for new arrivals.

Finally, they recommend a person-centered approach [72], i.e., one that considers the individual needs and preferences of the person with dementia by actively engaging residents and families in planning and decision-making.

Family members play a critical role in maintaining emotional connectedness and psychosocial health [72]. They provide information, support for ADLs, continuity in care, and a voice in decision-making [73, 74]. Their presence improves resident improves resident psychological and psychosocial well-being, the accuracy of diagnosis, and care delivery [75].

The Collaborative Studies of Long-term care (CS-LTC) Dementia Care study had as a goal identifying dimensions of quality that reflect person-centered care. In the CS-LTC study, Zimmerman's research team and liaison panel identified six areas of care to measure quality of life in long term care residents with dementia: depression, behavioral symptoms, pain, food and fluid intake, activity involvement, and mobility [76]. These dimensions of quality are addressed in the evidence-based *Dementia Care Practice Recommendations for Assisted Living Residences and Nursing Homes* of the Alzheimer's Association [77]. In order to implement these best practices, the Alzheimer's Association recommends practices for comprehensive assessment and care planning that actively engages residents and families, as summarized in Table 3.

Transitions in the Long-term Care Resident

The resident with dementia who lives in a long-term care setting often continues to experience transitions in care settings. For example, they may move from home to a dementia-specific assisted living facility, relocate from assisted living to the nursing home, be transferred to the hospital then to a subacute unit followed by long-term-care. The trajectory of relocations may be multiple and varied and not necessarily proceed in a linear fashion [7].

Medical, functional, and behavioral problems are associated with transitions from assisted living. Kenny and colleagues [78] found that depression score, walking speed, balance, and mental status score were significantly associated with transition and in multivariate analysis, balance performance predicted transfer. These results suggest that fall risk should receive attention on admission to AL to potentially mitigate the need to transfer the resident. Consistent with these findings, a multidisciplinary geriatric team assessment of individuals newly admitted to two dementia-specific, AL communities found that

Table 3 Alzheimer Association dementia care practice recommendations for assisted living residences and nursing homes

Assessment content	
• Cognitive health	• Decision-making capacity
• Physical health	• Communication abilities
• Physical functioning	• Personal background
• Behavioral status	• Cultural preferences
• Sensory capabilities	• Spiritual needs and preferences

Assessment process
- Assessments should acknowledge that the resident's functioning might vary across different staff shifts
- Assessments should be conducted as required by regulations, when the person is hospitalized or significant change in condition
- Sources of assessment include:
  - Verbal information directly from residents and from family
  - Medical records
  - Observation of behavior (which can communicate and demonstrate preferences)
- Include consultants as needed
- Obtaining the most current advance directive information (e.g., durable health care power of attorney or living will) as well as information about a resident's preferences regarding palliative care and funeral arrangements to help ensure that the resident's wishes will be honored

Care Plans need to:
- Include the input of resident, the family, direct care staff and all staff who interact with resident
- Be accessible
- Be current and flexible, i.e., adapt to daily changes in a resident's needs and wishes
- Be function-focused. They should build on the person's strengths

falls were the primary reasons for transitions to the nursing home [79]. The team developed individualized interventions, not just specific for fall prevention, which demonstrated trends for decreasing hospitalization and death.

A move to another facility or unit can increase confusion and anxiety, and increase risk for falls [13]. Interventions that promote safety and comfort include emotional support and close oversight provided by family members, volunteers and assigned staff; involvement in structured activities; and personalizing the environment [77].

Hospitalization of the Long-term Resident with Dementia

Hospitalization can dramatically change the health, function, and quality of life for the long-term care resident with dementia. Several studies suggest that many hospitalizations of nursing home residents in general are inappropriate, avoidable, or related to conditions that could be treated outside the hospital setting. The societal costs are significant as they cost more than $4 billion per year [80–82]. The majority of hospitalizations of nursing home residents with advanced dementia are due to infections and thus were potentially avoidable, given that infections are often treatable in the nursing home [83]. Ouslander [84] identifies two factors that contribute to unnecessary hospitalizations: fiscal constraints (nursing homes are not incentivized to provide care for acute problems) and the paucity of health care professionals trained in geriatrics and evidence-based long-term care.

The Affordable Care Act mandates that nursing homes implement quality-assurance and performance-improvement activity, which can be useful in reducing unnecessary transfers. The Interventions to Reduce Acute Care Transfers (INTERACT) is a program that provides clinical tools, educational resources, communication strategies, and documentation standards that enhance the nursing home's ability to identify, evaluate, and manage conditions before they become serious enough to necessitate hospital transfer [85]. INTERACT has been shown to reduce unnecessary hospitalizations [86]. Rantz and colleagues [87] implemented the use of INTERACT in combination with health information technology and a transitions coach working with multidisciplinary teams in Missouri nursing homes. Outcomes included reduced hospitalizations, improved hospital transitions, improved communication, and reduced polypharmacy [87].

Transitions at End of Life

One of the 11 INTERACT modules addresses advance care planning offering resources to support comfort care plans as an alternative to hospitalization for residents at the end of life, when the risks associated with hospital care may outweigh the benefits [85]. Samala and colleagues [88] also recommend that as part of hospital discharge planning, attending physicians and case managers should facilitate the transition of patients with advanced dementia and no apparent rehabilitation potential to long-term care instead of skilled nursing facility care. They also recommend implementing a procedure to monitor residents with dementia using hospice admission criteria, as well as the mortality risk index, to evaluate for hospice readiness. Finally, the SNF nursing staff should be trained to provide basic hospice care to patients until they are fully transitioned to hospice [88]. See Chapters "Dementia Palliative Care" by Brody and "Hospice Dementia Care" by Powers for discussion of palliative care and hospice, respectively.

Conclusion and Future Directions

Over the past two decades there has increased awareness of the personal and societal costs of transitions of the older adult, magnified in the person with dementia. The emergence of patient-centered interventions, quality improvement initiatives, and evidence-based transitional models holds promise to improve quality of care and quality of life. In some cases, these approaches also demonstrate cost-savings. There remain however, research gaps in the area of transitions of care for persons with dementia. As stated on other chapters, populations that have been not well represented in dementia research in general (as well as transitional research specifically) include persons with young-onset dementia and intellectual disability, and patients and families with complex and/or difficult relationships [89–91]. Additionally there is the need to replicate interventional research in diverse ethnic groups.

The role of the diagnostic process (including timing and provider roles) and its influence upon the utilization of health and social services warrants close examination. Such an understanding would provide guidance to the development of care pathways that support customized, cost-effective programs that reflect patient/caregiver preference and help minimize disruptions in health and routines. Additionally, longitudinal studies would provide a more complete understanding of the transitions in care of people with dementia. Studies that follow people from dementia diagnosis, and are linked to administrative data sources would incorporate both clinical and social markers to determine how the natural history and clinical progression of dementia influences and impacts on pathways [92].

Additionally, research examining the experience and outcomes of transitions in and out of community-based care (including adult day care, home health, and long-term home care) is particularly relevant for person with dementia and their caregivers. The results are necessary to inform effective and fiscally responsible models of collaboration between providers.

Acknowledgements This work was supported by the Alzheimer's Association International Research Grant NIRG-12-242090.

References

1. Hersch G, Spencer J, Kapoor T. Adaptation by elders to new living arrangements following hospitalization: a qualitative, retrospective analysis. J Appl Gerontol. 2003;22:315–39.

2. Wilson S. The transition to nursing home life: A comparison of planned and unplanned admissions. J Adv Nurs. 1997;26:864–71.

3. Epstein-Lubow G, Fulton AT, Gardner R, Gravenstein S, Miller IW. Post-hospital transitions: special considerations for individuals with dementia. Med Health Rhode Island. 2010;93(4):125–7.

4. Bechtel C. If you build it, will they come? Designing truly patient-centered health care. Health Aff (Millwood). 2010;29(5):914–20.

5. Callahan CM, Arling G, Tu W, Rosenman MB, Counsell SR, Stump TE, et al. Transitions in care for older adults with and without dementia. J Am Geriatr Soc. 2012;60(5):813–20.

6. Aaltonen M, Rissanen P, Forma L, Raitanen J, Jylha M. The impact of dementia on care transitions during the last two years of life. Age Ageing. 2012;41(1):52–7.

7. Mead LM, Eckert K, Zimmerman S, Schumacher JG. Sociocultural aspects of transitions from assisted living for residents with dementia. Geron. 2005;45(1):115–23.

8. Shankar KN, Hirschman KB, Hanlon AL, Naylor MD. Burden in caregivers of cognitively impaired elderly adults at time of hospitalization: a cross-sectional analysis. J Am Geriatr Soc. 2014;62(2):276–84.

9. Boltz M, Chippendale T, Resnick B, Galvin J. Anxiety in family caregivers of hospitalized persons with dementia: contributing factors and responses. Alzheimer Dis Assoc Disord. 2015 [Epub ahead of print].

10. Lander SM, Brazill AL, Ladrigan PM. Intrainstitutional relocation: Effects of residents' behavior and psychosocial functioning. J Gerontol Nurs. 1997;23(1):35–41.

11. Rowles GD. Habituation and being in place. Occup Ther J Res. 2000;20 Suppl 1:52S–66.

12. Ryff CD, Essex MJ. The interpretation of life experience and well-being: the sample case of relocation. Psychol Aging. 1992;7:507–17.

13. Capezuti E, Boltz M, Renz S, Hoffman D, Norman RG. Nursing home involuntary relocation: clinical outcomes and perceptions of residents and families. J Am Med Dir Assoc. 2006;7:486–92.

14. Bredin K, Kitwood T. Decline in quality of life for patients with severe dementia following a ward merger. Int J Geriatr Psychiatry. 1995;10:967–73.

15. McAuslane L, Sperlinger D. The effects of relocation on elderly people with dementia and their nursing staff. Int J Geriatr Psychiatry. 1994;9:981–4.

16. Lyketsos CJ. Prevention of unnecessary hospitalization for patients with dementia. JAMA. 2012;307(2):197–8.

17. Rose K, Palan Lopez R. Transitions in dementia care: theoretical support for nursing roles. Online J Issues Nurs. 2012;17(2):4.

18. Lazaroff A, Morishita L, Schoephoerster G, McCarthy T. Using dementia as the organizing principle when caring for patients with dementia and comorbidities. Minn Med. 2013;96(1):41–6.

19. Monahan PO, Boustani MA, Alder C, Galvin JE, Perkins AJ, Healey P, Chehresa A, Shepard P, Corby Bubp C, Frame A, Callahan C. Practical clinical tool to monitor dementia symptoms: the HABC-monitor. Clin Interv Aging. 2012;7:143–57.

20. Heyn P, Abreu BC, Ottenbacher KJ. The effects of exercise training on elderly persons with cognitive impairment and dementia: a meta-analysis. Arch Phys Med Rehabil. 2004;85(100):1694–704.

21. Gray GE. Nutrition and dementia. J Am Diet Assoc. 1989;89(12):1795–802.

22. Garand L, Dew MA, Lingler JH, DeKosky ST. Incidence and predictors of advance care planning among persons with cognitive impairment. Am J Geriatr Psychiatry. 2011;19(8):712.

23. Callahan CM, Boustani MA, Unverzagt FW, Austrom MG, Damush TM, Perkins AJ, et al. Effectiveness of collaborative care for older adults with Alzheimer's disease in primary care a randomized controlled trial. JAMA. 2006;295(18):2148–57.

24. Boyd CM, Reider L, Frey K, Scharfstein D, Leff B, Wolff J, et al. The effects of guided care on the perceived quality of health care for multi-morbid older

persons: 18-month outcomes from a cluster and randomized controlled trial. J Gen Intern Med. 2010;25(3):235–42.

25. Wolff JL, Giovannetti ER, Boyd CM, Reider L, Palmer S, Scharfstein D, et al. Effects of guided care on family caregivers. Gerontologist. 2009;50(4):459–70.

26. Rantz MJ, Phillips L, Aud M, Popejoy L, Marek KD, Hicks LL, Zaniletti I, Miller SJ. Evaluation of aging in place model with home care services and registered nurse care coordination in senior housing. Nurs Outlook. 2011;59(1):37–46.

27. Counsell SR, Callahan CM, Clark DO, Tu W, Buttar AB, Stump TE, et al. Geriatric care management for low-income seniors: a randomized controlled trial. JAMA. 2007;298(22):2623–33.

28. Alzheimer's Association. 2015 Alzheimer's disease facts and figures. Alzheimer Dement. 2015;11(3): 332–384.

29. Feng Z, Coots LA, Kalaganova Y, Wiener JM. Hospital and ED use among medicare beneficiaries with dementia varies by setting and proximity to death. Health Aff. 2014;33(4):683.

30. Phelan EA, Borson S, Grothaus L, Balch S, Larson EB. Association of incident dementia with hospitalizations. JAMA. 2012;307:165–72.

31. Boockvar KS, Gruber-Baldini AL, Burton L, Zimmerman S, May C, Magaziner J. Outcomes of infection in nursing home residents with and without early hospital transfer. J Am Geriatr Soc. 2005; 53(4):590–6.

32. Kruse RL, Mehr DR, Boles KE, Lave JR, Binder EF, Madsen R, et al. Does hospitalization impact survival after lower respiratory infection in nursing home residents? Med Care. 2004;42(9):860.

33. Loeb M, Carusone SC, Goeree R, Walter SD, Brazil K, Krueger P, Marrie T. Effect of a clinical pathway to reduce hospitalizations in nursing home residents with pneumonia: a randomized controlled trial. JAMA. 2006;295(21):2503.

34. Zekry D, Herrmann FR, Grandjean R, et al. Demented versus non-demented very old inpatients: the same co-morbidities but poorer functional and nutritional status. Age Ageing. 2008;37:83–9.

35. Margiotta A, Bianchetti A, Ranieri P, Trabucchi M. Clinical characteristics and risk factors of delirium in demented and not demented elderly medical inpatients. J Nutr Health Aging. 2006;10(6):535–9.

36. Mecocci P, von Strauss E, Cherubini A, et al. Cognitive impairment is the major risk factor for development of geriatric syndromes during hospitalization: results from the GIFA study. Dement Geriatr Cogn Disord. 2005;20(4):262–9.

37. Watkin L, Blanchard MR, Tookman A, et al. Prospective cohort study of adverse events in older people admitted to the acute general hospital: risk factors and the impact of dementia. Int J Geriatr Psychiatry. 2012;1:76–82.

38. Fong TG, Jones RN, Shi P, et al. Delirium accelerates cognitive decline in Alzheimer disease. Neurology. 2009;72(18):1570–5.

39. Morycz RK. Caregiving strain and the desire to institutionalize family members with Alzheimer's disease. Res Aging. 1985;7:329–61.

40. Daiello LA, Gardner R, Epstein-Lubow G, Butterfield K, Gravenstein S. Association of dementia with early rehospitalization among medicare beneficiaries. Arch Gerontol Geriatr. 2014;59(1):162–8.

41. Hospitalization. Alzheimer's association website. http://www.alz.org/national/documents/topicsheet_hospitalization.pdf. Retrieved 23 Jan 2015.

42. Murphy-White M. Home to hospital. In: Boltz M, editor. Need to know: dementia transition series. https://s3.amazonaws.com/Resources2014/NeedToKnow+Dementia+Home+to+Hospital.pdf. Retrieved 23 Jan 2015.

43. Boltz M, Resnick B, Chippendale T, Galvin J. Testing a family-centered intervention to promote functional and cognitive recovery in hospitalized older adults. J Am Geriatr. 2014;62(12):2398–407.

44. Naylor MD, Brooten DA, Campbell RL, Maislin G, McCauley KM, Schwartz JS. Transitional care of older adults hospitalized with heart failure: a randomized, controlled trial. J Am Geriatr Soc. 2004;52(5): 675–84.

45. Naylor MD, Stephens C, Bowles KH, Bixby MB. Cognitively impaired older adults: From hospital to home. A pilot study of these patients and their caregivers. Am J Nurs. 2005;105(2):40–9.

46. Coleman EA, Parry C, Chalmers S, Min SJ. The care transitions intervention: results of a randomized controlled trial. Arch Intern Med. 2006;166(17):1822–8.

47. Cumbler E, Carter J, Kutner J. Failure at the transition of care: challenges in the discharge of the vulnerable elderly patient. J Hosp Med. 2008;3(4):349–52.

48. Popejoy LL, Galambos C, Vogelsmeier A. Hospital to nursing home transitions: perceptions of nursing home staff. J Nurs Care Qual. 2014;29(2):103–9.

49. King BJ, Gilmore-Bykovskyi AL, Roiland RA, Polnaszek BE, Bowers BJ, Kind AJ. The consequences of poor communication during transitions from hospital to skilled nursing facility: a qualitative study. J Am Geriatr Soc. 2013;61(7):1095–102.

50. Morriss RK, Rovner BW, German PS. Changes in behavior before and after nursing home admission. Int J Geriatr Psychiatry. 1994;9(12):965–73.

51. Howland RH. Risks and benefits of antipsychotic drugs in elderly patients with dementia. J Psychosoc Nurs Ment Health Serv. 2008;46(11):19–23.

52. Popejoy LL. Participation of older adults, families, and health care teams in hospital discharge destination decisions. Appl Nurs Res. 2011;24:256–62.

53. Lamberg J, Person CJ, Kiely DK, Mitchell SL. Decisions to hospitalize nursing home residents dying with advanced dementia. J Am Geriatr. 2005;53(8): 1396–401.

54. Mitchell SL, Kiely DK, Hamel MB. Dying with advanced dementia in the nursing home. Arch Intern Med. 2004;164:321–6.

55. Sampson EL, Blanchard MR, Jones L, Tookman A, King M. Dementia in the acute hospital: prospective

cohort study of prevalence and mortality. Br J Psychiatry. 2009;195(1):6.

56. Zekry D, Herrmann FR, Grandjean R, Vitale AM, De Pinho MF, Michel JP, et al. Does dementia predict adverse hospitalization outcomes? A prospective study in aged inpatients. Int J Geriatr Psychiatry. 2009;24(3):283–91.

57. Gruneir A, Miller SC, Feng Z, Intrator O, Mor V. Relationship between state medicaid policies, nursing home racial composition, and the risk of hospitalization for black and white residents. Health Serv Res. 2008;43(3):869–81.

58. Mehta Z, Giorgini K, Ellison N, Roth ME. Integrating palliative medicine with dementia care. Aging Well. 2012;5(2):18.

59. Zimmerman S, Anderson W, Brode S, et al. Comparison of characteristics of nursing homes and other residential long-term care settings for people with dementia [Internet]. Comparative effectiveness reviews, No. 79. Rockville, MD: Agency for Healthcare Research and Quality (US); 2012.

60. Smith GE, Kikmen E, O'Brien PC. Risk factors for nursing home placement in a population-based dementia cohort. J Am Geriatr. 2000;48:519–25.

61. Gaugler JE, Yu F, Krichbaum K, Wyman JF. Predictors of nursing home admission for persons with dementia. Med Care. 2009;47(2):191–8.

62. Zimmerman S, Sloane PD, Williams CS, et al. Residential care/assisted living staff may detect undiagnosed dementia using the minimum data set cognition scale. J Am Geriatr Soc. 2007;55(9):1349–55.

63. Zimmerman S, Sloane PD, Heck E, Maslow K, Schulz R. Dementia care and quality of life in assisted living and nursing homes. Gerontologist. 2005; 45(Special issue I):5–7.

64. Arrighi HM, Neumann PJ, Lieberburg IM, Townsend RJ. Lethality of Alzheimer disease and its impact on nursing home placement. Alzheimer Dis Assoc Disord. 2010;24(1):90.

65. Mitchell SL, Teno JM, Miller S, Mor V. A national study of the location of death for older persons with dementia. J Am Geriatr Soc. 2005;53(2):299–305.

66. National Center for Health Statistics. 2010 national survey of residential care facilities data dictionary: facility public-use file. Atlanta, GA: Centers for Disease Control and Prevention; 2010.

67. Huang YC, Chu CL, Ho CS, Lan SJ, Hsieh CH, Hsieh YP. Decision-making factors affecting different family members regarding the placement of relatives in long-term care facilities. BMC Health Serv Res. 2014;14:2.

68. Centers for Medicare and Medicaid Services. Nursing home compare. n.d. www.medicare.gov/NHCompare. Accessed 23 Jan 2015.

69. Alzheimer Association. Carefinder guidebook. http://www.alz.org/national/documents/brochure_carefinderguide.pdf

70. Sury L, Burns K, Brodaty H. Moving in: adjustment of people living with dementia going into a nursing home and their families. Int Psychogeriatr. 2013; 25(6):867–76.

71. Gaugler JE, Mittelman MS, Hepburn K, Newcomer R. Clinically significant changes in burden and depression among dementia caregivers following nursing home admission. BMC Med. 2010;8:85.

72. Yamamoto-Mitani N, Aneshensel CS, Levy-Storms L. Patterns of family visiting with institutionalized elders: the case of dementia. J Gerontol B Psychol Sci Soc Sci. 2002;57(4):S234–46.

73. Dempsey NP, Pruncho RA. The family's role in the nursing home: predictors of technical and non-technical assistance. J Gerontol Soc Work. 1994;21(1 and 2):127–46.

74. Hopp F. Patterns and predictors of formal and informal care among elderly persons living in board and care homes. Geron. 1999;39(2):167–76.

75. Janzen W. Long-term care for older adults. The role of the family. J Gerontol Nurs. 2001;27(2):36–43.

76. Maslow K, Heck E. Dementia care and quality of life in assisted living and nursing homes: perspectives of the Alzheimer's association. Geron. 2005;45 Suppl 1:8–10.

77. Alzheimer's Association. Dementia care practice recommendations for assisted living residences and nursing homes. Available at http://www.alz.org/national/documents/brochure_DCPRphases1n2.pdf

78. Kenny AM, Bellantonio S, Fortinsky RH, Dauser D, Kleppinger A, Robison J, Gruman C, Trella P, Walsh SJ. Factors associated with skilled nursing facility transfers in dementia-specific assisted living. Alzheimer Dis Assoc Disord. 2008;22(3):255–60.

79. Bellantonio S, Kenny AM, Fortinsky RH, Kleppinger A, Robison J, Gruman C, et al. Efficacy of a geriatrics team intervention for residents in dementia-specific assisted living facilities: effect on unanticipated transitions. J Am Geriatr Soc. 2008;56(3):523–8.

80. Mor V, Intrator O, Feng Z, Grabowski DC. The revolving door of rehospitalization from skilled nursing facilities. Health Aff (Millwood). 2010;29:57–64.

81. Saliba D, Kington R, Buchanan J, et al. Appropriateness of the decision to transfer nursing facility residents to hospital. J Am Geriatr Soc. 2000;48:154–63.

82. Ouslander JG, Lamb G, Perloe M, et al. Potentially avoidable hospitalizations of nursing home residents: frequency, causes, and costs. J Am Geriatr Soc. 2010;58:627–35.

83. Givens JL, Selby K, Goldfeld KS, Mitchell SL. Hospital transfers of nursing home residents with advanced dementia. J Am Geriatr Soc. 2012;60(5):905–9.

84. Ouslander JG, Berenson RA. Reducing unnecessary hospitalizations of nursing home residents. N Engl J Med. 2011;365:1165–7.

85. Ouslander JG, Lamb G, Tappen R, et al. Interventions to reduce hospitalizations from nursing homes: evaluation of the INTERACT II collaborative quality improvement project. J Am Geriatr Soc. 2011;59: 745–53.

86. Rantz M, Alexander G, Galambos C, Vogelsmeier A, Popejoy L, Flesner M, et al. Initiative to test a multidisciplinary model with advanced practice nurses to reduce avoidable hospitalizations among nursing facility residents. J Nurs Care Qual. 2013;29(1):1–8.

87. Fulton AT, Rhodes-Kropf J, Corcoran AM, Chau D, Castillo EH. Palliative care for patients with dementia in long-term care. Clin Geriatr Med. 2011;27(2):153–70.

88. Samala RV, Galindo DJ, Ciocon JO. Transitioning nursing home patients with dementia to hospice care: basics, benefits, and barriers. Ann Long-term Care. 2011;19(4):41–7.

89. Arai A, Matsumoto T, Ikeda M. Do family caregivers perceive more difficulty when they look after patients with early onset dementia compared to those with late onset dementia. Int J Geriatr Psychiatry. 2007;22: 1255–61.

90. Jubb D, Pollard N, Chaston D. Developing services for younger people with dementia. Nurs Times. 2003;99(22):34–5.

91. Peisah C, Brodaty H, Quadrio C. Family conflict in dementia: prodigal sons and black sheep. Int J Geriatr Psychiatry. 2006;21(5):485–92.

92. Runge C, Gilham J, Peut A. Transitions in care of people with dementia: a systematic review of the literature. http://www.healthinfonet.ecu.edu.au/key-resources/bibliography/?lid=20299 (2009). Accessed 23 Jan 2015.

Dementia Palliative Care

Abraham A. Brody

Introduction

Palliative care is defined as *"specialized medical care for people with serious illnesses. It focuses on providing patients with relief from the symptoms and stress of a serious illness. The goal is to improve quality of life for both the patient and the family"* [1]. The goal of palliative care is to provide interprofessional, holistic patient and family centered care that matches their wishes and goals of care to actual care provided. Since the majority of dementias are incurable, terminal, life-limiting illnesses, persons with dementia (PWD) should be provided with palliative care starting at the onset of diagnosis. As the disease progresses, the intensity and frequency of palliative care will proportionally increase, and the need for specialist palliative care services, including hospice care (see chapter "Hospice Dementia Care"), may become appropriate and necessary. This chapter will discuss specialist vs generalist palliative care, and how to provide generalist palliative care services other than behavioral symptoms, which are covered elsewhere (See chapters "Treatment of Dementia: Pharmacological Approach," "Treatment of Dementia: Non-pharmacological Approach,"

A.A. Brody, RN, PhD, GNP-BC (✉)
Hartford Institute for Geriatric Nursing,
NYU College of Nursing, New York, NY, USA
e-mail: Ab.Brody@nyu.edu

"Home-Based Interventions Targeting Persons with Dementia: What Is the Evidence and Where Do We Go from Here?," and "Interventions to Support Caregiver Well-Being").

Specialist Versus Generalist Palliative Care

Care provided by specialist, highly trained, palliative care clinicians, can be exceedingly useful, particularly in more complicated cases. However, there is currently a lack of access to palliative care specialists, particularly in outpatient, non-oncologic settings, where palliative care is only starting to emerge [2]. Therefore, good palliative care can and should be provided to PWD by an individual's primary care and/or dementia care team from the moment a diagnosis is made.

Drs. Quill and Abernathy in the New England Journal of Medicine developed a model to differentiate care that can and should be provided by generalists vs specialists and a rationale for this division [3]. One of the most significant reasons, other than access, for generalists to provide the majority of palliative care is that there is an existing therapeutic relationship between the primary team and the patient/family versus introducing a new clinician team into the mix. Palliative domains that should be, and sometimes are today, covered by the primary or dementia specialist teams with varying expertise

© Springer International Publishing Switzerland 2016
M. Boltz, J.E. Galvin (eds.), *Dementia Care*, DOI 10.1007/978-3-319-18377-0_15

include exploring PWD/family values and beliefs regarding their healthcare, their goals of care, advanced care planning, prognosis, managing distressing symptoms, and providing for the spiritual and psychosocial needs of the PWD and their caregiver. In this model, specialist palliative care should only become involved where more complex or refractory symptoms, family dynamics, and futility become involved. Taking into account their significant behavioral symptom management expertise, refractory behavioral symptoms are likely still best addressed by dementia care specialists, though other symptoms such as complex pain, nausea or dyspnea may better be handled by palliative specialists.

Prognostication

Unfortunately, unlike many other disease conditions, dementia is not a single disease and life expectancy is highly variable even within discreet forms of dementia (e.g., Alzheimer's, Vascular, etc.…). For some PWD and their families, the goals will be clear regardless of the prognosis (e.g., "focus on comfort" or "do everything") due to religious or personal beliefs. However, for most, prognostication can be highly useful in helping PWD and their families to perform advanced care planning and even short-term decision making. It is therefore the responsibility of the clinician to do their best to provide a timeline and layout of how the disease progresses so that patients and families have the information needed to make decisions regarding their care.

Table 1 provides the mean time from symptom onset to death for the most common forms of dementia. However, multiple studies have found that increased age, male gender, worse functional status and multiple medical comorbidities are significantly associated with decreased life expectancy [4]. Therefore when discussing life expectancy with PWD and their families, it is important to both tailor the expectancy to the individuals' overall medical condition, and make clear that while these are average expectancies, individuals may live significantly longer or shorter. Making this more difficult, no well-

Table 1 Mean time from symptom onset to death in PWD

Type of dementia	Time from onset to death
Alzheimer's disease	6.6 years [71]
Vascular dementia	3.0–4.3 years [72]
Mixed dementia	5.4 years [73]
Dementia with lewy bodies	4.4 years [74]
Frontotemporal dementia	
Behavioral variant	9 years
Semantic	12 years
Progressive non-fluent aphasia	9 years
Motor neuron disease	3 years [75]

validated, generalized calculators exist specifically for long-term dementia life expectancy. In persons with advanced dementia living in nursing homes, the ADEPT tool has been found to have good specificity, but poor sensitivity in determining 6-month mortality, and can be used as part of the decision making process in this population sub-set [5]. An additional generalized tool called ePrognosis (http://eprognosis.ucsf.edu), which does take memory and functional issues into account but is not dementia specific, may also be useful in helping to frame prognosis for PWD and their families, but again it is only moderately sensitive and specific.

Holding a Crucial Conversation/ Family Meeting

The discussion of a diagnosis and prognosis with PWD and their families or progression of the disease can be very difficult and prompt significant anxiety. It is therefore very important to take great care and move slowly as you go through this information. VitalTalk, a clinical education and implementation program developed by experts in the field, have created a series of best practices for discussing prognosis and holding crucial conversations with patients and their families [6]. One tool they highlight for holding these crucial conversations with patients and their families uses the "SPIKES" acronym (see Table 2) [7]. When having a visit/meeting with the PWD and possibly their family both for initial diagno-

Table 2 The SPIKES protocol for breaking bad news [7]

Setting	Quiet, private location, focused attention to the PWD and family
Perception	What does the PWD/family know/ understand about their illness
Invitation	Ask how the PWD/family prefer to discuss/receive information; Ask permission to discuss results
Knowledge	Provide a warning prior to discussing serious news, then share news in a jargon free, clear, straightforward and simple fashion
Empathy	Stop at this point and wait for the PWD/Family to digest and provide empathy to them. Afterwards, ask any questions they might have
Summary	Summarize what has been discussed and ask the PWD/Family to repeat back to ensure understanding. Then begin process to schedule follow-up

sis or to provide new, crucial information about their illness, the first step, **Setting**, is to find a quiet, private location, have tissues and enough chairs available, and be prepared to provide your full attention to the patient (e.g., pagers, cell phones off, etc.…). Regardless of whether you as an individual will be holding the discussion or as part of a team, it is important to know going into the visit what will be said, by whom and what the objectives of the meeting are.

The second step, **Perception**, is to find out what the PWD/family knows. Here is where you would ask the PWD/family what their understanding and perception of the illness is using probing questions such as "Tell me what you understand about your illness."

The third step, **Invitation**, is to (1) Ask the PWD/family if it is ok to continue and discuss the results of testing and the diagnosis, and (2) Ask how they would prefer to discuss the information you are about to provide (e.g., speaking in generalities vs specifics, if there is one person they would prefer the conversation to occur with).

The fourth step, **Knowledge**, is to provide the results. In this case, the clinician/team should do its best to avoid medical jargon. In cases where you have to share the diagnosis/prognosis first, the clinician/team should stop and allow time for the PWD/family to adjust to the news and reflect. If you keep talking after this initial news, the

PWD/family is unlikely to hear anything else you have said.

The fifth step, **Empathy**, is to wait patiently for the PWD/family, and then empathize about the news you have just shared with them. A period of silence at this point is ok while you are waiting for the PWD/Family to digest the information. After you have shared this moment, you can then provide additional details about the disease.

The sixth and final step is **Summary**, where you ask the PWD/family what they have learned/ understand about the disease and its progression. At this point, there may be some initial treatments that are started, or depending on the disease and the state of the PWD/family, you may just want to share that you will want to start discussing treatment options (if they exist) as well as goals of care and advanced care planning (see next section) at a follow-up appointment. Many, but not all PWD and family will need time to digest the information you have provided and perform their own research or formulate their own questions, and therefore, these topics are generally best left for a follow-up meeting that is held within the next several days if the urgency of the illness allows.

Advanced Care Planning

Advanced care planning (ACP) is the process of discussing the future needs and wishes of an individual related to their care. While it does not need to be specific to a particular illness or condition, many individuals have difficulty holding discussions on this topic in more abstract terms. This coupled with a general reticence amongst individuals to talk about death and declining health, and limited reimbursement for primary care providers to hold these discussions, leads to very few individuals beginning advanced care planning discussions early in life or even early on in the process of a disease [8].

Particularly in dementia, where individuals will lose the capacity to make decisions over time, it is important for the primary care team to understand the PWD's wishes for their care, as well as for the PWD to designate a healthcare proxy and discuss with their healthcare proxy their wishes. This way, as the PWD declines, there is little ambiguity to their wishes and thus less chance of significant conflict or disagreement about goals of care.

Within the first several visits following diagnosis, the care team should work with the PWD to develop a plan of care and assign a healthcare proxy. Studies have found that PWD are able to develop their own advanced care plan with mild dementia [9, 10] and can still designate a healthcare proxy with moderate dementia [11]. The earlier this process starts however, the more likely it is that the PWD's wishes will be met, and the worse the cognitive function at initial discussion, the more likely the PWD will opt for aggressive life sustaining treatment [12]. Similarly, family members are more likely to opt for more aggressive treatment than the PWD might [11].

Discussions around advanced care planning should include when CPR or intubation should be performed, types of medical interventions that would be wanted [e.g., oxygen, suctioning, antibiotics, non-invasive airway (bipap)] and in what instances they would want them, whether the PWD would want to go to the hospital and for what conditions, where they would want care as their disease advances and when they are dying (home, assisted living, nursing home, etc....), and whether they would want artificial nutrition and hydration and if so in what instances (See Box 1). The latter is particularly important as in some states, such as New York, the law does not allow a healthcare proxy to make decisions about artificial nutrition and hydration unless an explicit statement has been made about their wishes on this subject by the PWD.

> **Box 1: Key Topics in Advanced Care Planning Discussions**
> - Healthcare Proxy Designation
> - Resuscitation Status (Inpatient and Outpatient)
> - Aggressiveness of Care
> - Hospitalization
> - Medical Interventions Wanted
> - Artificial Nutrition and Hydration
> - Preferred Living Setting

> **Box 2: Types of Advance Directives**
> - Healthcare Proxy
> - Living Will
> - Pre-Hospital DNR
> - Five Wishes
> - Physician Orders for Life Sustaining Treatment (POLST) called MOLST or MOST in some states

Part of the clinician team's time in working with the PWD following diagnosis should be spent in developing both an advanced care plan and assisting the PWD and family to complete the necessary legal documents/advanced directives to put in place (See Box 2). The simplest document is the healthcare proxy. Every PWD should have a healthcare proxy completed with, if possible, both a primary and backup proxy. A backup proxy should be provided as often issues may arise with communication with the primary. For instance, the PWD's spouse is their primary proxy, but she is a frail elder and has a fall leading to a hip fracture. Simultaneously an acute event in the PWD requires a proxy to be available to make a treatment decision. A backup proxy, such as an adult child, could then make the decision as the primary proxy is not contactable or not competent at that moment to make a decision. The PWD should also have a discussion facilitated with the proxy(s) regarding their wishes or when discussing the plan initially. This will make it more likely for the proxy to follow the PWDs wishes.

Another useful document that can be filled out in place of a healthcare proxy is the Physicians Orders for Life Sustaining Treatment or POLST form (called MOLST in some states) [13]. This form, approved for use in some ways in 45/50 U.S. states [14], includes both a healthcare proxy with legally binding medical orders that are transferrable across settings regarding PWD wishes for intensity of care, code status, artificial nutrition and hydration, and healthcare proxy designation. Some states also have additional fields. Studies have found the POLST forms are highly respected and followed compared to other advanced directives such as living wills or healthcare proxy alone [8, 15].

Other forms of advance directives, can be useful but are much less likely to be followed unless a case end in a court battle. Living wills are written by an individual with a lawyer and are therefore often difficult to interpret in various more complex medical situations. Another form, Five Wishes, includes both the traditional living will and healthcare proxy, along with wishes for post-death ceremonies and remembrance. The document is long, and may be better as a conversation guide for PWD and their families than as an actual legal document. Overall, regardless of what form of documentation to be used, the key is to start advanced care planning conversations with the PWD and their family/proxy early so that their wishes can be determined, shared with the appropriate healthcare team members and family members, and documented prior to loss of capacity. The conversations should be ongoing as condition changes to the greatest extent possible as the PWD's condition worsens.

Polypharmacy and Discontinuation of Medications

As a PWD's conditions advance, clinicians need to continually re-evaluate the treatments the PWD is receiving. Of greatest concern, particularly in geriatrics, is that of polypharmacy. Many medications can have significant side effects in older adults, and the polypharmacy experience by many older adults only makes this worse. Clinicians need to take into account life expectancy and relative benefit versus harm. Included here is a list of medications that can potentially be withdrawn or decreased as PWD decline (See Box 3).

One of the easiest medications to withdraw as PWD decline is statins. Statins can cause significant myalgias, and though they in general have significant efficacy for cardiovascular disease, the likely benefits in persons with severe dementia are minimal and the recommendation is therefore to discontinue at this stage so long as there hasn't been a recent acute coronary syndrome or cerebrovascular accident [16].

> **Box 3: Potentially Withdrawable Medications in Persons with Advanced Dementia**
> - Statins
> - Bisphosphonates
> - Vitamins and Supplements
> - Antihypertensives
> - Antiglycemics
> - Acetylcholinesterase Inhibitors
> - Antipsychotics
> - Antispasmodics

Similarly, given the time to effect for bisphospinates for osteoporosis, these medications are of limited benefit in severe dementia, though should be maintained in earlier stages [17]. Additionally, in older adults in general, but especially at the severe stage, tight control of blood pressure (SBP<140 vs <160) and diabetes mellitus(HbA1c <7 % vs 8 %) may lead to more problems and adverse events than benefits [18], including increased worsening of cognition [19], and an easing of antihypertensive and antiglycemics should be considered. Especially in PWD with poor PO intake, antiglycemics other than metformin can lead to hypoglycemia, and metformin can cause decreased PO intake and digestive symptoms [20]. Finally in PWD with poor PO intake or who have had highly variable INR levels requiring frequent adjustment, discontinuation of anticoagulation therapy may be appropriate as the risks of supratherapeutic levels may be worse than the risk of an embolic event [21].

Another class of drugs to examine are anticholinergic medications, which are often inappropriate in older adults in general [22], but particularly so in PWD as they can cause increased confusion and falls. These medications should be reduced where possible in all older adults, and particularly in PWD. Some anticholinergics such as antispasmodics for urinary incontinence are often prescribed in older adults. These medications can be reduced early on, however if the PWD or their family insists on maintaining a medicine in this class for functional reasons, once the PWD becomes incontinent of urine, the medication can be withdrawn as there is no further reason to maintain the PWD on it.

The appropriateness of withdrawal of acetylcholinesterase inhibitors and memantine are more difficult to determine. Acetylcholinesterase inhibitors such as donepezil and galantamine are approved for treating mild to moderate Alzheimer's disease though there is some evidence for their use in vascular and Lewy Body dementia. Once a drug in this class is removed, any benefit from the drug is negated and the PWD could decline precipitously. While its efficacy at the end of life is likely limited, there are no current studies to this effect. At the end stage of dementia, if disturbing symptoms exist such as GI disturbance or diarrhea, removal should be considered weighing the unknown benefits of the drug vs the side effects and cost. Similarly, while memantine is indicated in moderate to severe stage disease, there is limited evidence for its use at the end stage, once a PWD has reached FAST 7C level or higher. However, there is also limited evidence for its withdrawal, and therefore a discussion of the pros and cons of withdrawal should be undertaken with the healthcare proxy.

Finally, without discussing the merits of using antipsychotics for behavioral and psychological symptoms of dementia in PWD here (See chapter "Treatment of Dementia: Pharmacological Approaches"), there is evidence that these medications can often be withdrawn without negative effect, and may even improve functional and cognitive status [23]. Additionally, in cases where a PWD is entering the final stage of the disease and no longer have any significant functional or cognitive capacity, even if the PWD had prior hallucinations or delusions that became well controlled with antipsychotics, at this point in the disease, the PWD may no longer be having these symptoms and a test of withdrawing antipsychotics should be considered.

Functional Decline

As part of their condition, PWD have significant decline in physical function over time. While physical activity programs, acetylcholinesterase inhibitors and memantine can slow this decline to varying degrees, over time, regardless of any treatment provided, PWD will develop significant functional debility. While every attempt should be made to maximize function for as long as possible (see chapters "Home-Based Interventions Targeting Persons with Dementia: What Is the Evidence and Where Do We Go from Here", "Experiences and Perspectives of the Family Caregiver of the Person with Dementia"), at some point most PWD will develop such severe functional limitations that they will be unable to perform any of their activities of daily living (feeding, toileting, dressing, grooming, maintaining continence, bathing, walking). The most concerning palliation issues related to these functions are artificial nutrition and hydration, pressure ulcers, and contractures, which are discussed in greater detail below.

Artificial Nutrition and Hydration

At some point in advanced dementia, PWD will lose the ability to feed themselves. They may also develop dysphagia as the body begins to unlearn the mechanism behind swallowing. These two related issues can lead to the suggestion of tube feeding in PWD. Many families take advantage of this option if it is presented as it has face validity to the family. The family may be concerned about their loved one starving to death or having significant feelings of thirst, or that because of their religious or cultural beliefs that they have to "do everything" to keep their loved one alive. While hopefully this can be addressed early on or prevented through a frank discussion during advanced care planning shortly after diagnosis, this often does not occur.

Multiple studies have shown there is a lack of efficacy for tube feeding in PWD [24], and in fact may have poorer outcomes, agitation, and reduced survival compared to those who are not tube-fed [25, 26]. Rather, hand feeding patients by spoon in a fully upright 90° position has been shown to be efficacious across settings for maintaining intake and preventing aspiration [27]. If the patient continues losing weight even with hand feeding, trying higher calorie foods such as an "ice cream diet" may be helpful.

The major limitation of hand feeding is that it is time consuming, taking up to 30 min per meal. Therefore, many families can feel pressured into having a PEG tube due to lack of resources in the care setting, not the needs and wishes of the PWD. By having a discussion outlining the negatives of tube feeding before the PWD declines however, or even if they have declined but not to the point of this being an issue, a clear decision can be made without the pressure of an institution or a poorly placed gastroenterology consult in the inpatient setting if the PWD is for some reason hospitalized. To be unequivocal, tube feeding is not appropriate under the majority of circumstances in PWD, and the American Geriatrics Society amongst others have developed policy statements against their use [28].

Pressure Ulcers

In the advanced stages, PWD are at high risk for developing pressure ulcers due to a mixture of decreased mobility and nutrition, and increased skin moisture secondary to incontinence. It is important as a first line, to educate caregivers to provide care that can limit pressure ulcers as much as possible. This includes when possible performing frequent toileting, or barring that possibility frequent changes of incontinence briefs along with moisture absorbing powder to keep the skin dry. Additionally, caregivers, should do their best to maintain nutrition through hand feeding as discussed above, and taught in bed-bound patients to reposition the PWD every 2 h and how to prevent bony prominences from pressing against each other or a hard surface. In PWD who are at high risk for pressure ulcers due to nutritional status, limited mobility and moisture, the provider can order a hospital bed, and in certain cases either a mattress overlay or powered mattress overlay depending on the insurance company and their criteria for each.

Once a pressure ulcer has formed, it can be incredibly difficult to heal, especially without fixing underlying nutritional and moisture issues. In addition to prescribing a dressing appropriate to the stage, size, shape, depth, and tissue damage of the wound, clinicians must work with caregivers to assist them in reducing moisture and pressure to the affected area. Additionally, clinicians should assess for pain related to the pressure ulcer and prescribe analgesics and perform non-pharmacologic interventions as appropriate (see Pain section below).

Contractures

Contractures are shortening of the muscle or joint. There are different underlying pathophysiologies behind various contractures, and some are preventable, while others are not. One of the most common forms of contracture found in advanced dementia is however preventable, the fixed contracture. This type of contracture is caused by limited movement in advanced dementia patients caused by functional decline. Upwards of 75 % of non-ambulatory PWD were found in one study to have developed a contracture [29]. As PWD decline to the point where they have limited activity, it is therefore important to educate their caregiver(s) on performing range of motion exercises over the full range of motion of the muscle/joint in both the lower and upper extremities and digits of the feet and hands. In PWD living in community based setting, a home physical therapy consult can be ordered to perform training with the primary caregiver, and in the nursing home setting, ordering ROM exercises may help with limiting the formation contractures [30].

Once contractures do form they can cause pain with movement and positioning, and patients should be assessed for pain and if present appropriate analgesics provided. Additionally, physical therapy should be consulted to prevent the contracture from becoming worse. In some hand contractures, botox injection may also be performed in order to assist with releasing the contracture [31].

Identification and Management of Non-behavioral Symptoms

While behavioral and psychological symptoms of dementia are the core distressing symptoms for PWD and their families, often times these symptoms are manifestations of other needs that the PWD cannot relate due to their lack of cognition. While other chapters in this book focus on the identification and management of behavioral and psychological symptoms of dementia (See chapters "Hospice Dementia Care", "Treatment of Dementia: Pharmacological Approach," "Treatment of Dementia: Non-pharmacological Approach," "Home-Based Interventions Targeting Persons with Dementia: What Is the Evidence and Where Do We Go from Here?," and "Interventions to Support Caregiver Well-Being"), additional symptoms are frequently present in PWD that can lead to significant discomfort, such as pain, dyspnea, fever, and GI disturbances. These symptoms can initiate or worsen behavioral and psychological symptoms, and are discussed in this section.

Pain

Pain is highly prevalent in PWD; in the community dwelling and nursing home population as high as 80 % and 75 % respectively experience pain [32, 33]. Moreover, caregiver-rated pain has been found to have limited congruence [33], and be affected by the caregiver's own pain [34]. Given both the difficulty of rating the subjective experience of another, and the physiologic changes that cause the pain experience to differ substantially in PWD [35], it should come as no surprise that pain is both underreported and undertreated in this population, particularly as dementia becomes more severe [32, 36, 37].

When assessing PWD for pain, it is important to keep several factors in mind. *First*, while pain is not caused by dementia, most older adults have other concurrent chronic conditions that can cause pain (see Box 4). Therefore, it is important when assessing PWD for pain to consider whether they have a potentially painful pathophysiologic condition.

> **Box 4: Potentially Painful Conditions Commonly Found in Older Adults**
> - Rheumatoid or Osteoarthritis
> - Gout
> - Pressure Ulcers
> - Cancer
> - Post Herpetic Neuralgia
> - Back Pain
> - Vertebral Fractures
> - Diabetic Neuropathy

Second, as many PWD lose short term memory, their ability to report pain if they are not currently experiencing it decreases. Therefore, it is important to assess the PWD for pain both at rest and with movement. When observing movement, it is important to watch their gait if walking, and any bracing, physical or verbal aggression, moaning or other verbal expressions and facial expressions, as these may be cues or clues that the PWD is experiencing pain.

Third, older adults do not always use the word "pain" to refer to uncomfortable sensation, and therefore numerous descriptors should be used when inquiring about a PWD's pain (e.g., dullness, soreness, achiness, the arthritis) [38].

Fourth, while the reliability decreases with time, it is important to still obtain a self report. Studies have found that individuals with mild to moderate dementia can still reliability complete a self report using standard scales such as the faces pain scale, numerical rating scale, or verbal descriptor scale [39]. However, the first time you work with an individual, using more than one scale might be beneficial in order to both take the PWD's preference into account and because they may have better ability to complete one over another. Also, as discussed above, make sure to perform the scale both at rest and with movement. Should an individual have moderate-severe dementia, they may no longer be able to self report, and in addition to a self report, an observational pain scale such as the PAINAD [40] should be used to assess for pain. While no observational instrument currently available is perfect, they can at least provide for baseline and change over time to have a more constant and objective assessment/measurement of pain.

Finally, once pain is identified, the question becomes, how to treat the pain. In PWD, it is best, if possible to not use opioids as they lead to increased falls and delirium in this population [41, 42]. However, if severe pain is present in a PWD, it can actually increase the risk of delirium and thus falls, and therefore it is a difficult balancing act [42]. Additionally, while treating the pain, it is important to concomitantly treat other symptoms that can worsen/aggravate pain, such as depression, sleep disturbance, fatigue, and anxiety, otherwise regardless of how optimal the pain treatment regimen is, the pain may not fully subside.

The first step in most pain, so long as it is not severe or from a traumatic event should be to perform a mixture of non-pharmacologic interventions along with around the clock acetaminophen not to exceed 3 g/day. The reason not to prescribe any pain medicines as needed to PWD is generally they will not ask for them and they will simply not be given, regardless of the setting [43]. Non-pharmacologic measures appropriate for all patients include music therapy, heat/cold, massage, spiritual practice, therapeutic touch, and healing touch, physical therapy, and exercise. Additionally, the following modalities may be appropriate in those with only mild to moderate dementia: TENS units, guided imagery, relaxation, acupuncture, chiropractic services and Reiki.

It is common however, that acetaminophen and non-pharmacologic measures alone are not enough to treat a PWD's pain, and the provider will need to begin low dose opioid therapy [44]. It is best to start with low doses of oxycodone 2.5 mg Q6h or Percocet ½ tab Q6h. If Percocet is used, acetaminophen should either be discontinued or decreased to remain below 3 g/day of total acetaminophen. Other combo products such as hydrocodone are more constipating and take additional steps to metabolize in the body and therefore are not as good a choice in this population. Additionally, tramadol (Ultram, Ultracet) and propoxyphene (Darvocet, Darvon) should be avoided as they have higher side effect profiles in this population [22, 45]. Opioids can be titrated up slowly as needed.

Whenever an opioid is started in this population, significant caregiver education needs to be performed regarding the side effects of the medication including sedation, respiratory depression, dizziness, gait instability and they need to be monitored for these effects. Additionally, a bowel regimen will need to be started and a stool log should be created. A preferential bowel regimen would include polyethylene glycol 17 g/day. Other options include Senna 1–2 BID, lactulose 15–30 mL daily. Docusate sodium is not recommended as its efficacy is limited and it can cause GI disturbance/discomfort [46].

Dyspnea

Dyspnea can be a significant concern in PWD [47], particularly those who also suffer from asthma, COPD, or CHF. Limited research has been performed specific to this population, however, continuing to treat the underlying disease and ensuring adherence with the complex regimens inherent in treating these diseases is the greatest concern. As their underlying disease worsens, it may be appropriate to prescribe oxygen or low dose opioids, and at the end of life high dose opioids may become appropriate [48]. As discussed above, the benefits of opioids need to be weighed against their risks and if started, a bowel regimen and rigorous caregiver education needs to be performed as well.

Fever

Over the last 3 months of life, approximately one-third of PWD will experience a febrile episode [49], most as result of pneumonia. In general the mortality of pneumonia in severe dementia may be as high as 53 % [50]. One study has found that aggressive treatment of fever with antibiotics as an inpatient did not improve symptoms or survival in individuals with advanced dementia [51]. Another study found use of opioids and antipyretics to be superior to aggressive treatment in this population [52]. While it is still likely appropriate to treat with antibiotics in most PWD other than in severe dementia, this decision should be made on a case by case basis with the PWD or their proxy, and is further reason to hold advanced care planning discussions as early as possible in the disease trajectory.

Avoidance of Hospitalization

In general many hospital admissions can be prevented in PWD, and this is to the benefit of the PWD, their family, and the healthcare system as a whole. Unfortunately, emergency rooms and hospitals in general are not setup to provide appropriate care for PWD, and therefore they exhibit worse outcomes and care when admitted in this setting [53–55]. Many conditions that lead to hospitalization can be treated on an outpatient basis, though those living in rural areas may have limited access to necessary outpatient care and are therefore more likely to be hospitalized for ambulatory care sensitive conditions [56].

Two of the most significant causes of hospitalization are respiratory and urinary tract infections [57]. In many cases, these infections can be identified through diagnostics performed either at the PWD place of living or in an outpatient office and treatment performed without need of admission. However, oft times it is easier for the family/caregiver to call 911 and send to the emergency room, especially since the first sign of these conditions is generally delirium and caregivers can panic. Therefore, it is important to perform caregiver education to help them understand the signs and symptoms of delirium. Proactive development of a plan prior to an event with the primary care team for home or office based diagnosis and treatment should be performed. This generally involves researching the community based resources that are available including home lab and diagnostic services, pharmacies, and home health agencies to understand their response times and availability. Additionally, studies have shown that significant changes in routine and environment increase

risk for admission, so limiting these changes to the extent possible is also important [57].

Another significant cause of admissions is falls/syncope [57]. Even more concerning is that a large proportion of individuals admitted for a fall will be discharged to a nursing home and may never return to the community [58]. Therefore, everything should be done to reduce the risk of a fall or injury from falling. Evidence based practices include doing as many of the following as possible: having an occupational therapist perform a home safety evaluation, development of a continuous physical exercise regimen, ensuring Vitamin D supplementation where it is low, treating osteoporosis in cases where the PWD has the condition, and maintaining adequate nutrition to the degree possible [59].

When a fall is not preventable, the question becomes when is an ER visit necessary. When there is no significant pain, mobility change, head injury, or significant skin wound, an office or home based evaluation may be adequate. In cases where a visit to the emergency room is less avoidable, attempting to discharge directly from the ER or as soon as possible after admission may limit delirium and other iatrogenic adverse events. Being proactive and having advanced care planning discussions early may also reduce the length of hospitalization and intensity of care depending on the situation, as the goals of care are clearer from the onset [60]. Hospital at home may also be a good option in these cases where it is available as it has shown reduction in behavioral disturbances, and family caregiver stress [61].

Caregiver Burden, Stress and Burnout

Any palliative intervention seeks to look at the whole person as well as the system in which they reside. Therefore, just as important as assessing the PWD is assessing their primary caregiver. If the caregiver becomes burdened, stressed, and/or burned out, their ability to care for the PWD diminishes to the point where they are at risk for institutionalization [62]. While caregiving and interventions to support the caregiver are discussed elsewhere (See chapters "Experiences and Perspectives of the Family Caregiver of the Person with Dementia" and "Interventions to Support Caregiver Well-Being"), it is important when viewing the PWD and their support system through a palliative lens to (1) Assess the caregiver for burden stress and burnout using a standardized instrument such as the Caregiver Burden Inventory [63] or Caregiver Strain Index [64]. (2) Assess the caregiver for depression using a standardized instrument such as the PHQ-9 [65] or Geriatric Depression Scale [66]. (3) Provide options for relieving some of these feelings and actively treating any depression that develops. Support from the Alzheimer's Association, caregiver support groups, adult day health programs, temporary or permanent part or full-time paid caregivers (financial resources permitting), and respite care should all be considered. In addition the PWD's provider should attempt to reduce behavioral and psychological symptoms the PWD may have in order to reduce caregiver burden and burnout.

Spiritual Support

Spiritual support can be an important element for both the PWD and their caregiver, whether or not they have been actively involved in organized or independent practice in recent years, so long as their spiritual beliefs remain. Increased religiosity is associated with slowed cognitive decline and improved behavioral and psychological symptoms [67]. It has also been found to improve coping with illness and perceived quality of life [68]. In the family caregiver of the PWD, it also has similar effects, reducing stress [69] and improving their mental health [70]. Therefore, the clinician should seek, where appropriate, to integrate spiritual care or at a minimum suggest it for both the PWD and their family. Spiritual care can be practiced independently, through chaplaincy or organized religious congregations whether through an existing relationships or returning to practicing. One benefit of becoming

part of an organized religious congregation however is the additional support that can be provided to both the PWD and their caregiver, including home visits, parish nurses, and support groups.

Conclusion

Palliative care is not just specialty care but a holistic model that should be integrated into care for all PWD and their families. By providing comprehensive generalist palliative care from the moment a PWD is diagnosed, including advanced care planning, symptom management, management of functional decline, spiritual care, and attention to the needs specific to community based PWD, providers caring for this vulnerable population and their families can reduce symptoms, caregiver burden, strain and burnout, institutionalization, and hospitalization.

References

1. Center to Advance Palliative Care. What is palliative care; 2012 [13 Aug 2014]. Available from: http://get-palliativecare.org/whatis/
2. Hughes MT, Smith TJ. The growth of palliative care in the United States. Annu Rev Public Health. 2014; 35:459–75.
3. Quill TE, Abernethy AP. Generalist plus specialist palliative care--creating a more sustainable model. N Engl J Med. 2013;368(13):1173–5.
4. Lee M, Chodosh J. Dementia and life expectancy: what do we know? J Am Med Dir Assoc. 2009;10(7): 466–71.
5. Mitchell SL, Miller SC, Teno JM, Kiely DK, Davis RB, Shaffer ML. Prediction of 6-month survival of nursing home residents with advanced dementia using ADEPT vs hospice eligibility guidelines. JAMA. 2010;304(17):1929–35.
6. Back AL, Arnold R, Edwards K, Tulsky J. Talking map for the family conference [14 Dec 2014]. Available from: http://vitaltalk.org/clinicians/
7. Baile WF, Buckman R, Lenzi R, Glober G, Beale EA, Kudelka AP. SPIKES-A six-step protocol for delivering bad news: application to the patient with cancer. Oncologist. 2000;5(4):302–11.
8. Covinsky K, Fuller J, Yaffe K, Johnston C, Hamel M, Lynn J, et al. Communication and decision-making in seriously ill patients: findings of the SUPPORT project.

The study to understand prognoses and preferences for outcomes and risks of treatments. J Am Geriatr Soc. 2000;48 Suppl 5:S187–93.

9. Fazel S, Hope T, Jacoby R. Assessment of competence to complete advance directives: validation of a patient centred approach. BMJ. 1999;318(7182):493–7.

10. Gregory R, Roked F, Jones L, Patel A. Is the degree of cognitive impairment in patients with Alzheimer's disease related to their capacity to appoint an enduring power of attorney? Age Ageing. 2007;36(5): 527–31.

11. Mezey M, Teresi J, Ramsey G, Mitty E, Bobrowitz T. Decision-making capacity to execute a health care proxy: development and testing of guidelines. J Am Geriatr Soc. 2000;48(2):179–87.

12. Fazel S, Hope T, Jacoby R. Effect of cognitive impairment and premorbid intelligence on treatment preferences for life-sustaining medical therapy. Am J Psychiatry. 2000;157(6):1009–11.

13. Tolle SW, Tilden VP, Nelson CA, Dunn PM. A prospective study of the efficacy of the physician order form for life-sustaining treatment. J Am Geriatr Soc. 1998;46(9):1097–102.

14. The National POLST Paradigm. POLST programs in your state [16 Dec 2014]. Available from: http://www.polst.org/programs-in-your-state/

15. Hickman SE, Nelson CA, Moss AH, Tolle SW, Perrin NA, Hammes BJ. The consistency between treatments provided to nursing facility residents and orders on the physician orders for life-sustaining treatment form. J Am Geriatr Soc. 2011;59(11):2091–9.

16. Parsons C, Hughes CM, Passmore AP, Lapane KL. Withholding, discontinuing and withdrawing medications in dementia patients at the end of life: a neglected problem in the disadvantaged dying? Drugs Aging. 2010;27(6):435–49.

17. Bjorkman M, Sorva A, Risteli J, Tilvis R. Vitamin D supplementation has minor effects on parathyroid hormone and bone turnover markers in vitamin D-deficient bedridden older patients. Age Ageing. 2008;37(1):25–31.

18. Huang ES, Zhang Q, Gandra N, Chin MH, Meltzer DO. The effect of comorbid illness and functional status on the expected benefits of intensive glucose control in older patients with type 2 diabetes: a decision analysis. Ann Intern Med. 2008;149(1):11–9.

19. Nilsson SE, Read S, Berg S, Johansson B, Melander A, Lindblad U. Low systolic blood pressure is associated with impaired cognitive function in the oldest old: longitudinal observations in a population-based sample 80 years and older. Aging Clin Exp Res. 2007;19(1):41–7.

20. Makimattila S, Nikkila K, Yki-Jarvinen H. Causes of weight gain during insulin therapy with and without metformin in patients with Type II diabetes mellitus. Diabetologia. 1999;42(4):406–12.

21. Onder G, Landi F, Fusco D, Corsonello A, Tosato M, Battaglia M, et al. Recommendations to prescribe in complex older adults: results of the CRIteria to assess appropriate Medication use among Elderly complex patients (CRIME) project. Drugs Aging. 2014;31(1): 33–45.

22. American Geriatrics Society Beers Criteria Update Expert P. American Geriatrics Society updated Beers Criteria for potentially inappropriate medication use in older adults. J Am Geriatr Soc. 2012;60(4): 616–31.

23. Ballard C, Lana MM, Theodoulou M, Douglas S, McShane R, Jacoby R, et al. A randomised, blinded, placebo-controlled trial in dementia patients continuing or stopping neuroleptics (the DART-AD trial). PLoS Med. 2008;5(4):e76.

24. Finucane TE, Christmas C, Travis K. Tube feeding in patients with advanced dementia: a review of the evidence. JAMA. 1999;282(14):1365–70.

25. Mitchell SL, Kiely DK, Lipsitz LA. Does artificial enteral nutrition prolong the survival of institutionalized elders with chewing and swallowing problems? J Gerontol A Biol Sci Med Sci. 1998;53(3):M207–13.

26. Meier DE, Ahronheim JC, Morris J, Baskin-Lyons S, Morrison RS. High short-term mortality in hospitalized patients with advanced dementia: lack of benefit of tube feeding. Arch Intern Med. 2001;161(4):594–9.

27. DiBartolo MC. Careful hand feeding: a reasonable alternative to PEG tube placement in individuals with dementia. J Gerontol Nurs. 2006;32(5):25–33. quiz 4–5.

28. American Geriatrics Society Ethics C, Clinical P, Models of Care C. American Geriatrics Society feeding tubes in advanced dementia position statement. J Am Geriatr Soc. 2014;62(8):1590–3.

29. Souren LE, Franssen EH, Reisberg B. Contractures and loss of function in patients with Alzheimer's disease. J Am Geriatr Soc. 1995;43(6):650–5.

30. Frank C, Akeson WH, Woo SL, Amiel D, Coutts RD. Physiology and therapeutic value of passive joint motion. Clin Orthop Relat Res. 1984;185:113–25.

31. Urban M, Rutowski R, Urban J, Mazurek P, Kulinski S, Gosk J. Treatment of camptodactyly using injection of botulinum neurotoxin. Adv Clin Exp Med. 2014;23(3):399–402.

32. Husebo BS, Strand LI, Moe-Nilssen R, Borgehusebo S, Aarsland D, Ljunggren AE. Who suffers most? Dementia and pain in nursing home patients: a cross-sectional study. J Am Med Dir Assoc. 2008;9(6): 427–33.

33. Shega JW, Hougham GW, Stocking CB, Cox-Hayley D, Sachs GA. Pain in community-dwelling persons with dementia: frequency, intensity, and congruence between patient and caregiver report. J Pain Symptom Manage. 2004;28(6):585–92.

34. Orgeta V, Orrell M, Edwards RT, Hounsome B, Woods B, Team R. Self- and carer-rated pain in people with dementia: influences of pain in carers. J Pain Symptom Manage. 2014 Dec 24. pii: S0885-3924(14)00917-8. doi: 10.1016/j.jpainsymman.2014.10.014. [Epub ahead of print].

35. Rainero I, Vighetti S, Bergamasco B, Pinessi L, Benedetti F. Autonomic responses and pain perception in Alzheimer's disease. Eur J Pain. 2000;4(3): 267–74.

36. Fisher SE, Burgio LD, Thorn BE, Allen-Burge R, Gerstle J, Roth DL, et al. Pain assessment and management in cognitively impaired nursing home residents: association of certified nursing assistant pain report, Minimum Data Set pain report, and analgesic medication use. J Am Geriatr Soc. 2002;50(1): 152–6.

37. Cohen-Mansfield J. The adequacy of the minimum data set assessment of pain in cognitively impaired nursing home residents. J Pain Symptom Manage. 2004;27(4):343–51.

38. Herr KA, Garand L. Assessment and measurement of pain in older adults. Clin Geriatr Med. 2001;17(3):457–78. vi.

39. Pautex S, Herrmann F, Le Lous P, Fabjan M, Michel JP, Gold G. Feasibility and reliability of four pain self-assessment scales and correlation with an observational rating scale in hospitalized elderly demented patients. J Gerontol A Biol Sci Med Sci. 2005; 60(4):524–9.

40. Warden V, Hurley AC, Volicer L. Development and psychometric evaluation of the Pain Assessment in Advanced Dementia (PAINAD) scale. J Am Med Dir Assoc. 2003;4(1):9–15.

41. Kelly KD, Pickett W, Yiannakoulias N, Rowe BH, Schopflocher DP, Svenson L, et al. Medication use and falls in community-dwelling older persons. Age Ageing. 2003;32(5):503–9.

42. Clegg A, Young JB. Which medications to avoid in people at risk of delirium: a systematic review. Age Ageing. 2011;40(1):23–9.

43. Nygaard HA, Jarland M. Are nursing home patients with dementia diagnosis at increased risk for inadequate pain treatment? Int J Geriatr Psychiatry. 2005;20(8):730–7.

44. Buffum MD, Sands L, Miaskowski C, Brod M, Washburn A. A clinical trial of the effectiveness of regularly scheduled versus as-needed administration of acetaminophen in the management of discomfort in older adults with dementia. J Am Geriatr Soc. 2004;52(7):1093–7.

45. Won AB, Lapane KL, Vallow S, Schein J, Morris JN, Lipsitz LA. Persistent nonmalignant pain and analgesic prescribing patterns in elderly nursing home residents. J Am Geriatr Soc. 2004;52(6):867–74.

46. Tarumi Y, Wilson MP, Szafran O, Spooner GR. Randomized, double-blind, placebo-controlled trial of oral docusate in the management of constipation in hospice patients. J Pain Symptom Manage. 2013; 45(1):2–13.

47. Teno JM, Gozalo PL, Lee IC, Kuo S, Spence C, Connor SR, et al. Does hospice improve quality of care for persons dying from dementia? J Am Geriatr Soc. 2011;59(8):1531–6.

48. Hendriks SA, Smalbrugge M, Hertogh CM, van der Steen JT. Dying with dementia: symptoms, treatment, and quality of life in the last week of life. J Pain Symptom Manage. 2014;47(4):710–20.

49. Mitchell SL, Teno JM, Kiely DK, Shaffer ML, Jones RN, Prigerson HG, et al. The clinical course of advanced dementia. N Engl J Med. 2009;361(16): 1529–38.

50. Morrison RS, Siu AL. Survival in end-stage dementia following acute illness. JAMA. 2000;284(1): 47–52.

51. Hurley AC, Volicer BJ, Volicer L. Effect of fever-management strategy on the progression of dementia of the Alzheimer type. Alzheimer Dis Assoc Disord. 1996;10(1):5–10.

52. Hurley AC, Volicer B, Mahoney MA, Volicer L. Palliative fever management in Alzheimer patients. Quality plus fiscal responsibility. ANS Adv Nurs Sci. 1993;16(1):21–32.

53. Laditka JN, Laditka SB, Cornman CB. Evaluating hospital care for individuals with Alzheimer's disease using inpatient quality indicators. Am J Alzheimers Dis Other Dement. 2005;20(1):27–36.

54. Afzal N, Buhagiar K, Flood J, Cosgrave M. Quality of end-of-life care for dementia patients during acute hospital admission: a retrospective study in Ireland. Gen Hosp Psychiatry. 2010;32(2):141–6.

55. Clevenger CK, Chu TA, Yang Z, Hepburn KW. Clinical care of persons with dementia in the emergency department: a review of the literature and agenda for research. J Am Geriatr Soc. 2012;60(9):1742–8.

56. Thorpe JM, Van Houtven CH, Sleath BL, Thorpe CT. Rural-urban differences in preventable hospitalizations among community-dwelling veterans with dementia. J Rural Health. 2010;26(2):146–55.

57. Toot S, Devine M, Akporobaro A, Orrell M. Causes of hospital admission for people with dementia: a systematic review and meta-analysis. J Am Med Dir Assoc. 2013;14(7):463–70.

58. Rowe MA, Fehrenbach N. Injuries sustained by community-dwelling individuals with dementia. Clin Nurs Res. 2004;13(2):98–110. discussion 1–6.

59. Gillespie LD, Robertson MC, Gillespie WJ, Lamb SE, Gates S, Cumming RG, et al. Interventions for preventing falls in older people living in the community. Cochrane Database Syst Rev. 2009;2:CD007146.

60. Brumley R, Enguidanos S, Jamison P, Seitz R, Morgenstern N, Saito S, et al. Increased satisfaction with care and lower costs: results of a randomized trial of in-home palliative care. J Am Geriatr Soc. 2007;55(7):993–1000.

61. Tibaldi V, Aimonino N, Ponzetto M, Stasi MF, Amati D, Raspo S, et al. A randomized controlled trial of a home hospital intervention for frail elderly demented patients: behavioral disturbances and caregiver's stress. Arch Gerontol Geriatr Suppl. 2004;9:431–6.

62. Hébert R, Dubois M-F, Wolfson C, Chambers L, Cohen C. Factors associated with long-term institutionalization of older people with dementia: data from the Canadian Study of Health and Aging. J Gerontol A Biol Sci Med Sci. 2001;56(11):M693–M9.

63. Novak M, Guest C. Application of a multidimensional caregiver burden inventory. Gerontologist. 1989;29(6):798–803.

64. Robinson BC. Validation of a caregiver strain index. J Gerontol. 1983;38(3):344–8.

65. Kroenke K, Spitzer RL, Williams JB. The PHQ-9: validity of a brief depression severity measure. J Gen Intern Med. 2001;16(9):606–13.

66. Dunn VK, Sacco WP. Psychometric evaluation of the geriatric depression scale and the zung self-rating depression scale using an elderly community sample. Psychol Aging. 1989;4(1):125–6.

67. Coin A, Perissinotto E, Najjar M, Girardi A, Inelmen EM, Enzi G, et al. Does religiosity protect against cognitive and behavioral decline in Alzheimer's dementia? Curr Alzheimer Res. 2010;7(5):445–52.

68. Katsuno T. Personal spirituality of persons with early-stage dementia: is it related to perceived quality of life? Dementia. 2003;2(3):315–35.

69. Marquez-Gonzalez M, Lopez J, Romero-Moreno R, Losada A. Anger, spiritual meaning and support from the religious community in dementia caregiving. J Relig Health. 2012;51(1):179–86.

70. Hebert RS, Dang Q, Schulz R. Religious beliefs and practices are associated with better mental health in family caregivers of patients with dementia: findings from the REACH study. Am J Geriatr Psychiatry. 2007;15(4):292–300.

71. Wolfson C, Wolfson DB, Asgharian M, M'Lan CE, Østbye T, Rockwood K, et al. A reevaluation of the duration of survival after the onset of dementia. N Engl J Med. 2001;344(15):1111–6.

72. Knopman DS, Rocca WA, Cha RH, Edland SD, Kokmen E. Survival study of vascular dementia in Rochester, Minnesota. Arch Neurol. 2003;60(1):85–90.

73. Fitzpatrick AL, Kuller LH, Lopez OL, Kawas CH, Jagust W. Survival following dementia onset: Alzheimer's disease and vascular dementia. J Neurol Sci. 2005;229–230:43–9.

74. Oesterhus R, Soennesyn H, Rongve A, Ballard C, Aarsland D, Vossius C. Long-term mortality in a cohort of home-dwelling elderly with mild Alzheimer's disease and Lewy body dementia. Dement Geriatr Cogn Disord. 2014;38(3–4):161–9.

75. Onyike CU, Diehl-Schmid J. The epidemiology of frontotemporal dementia. Int Rev Psychiatry. 2013;25(2):130–7.

Hospice Dementia Care

Richard E. Powers and Heather L. Herrington

Introduction

Hospice care for persons with dementia is slowly evolving as the public understands of the nature of the disease, clinicians improve their abilities to assess prognosis for late stage dementia and funders understand the financial wisdom of hospice care. Medicare utilization of hospice services in 2009 by patients with dementia increased to 6 % of hospice admissions for persons with Alzheimer's disease and 11 % of all admissions for persons with dementia other than Alzheimer's disease e.g., Lewy body dementia. Length of stay in hospice for persons with Alzheimer's disease expanded from 67 days in 1998 to 106 days in 2009 [1]. The LOS for non-AD dementia increased from 57 days to 92 days. The extended LOS has produced a tenfold increase in Medicare expenditures from $184 to $1,880 per recipient with dementia. The number of hospice agencies that serve patients with dementia increased from 21 % of providers in 1994 to 94 % in surveys from 2008 [2]. A survey of 16,347 nursing homes in the US revealed a significant increase in the number of demented residents who used hospice from 26.5 % in 2003 to 34.4 % in 2007 [3]. Most patients with dementia have complex care needs in the final stages of the illness. In contrast to the hospice expenditure, the cost of assisted living care is approximately $3,600 per month while the cost of nursing home care is about $255 per day. Long term care for dementia in any setting is expensive however the modest cost of hospice care coupled with potential savings from avoiding unnecessary hospital admissions points to the relative value of hospice care [1]. For-profit hospice agencies are more likely to take patients with dementia; these individuals frequently have lower "skilled needs" and longer length of stay [4].

Most dementias that occur in older adults are lethal. The majority of deaths in patients with dementia are from complications caused by the neurological damage as opposed to death from the direct damage to the brains such as that seen in cerebral anoxia or trauma. Patients with dementia may die at home, in a nursing home, in an assisted living facility, in a hospital or in an inpatient hospice program. Many (40 %) non-demented hospice recipient's exhibit some signs of cognitive impairment during hospice care [5]. Most dementias are clinically dynamic and gradually change over time however some forms of dementia can progress quite rapidly as seen in diseases such as Creutzfeldt-Jacob disease.

R.E. Powers, MD (✉)
Division of Neuropathology, Department of Pathology and Psychiatry, UAB School of Medicine, Birmingham, AL, USA

Post-Traumatic Stress Disorder Program, Veterans Administration Hospital, Birmingham, AL, USA
e-mail: richardpowersmd@gmail.com

H.L. Herrington, MD
Department of Medicine, University of Alabama at Birmingham, Birmingham, AL 35294, USA
e-mail: hherrington@uabmc.edu

© Springer International Publishing Switzerland 2016
M. Boltz, J.E. Galvin (eds.), *Dementia Care*, DOI 10.1007/978-3-319-18377-0_16

Dementia usually causes cognitive, behavioral and psychiatric manifestations with no two patients having the same constellation of symptoms or speed of progression. The person to person clinical heterogeneity of medical and behavioral features can pose a specific challenge to the hospice team in assessing, treating and adapting care strategies for each individual patient. Despite these obstacles, hospice continues to be the strategy of choice for persons with dementia who are in the final phases of their illness or demented patients who are dying from other causes such as cancer or cardiovascular disease. This chapter begins where the palliative care section ends and provides a roadmap to all members of the hospice team in caring for the patient, the family caregivers and the dedicated health care providers who know this patient very well. The historical perspective about end of life care for patients with dementia reveals significant suffering during the dying process with a report from 2005 entitled, "Dying dementia patients, Too much suffering, too little palliation," This report stated that 63 % of patients die with high suffering and 29.6 % intermediate suffering but only 7 % die with low suffering [6]. Since that time, academic and industry leaders have attempted to understand the challenges to hospice for dementia, construct evidence based practices and create best practices within the industry. This effort is a work in progress.

Profile of the Hospice Patient with Dementia

Dementia is a common diagnosis in nursing homes where many end of life studies are conducted. National studies show that one third of persons over age 65 will receive Medicare-funded nursing home care in the last 6 months of their life [7]. In one nursing home study, 54.8 % of nursing home residents with dementia died over an 18 month period and at least 40.7 % of residents had at least one burdensome intervention in the last 3 months of life [8]. Similar detailed studies are not available for home-based care or assisted living. Recent Medicare data sug-

gests that more elders are dying at home and fewer are dying in the hospital but more elders are receiving ICU care within the last 6 months of their lives [9]. Most patients with dementia spend the last months of their lives in nursing homes. Nursing home outcome studies provide some research advantages as patients receive a standardized assessment on admission termed the Minimum Data Set and medical care is somewhat standardized by federal regulations. However, nursing home outcomes studies are not fully representative of the community population that is dying with dementia. For instance, many residents of assisted living have dementia. A study of hospice services for assisted living residents who are "dual eligible" i.e. who qualify for both Medicaid and Medicare, revealed that most (58 %) were demented and hospice care may reduce the likelihood of nursing home transfer or hospital admission of these residents [10]. Developing a comprehensive picture for end of life care is another work in progress.

Dementia can produce a range of cognitive deficits, functional impairments, psychiatric symptoms and behavioral challenges depending on the type of neurodegenerative disorder. For example, the cognitive symptoms of Alzheimer's disease are usually progressive over time while deficits in post-traumatic dementia can be stable. An important principle of hospice care for persons with dementia is that the team will treat the person rather than the diagnosis. No assumption should be made about a patient's needs or abilities until a multidisciplinary team completes a thorough assessment of the patient's deficits and abilities. Frail older patients often have other comorbidities such as sensory deficits like impaired hearing or eye sight as well as academic limitations that can mislead the treatment team into believing that the patient is more severely impaired than the actual clinical reality. The patient should be defined by abilities rather than deficits. For example, a patient who cannot speak but can sing may benefit for musical programs or the chaplain singing hymns. All aspects of care must accommodate the neurological and psychiatric status of the patient. For example, patients with receptive aphasia need visual cues and non-verbal communication to reassure them about your good intentions. And finally, family interactions must be sensitive to the unique relationship between the caregivers and the patients as well as mindful of distant caregivers who may not understand the disease process or the clinical realities of care. For example, the caregiver may be a unique resource of advice on methods to get a patient to swallow, turn in bed or not resist during changes. The distant caregiver who sees a patient once a year many not understand the progression of symptoms in the patient.

Dementia can afflict patients across a wide range of ages from early onset patients who may be dying in their mid to late fifties to the very old. Centenarians are very likely to develop dementia and frailty. In one survey, community dwelling individuals over age 85 were highly likely (80 %) to die away from their home with a high likelihood of hospitalization [11]. Little is reported about the dying process for early onset dementia and the role of hospice in sustaining their quality of life. Unlike the very old who have often outlived friends and family, the early onset patients often have young families that are severely impacted by the disease and loss.

Goals of Hospice Dementia Care

The ultimate goals for hospice dementia care are to sustain function and quality of life for as long as possible and then allow patients to die in their preferred location with comfort and dignity. The quality of death for the general population incorporates seven broad domains that include the physical, psychological social, spiritual, existential, health care, life closure, death preparation and circumstances of death [12]. Some of these domains may no longer apply to persons with severe dementia who may have already experienced psychological, existential or cognitive death. Clinicians and researchers with expertise in death in dementia usually agree that a holistic approach to hospice care should include physical, psychological, social, emotional and cultural needs of the patient as well as attention to the welfare of the caregiver [13]. Cognitively intact older

persons have opinions about the future direction of their life and the hoped-for circumstance of their death. Research and ethical issues such as defining choices in healthy persons versus dying patients complicate studies to identify the preferences of older persons on the location of death [14], Surveys of different countries with different cultures show that the general population of older persons prefers to die in their own home [15]. This cross cultural consistency suggests that wishing to remain at home with your family, pets and familiar surroundings is a consistent human theme. Hospice services can affirm that wish and operationalize those preferences. Patients who are enrolled in hospice are significantly more likely to die in their chosen location [16].

Death and the Active Dying Process in Dementia

The concept of death in dementia is more complex than other diseases because many patients retain some physical or medical vigor while their brain slowly dies. A recent international consensus operational definition of death reads, "Death is the permanent loss of capacity for consciousness and all brain stem functions. This may result from permanent cessation of circulation or catastrophic brain injury. In the context of death determination, 'permanent' refers to loss of function that cannot resume spontaneously and will not be restored through intervention" [17]. Although some court rulings have obscured the linkage of brain death to actual death, the consensus of clinical and ethical experts defines brain death as synonymous with death [18]. Many patients with advanced dementia do not fall neatly into this definition since they may retain stable general health and exhibit varying patterns of cognitive deficits. The permanent aspect can sometimes be questioned based on clinical fluctuations that can occur when a dementia patient may seem to occasionally function above their baseline. A patient may be completely unresponsive on one occasion and seem to recognize family on other occasions. The definition of death in dementia is often linked to brain death and should be distinguished from coma or persistent vegetative state where brain damage may remain stable or improve over time. Most dementias are neurodegenerative disorders that will progress over time and continuously reduce brain function. The clinical features of end-stage dementia include loss of all higher cognitive function and pathological features often include brain volume reduction from 1,400 g to 800 or 900 g; changes that resemble alterations described in brain death despite the survival of autonomic centers in the brain stem (Fig. 1). A family member may have an isolated interaction with the end stage patient when the patient seems more responsive and seems to acknowledge their presence. This brief behavioral change can be misinterpreted as latent cognitive ability suggesting that the patient might "wake-up." The family member's hopes may be raised and the decision to forgo heroic measures may be questioned by the caregiver. Proactive and interactive education about the brain changes caused by dementia can be helpful in allaying concerns about whether the patient has irreversibly lost function.

The death process for persons with advanced stage dementia often includes a major health event in the last 30 days such as pneumonia or other infections. Nursing home residents acutely dying with dementia exhibit problems with mobility 81 %, sleep 63 % and pain 71 % [19]. Individuals dying at home were described as suffering from weakness 94 % and fatigue 94 % in the last 2 days of life. They also described loss of appetite 86.4 %, dyspnea 56.7 %, anxiety 61 % and pain 52.5 % during the last few days of life [20]. Within the last week, swallowing problems and pain are common symptoms with up to 26 % developing decubiti. In this Belgium study, physical restraints were employed in 21 % of residents and 10 % died outside the home, inferred to be in the hospital [21]. A single descriptive study of patients in the last few days of their lives with very severe dementia as defined by mini-mental status scores of zero found that the majority subjects reported no pain on the PAINAD scale (63.9 %). Most died quietly and few 8 % were aware of their symptoms [22]. The limited data

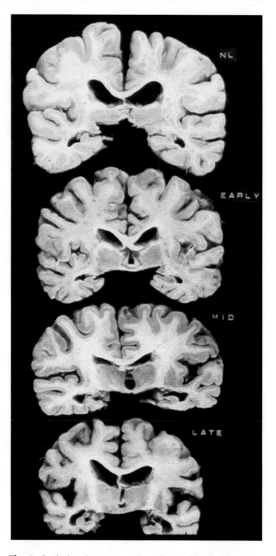

Fig. 1 Includes three coronal sections of brains from age matched individuals with Alzheimer's disease that are contrasted to the normal brain (*top*). The sections depict the progression of atrophy and ventriculomegaly present in the early, middle and later stages of the disease. The late stage brain came from an individual with dementia for 8 years and this subject had severe cognitive impairment

on the final days of patients with advanced dementia who died from dehydration or cachexia suggests no excess patient suffering in a properly managed clinical setting [22]. The limited published data suggests that dying dementia patients can experience significant distress in the last 30 days of life with symptoms that lessen during the last few days of life.

Clinical Aspects of Hospice Care for Dementia Other Than Alzheimer's Disease

Vascular dementia, alcohol related dementia, Lewy body disease and Frontotemporal dementia are four common causes of cognitive loss in older persons. The clinical features of these dementias are discussed elsewhere in the book. The natural history of late stage dementias other than Alzheimer's disease is poorly defined. Most common dementias are progressive although alcohol related dementia may stabilize in some patients who become abstinent. Biomarkers are not helpful in defining the life expectancy or clinical course for these dementias.

Parkinson's disease is a movement disorder that afflicts up to 1 % of elders. Many patients with PD develop cognitive symptoms in later life and the clinical onset of Parkinson's disease reduces expected survival by about 5 % per year of disease [23]. Patients with movement disorders frequently develop depression and other psychiatric complications. The hospice admission process for a patient with Parkinson's disease and dementia should include the exclusion of psychotic depression as a cause of "terminal decline." Therapy-resistant depression in patients with Parkinson's disease can worsen motor symptoms and aggressive therapy to include electroconvulsive therapy (ECT) may reverse the changes. End of life care for patients with Parkinson's disease is complicated by the presence of extrapyramidal features and the complexity of pharmacology that reduces rigidity and improves mobility. Proper end of life management of patients with Parkinson's disease may improve bowel function, dysphagia, anxiety, pain and drowsiness [24]. Dementia in the parkinsonian patient is calculated to precede death by 3.3 years [25]. Biomarkers cannot predict dementia or speed of cognitive decline in patients with Parkinson's disease. Some patients may have deep brain stimulators implanted. The decision to reduce or stop medications that sustain motor function requires thoughtful consideration and careful follow-up. The treating neurologist can provide helpful advice. Palliative care has been shown to be effective for persons with Parkinson's disease [24] but little is written specifically on hospice care for individuals with Parkinson's disease or Lewy body dementia. Family caregivers for persons with Parkinson's disease experience both anticipatory and post death bereavement as can be seen in other neurodegenerative disorders [26]. The reduction or discontinuation of psychotropic medications should include careful monitoring for the reoccurrence of distressing symptoms such as visual hallucinations.

FTD has the highest mortality risk followed by Lewy body dementia, vascular dementia and then Alzheimer's disease. Similar statistics are not available for other diseases although prion diseases are known to have short survivals i.e., less than 2 years [27]. The three major dementias, AD, VAD and DLB do not produce late-stage functional decline with clinically discernable differences although subtle differences are noted by researchers [28].

Basic Requirements for a Hospice Program to Serve Persons with Dementia and Their Families

Hospice services for persons with dementia may be provided in many locations, including the patient's home, an assisted living area, their nursing home room or an inpatient hospice program. The decision to use hospice may come as part of a discharge plan following an acute hospitalization for the patient or as part of a conversation between caregiver and primary care provider. Each location can have a unique set of challenges for the patient, the caregiver and the provider team. The basic features of effective dementia care across all hospice settings are similar and are described in Table 1.

Defining Patient and Family Wishes

Excellent hospice care begins with knowledgeable physicians or nurse practitioners talking to patients and family caregivers across the course

Table 1 Features of effective dementia care across hospice settings

Define the wishes of the patient and the family
Employ an integrated interdisciplinary team
Assure knowledge and practice competency for hospice skills, and cognitive and neuropsychiatric disorders among all team members
Adjust care to the comfort and wellness needs of the patient
Understand the cognitive, psychiatric and behavioral needs of each patient
Construct treatment goals and a plan of care that is unique to each individual
Avoid disruptive transitions of care
Maximize patient comfort and dignity
Communicate effectively with the local and distant caregivers
Address caregiver grief during the anticipatory and the post mortem phase

of a chronic illness. Unlike hospice provided to cancer patients or others dying from medical diseases, hospice care for dementia patients requires two distinct skill sets that meet both the medical and the neuropsychiatric needs of the patient and family [13]. Good planning requires that the family and clinician solicit information about the patient's preference on how they want to spend the last days of their life while the patient retains the capacity to provide this guidance. The clinical team should strive to accomplish those goals defined by the patient (see Chapter "Experiences and Perspectives of Family Caregivers of the Person with Dementia" for further discussion). Caregivers often avoid these complicated and difficult discussions with the patient from fear that the patient is not ready to make such decisions. Families often continue to avoid the subject until an emergency arises such as a catastrophic health problem that requires aggressive medical interventions. Advanced planning for dementia care usually requires a complex discussion with a primary care provider (PCP) who may have limited information about the expected complications in advanced disease. The PCP also often has limited understanding of the potential pitfalls for the future use of futile aggressive interventions such as PEG tubes as well as the concern that such advice may suggest a tacit endorsement of euthanasia. Many physicians (33 %) report lack of time as a major issue. Family factors dominated the family's attitude toward initiating advanced care planning [29].

The expected clinical course is difficult to predict in all patients but most families will deal with questions about aggressive measures to sustain life such as pacemaker insertion, dialysis, artificial feeding, hospitalization and place of death. Many patients also have clear ideas about arrangements for death such as place of burial or type of ceremony. The individual natural history can impacted by type of neurodegenerative disease, age of patient, medical comorbidities, psychosocial resource for both the patient as well as caregiver, family understanding about the disease and family understanding about the nature of hospice care. Racial disparities in the quality of care for advanced dementia exist. A non-white patient is at significantly greater risk for tube feedings, hospitalization and absence of an advanced directive [30].

Local medical practices and beliefs can also impact some aspects of care or recommendations made to the family. For example, significant regional variations exist in the US on the use of hospice versus the use of acute hospitalization at the end of life. A survey of Medicare expenditures reveals that patients in the southeast US are less likely to use hospice than recipients who reside in other regions of the country [31]. These differences may occur as the result of regional variations of medical provider attitudes or regional cultural issues that place pressure on family caregivers to employ heroic measures rather than comfort care. The family should be encouraged to consider end of life issues and seek guidance from the patient while the patient still has the capacity to provide input, such as individuals with mild cognitive impairment or mild dementia. This may reduce later burdens when family can limit aggressive or heroic care based on the patient's wishes. Likewise, it provides an opportunity for distant caregivers to participate in care planning in a non-crisis environment [30].

Research on advanced care planning for persons with end-stage dementia suggests that the wishes of the caregivers and the opinion of the treatment team may play a greater role as opposed to the expressed directions of the patient [32]. Older age, male gender, availability of hospital or nursing home beds and hospice enrollment can impact the end-of-life outcome in the general population of older patients [33]. A patient's desire to die at home may be impossible if the care needs exceed the capacity of home services and the resources of the caregivers. Financial issues may require placement in a nursing home or the person with dementia may live alone and not have family to assist with care. The team should understand the wishes of the patient and attempt to honor those directives but in some instances those wishes may not be realistic for the existing situation. For example, the death of a caregiver around the time a patient enters the dying phase of the illness may limit options for the remaining family. The team should strive to abide by the family wishes unless specific obstacles exist.

The Hospice Interdisciplinary Team

A broad range of professionals can be involved with hospice care for the person with dementia. The team may include nurses, doctors, direct care providers, nurse practitioners, nutritionists, social workers, chaplains, recreational therapists, speech pathologists, elder lawyers, and most importantly the family caregiver. Each member of the team has unique skills that can improve the quality of life for both the patient and the family although each individual patient may not need assistance from all these individuals. Members of the team must achieve basic neuropsychiatric knowledge and skill proficiency across all stages for the common types of dementia. Direct, hands-on care providers should understand the patient's cognitive deficits as well as the behavioral consequences of those clinical challenges. Behavioral intervention are always preferable to pharmacological interventions and all staff

that touch the patient must understand normal brain function, behavioral manifestations of brain damage and behavioral strategies to reduce problems such as screaming, hitting, resisting, or refusing to eat.

Educating family care givers about the natural history of dementia is an important component to hospice care. In one study, 28 % of responding families were unaware that their nursing home resident had dementia with almost one fifth of that group having family-members with severe dementia. Nursing home residents with longer stays were more likely to go unrecognized by the family who may believe that dementia is a "normal" part of aging [34]. This lack of recognition can impact the family's ability to assist with care plans and develop advanced directives for the patient. Distant caregivers have not been studied but logic would suggest that persons who are distant from the individual and spend little time with the resident would be less informed about their level of disability. Family knowledge may also impact patient outcomes. Families that perceive dementia as a fatal disease have outcomes where the patient has higher levels of comfort during the dying process. Many (43 %) family caregivers of nursing home residents recognized dementia as a fatal disease while some (28 %) did not know [35]. Such basic knowledge about the natural history may improve patient outcome and reduce caregiver distress.

Knowledge and Competency of the Hospice Team

Education is an important tool for team building, improving care and quality of life of patients with dementia in all stages of the disease. Inter professional education and dissemination about best practices for managing dementia can improve patient-centered care. Dissemination of existing or available educational programs is strongly encouraged for all professionals [36]. The value of education assures that all staff understands the basic clinical features of dementia, the natural history and the management strategy. A consistent message and treatment philosophy communicated to the caregiver or other involved family members can prevent family confusion and promote family confidence. The dementia knowledge level of direct care hospice workers has not been carefully studied. The clinical manifestations of dementia may be confusing to the direct care worker as the patient may appear physically healthy yet the team is discussing a terminal illness. The patient with swallowing dyspraxia may be able to bite and spit but not chew. The staff may not understand that a PEG tube will not protect against aspiration. Each team member should understand the brain pathology caused by neurodegenerative disease and the logic of the hospice management strategies that are used by the team.

Quality measures to define a "good death" [12] for demented patients in hospice may be limited by communication deficits experienced by the patients. However available studies suggest that the quality measures employed in regular hospice care also apply to care for patients with dementia [37]. Data from the National Home and Hospice Care Survey showed that dementia patients were older, more likely to be widowed, more likely to receive care in a nursing home with only 24 % receiving care in a private setting. Dementia patients were more likely to get tube feeding but had fewer identified pain complaints. Some (14 %) had stage 2 or greater decubiti. Some (24 %) received antibiotics in the last 7 days of care. Most (88 %) had a DNR order. The presence of advanced care planning often serves as a quality measure in hospice care. The chances of having better emotional well-being were three times higher in patients with written advanced directives especially when a DNR order was written [38]. Basic quality measures would assess the use of advanced care planning, the prevention of disruptive transitions of care, the management of pain and distress, the use of dementia-appropriate behavioral interventions, the reduction of polypharmacy and the ability to support caregivers throughout the entire process. The expected outcome for the average hospice agency is to "dementia-proof" basic hospice services [13].

Maintaining environmental consistency and avoiding disruptive transitions of care may improve quality of life for patients dying with dementia. The number of disruptive transitions of care is a common benchmark of quality of care. Many older persons, especially those with dementia, spend the last months of their life in nursing homes where national trend data suggests a substantial likelihood of transfer to an acute care facility (prior to death.). The number of nursing home residents who die in hospital has been steadily rising in the United States from 16 % in 1990 to 25 % in 2001 with a projection of 40 % in 2020 as the Baby boomers begin to die [39]. A similar phenomenon is seen in other western health systems such as Germany and Canada as population's age. The number of nursing home residents with advanced dementia who were hospitalized in the ICU within 4 months of death rose from 6.1 % in 2000 to 9.5 % in 2007. Significant geographical variation occurred with 0.8 % in Montana versus 22 % in the District of Columbia [40]. Southern residents in the United States are more likely to have problematic changes such as the use of feeding tubes, intensive care unit admission, stage 4 decubiti, and late entry into hospice [41]. In other countries with advanced health care systems, the national trend is moving towards hospice over hospital care [42].

Families usually want to find the "best" provider and hospice providers usually like to show established quality measures that support their excellence of services. Specific standards do not exist for hospice care of persons dying from dementia or people dying with dementia. There is no documentation on the number of hospice programs in the US that have definable expertise in dementia care and these organizations have no method to document that expertise even if they have excellent programming. Family caregivers and referring physicians may have limited methods to judge the ability of a hospice agency to manage a patient dying with dementia. The National Hospice and Palliative Care Organization has published best practices but there is not a comprehensive rating system, similar to that established for nursing homes by Center for Medicare and Medicaid Services (CMS) for hospice in general and for dementia care in particular.

Managing Referrals and Eligibility for Hospice Services

Referrals to hospice require the ordering of a consultation by a physician who is often a primary care provider. Many primary care providers view dementia care as frustrating and the diagnosis of dementia may be missed or delayed. Physicians may be poorly reimbursed to engage in conversations with families and patients about advanced wishes despite the fact that such discussions are helpful to both the patient and the family [43]. The development of person-centered care requires education and commitment by the clinicians and health care system however these policies and resources are rarely present [44]. Although recent trends suggest more clinicians are suggesting hospice care to family caregivers, previous study in the state of Michigan showed that 10.7 % of homecare patients dying with advanced dementia and 5.7 % of nursing home residents were referred for hospice service [45]. Surveyed agencies have consistently identified several barriers to referral that include problems with predicting survival, lack of understanding about the terminal nature of Alzheimer's disease and other dementia and uncertainty about Medicare regulations on the matter.

Determination of hospice eligibility for a diagnosis of dementia is a major concern for families and health care professionals. The FAST scale is the accepted clinical staging instrument but the primary care provider must request the service and affirm that the patient has a terminal illness with a life expectancy of 6 months or less [46]. The FAST has seven major stages and 16 sub-stages that evaluate activities of daily living (ADL) and communication. Stage six quantifies many ADL impairments. Stage seven includes the following criteria: speech is limited to five words, all intelligible vocabulary is lost, not able to ambulate, cannot sit independently, unable to smile, and unable to control movement of head. The medical director for the hospice agency will also affirm the prognosis but the primary care provider is the critical first step. The prediction of whether a person with dementia will die within 6 months or 1 week is fraught with difficulties and limitations [47]. Significant health problems in the final stage can reduce 6 month survival with a 6 month mortality of 53 % for pneumonia compared to 13 % for intact elders and 55 % for hip fracture compared to 12 % for intact individuals [48]. The expected survival of a patient with dementia can be influenced by multiple clinical factors including the type of dementia, associated medical morbidities, functional level, current care environment, and the wishes of the family. Studies show that most (77 %) patients who meet FAST 7 criteria died within 6 months and most (71 %) survivors continued to meet Medicare criteria for hospice care. The mean survival ranged from 3.1 to 4.2 months [49]. Other simple instruments used for predictions such as the Minimum Data Set have been shown similar predictive value [50].

A single study suggests that death may be predicted with accuracy up to 95 % over a multiyear span using a research tool but the algorithm is complicated and incorporates as many as 16 covariates [51]. Common features include gender, functional capacity and behavioral or psychiatric features. The ADEPT, advanced dementia prognostic tool, uses data from 12 items from the Minimum Data set to predict 6 month survival in nursing home residents with better accuracy than existing criteria used by the Centers for Medicare Medicaid Services [52]. Simple instruments such as the FAST have limited predictive value and cognitive testing such as the mini mental status examination have less predictive value. Delayed admission to hospice can reduce the benefit to the patient but predicting immanent death in dementia is challenging. A past history of rapid decline based on functional assessment or MMSE score loss is somewhat indicative of future rapid decline but no specific clinical feature is absolutely predictive at any stage in the illness.

Standardized testing can predict 1 week mortality in some medical conditions such as pulmonary disease but available instruments are less precise in diseases such as cancer or dementia [53].

The prognostic uncertainty for dementia is a major reason why doctors avoid raising the issue with families since the ultimate decision rests with the patient and the family. This trigger point for discussion with the caregiver about hospice or palliative care varies according to the clinical and psychosocial features for each individual. The topic may need to be approached on several occasions before the conversation between the clinician and the family is completed. Increased dependence, decreased global cognitive function and the presence of at least one neuropsychiatric symptom suggests but does not predict the need to initiate the discussion [54]. Predicting hospice survival can be difficult. A review of 13,479 general hospice recipients showed that 14 % were discharged for not meeting clinical criteria and a quarter was enrolled for 5 days or less [55]. A study of 24,111 hospice recipients with dementia revealed that 5 % were discharged alive because their condition stabilized or improved and they no longer met criteria. Of those discharged alive, 75.5 % were still alive in 1 year. Of those who died, the median life expectancy was almost 6 months [2] Dementia patients are more likely to exceed the 6 month limit in comparison to persons with other diseases such as cancer. The medical benefit comes under Part A of the Medicare benefit and includes two 90 day certification periods followed by 60 day recertification periods. These individuals are more likely to require a face to face assessment for recertification as per the guidance from the Centers for Medicare and Medicaid Services issued in 2011 [56].

Pathobiology of Late Stage Dementia

Brain imaging, molecular markers such as cerebrospinal fluid levels of beta amyloid or tau and genetic markers such as APOE typing are now used to enhance diagnostic accuracy for demen-tia. These adjunctive tests can assist with predicting some risks for developing dementia or the likelihood of transition from mild cognitive impairment to dementia [57]. However, the use of biomarkers to predict speed of progression in mid to late stage is far less developed and the clinician must rely on their clinical judgment to estimate stage and life expectancy. The inaccuracy of biomarkers at predicting life expectancy can be understood in the context of brain pathology in advanced dementia.

The microscopic and molecular neuropathology differs for each of the common clinical forms of dementia. Alzheimer disease produces at least four types of brain pathology including senile plaques, neurofibrillary tangles, neuronal loss and synaptic depletion. Microscopic damage is poorly correlated to clinical staging or proximity to death. Amyloid may accumulate as plaques or within blood vessels however the quantity of brain amyloid does not predict the stage of disease or speed of progression in later stages [58]. White matter damage may occur as either a primary or secondary event however estimates of white matter volume loss are not shown to predict speed of progression or proximity to death.

The clinical definition of brain death for persons with massive neurological injury resulting from a defined insult such as head trauma or cerebral anoxia has been extensively discussed in the published literature. Specific neurological finding such as seizures, spasticity or coma do not predict impending death in persons with dementia. There is no evidence that electrical silence on EEG or reduced cerebral blood flow can predict impending death. Most common dementias damage higher cortical association cortices while sparing primary motor or sensory cortices as well as brain stem centers that manage autonomic drive. This pattern of damage results in loss of cognitive function with relative sparing of respiratory and cardiovascular control. Likewise, the involuntary activity such as turning to sound or groaning during repositioning does not suggest or confirm any form of cognitive awareness of surroundings.

The postmortem pathological heterogeneity of dementia reflects the range of clinical features

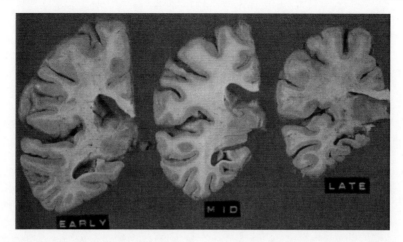

Fig. 2 Contrasts coronal hemispheric section from three individuals with Alzheimer's disease who had early, mid-stage disease and late stage disease on the right. There is progressive atrophy of the temporal lobes along with progressive dilation of the inferior horn of the lateral ventricle caused by volume loss of the mesial temporal lobe structures

seen with end-stage dementia. Most common brain pathologies do not reach a plateau but rather the disease progression causes more atrophy and ventriculomegaly (Fig. 2). Vascular dementia has no consensus quantity or location of vascular pathology to predict cognitive loss or severity of dementia. Quantitative methodology to measure the volume of brain damage caused by vascular disease using in vivo brain imaging or post mortem brain examination may not capture common types of subtle disease such as hypertensive leukoencephalopathy. Vascular damage is a common second pathology in mixed dementias. Lewy body dementia is defined by cortical Lewy bodies that contain synuclein and alcohol related dementia involves a mixture of pathologies that are non-specific. The most common pathological finding in a community sample of persons with dementia is the presence of two or more pathologies referred to as mixed dementia. This clinicopathological heterogeneity reduces the likelihood that biomarkers or brain imaging will predict life expectancy or intensity of damage. The pathological causes of dementia in younger individual are more heterogeneous and often include alcohol-related dementia, traumatic brain injury, multiple sclerosis HIV infection and others.

The Neuropathology of Late Stage Dementia Other Than Alzheimer's Disease

The gross appearance of an advanced stage dementia other than Alzheimer's disease often includes severe atrophy and ventriculomegaly. Some brains such as FTD may have severe regional atrophy and vascular dementia may include extensive infarctions but many cases may be indistinguishable from advanced Alzheimer's disease. The neuropathology of advanced stage Parkinson's disease may include both synuclein and tau based pathology. Available late stage clinicopathological studies indicate that cortical lewy bodies and dystrophic neuritis are present in the rostral areas of the brain in end stage disease. The severity of the rostral pathology was related to the severity of dementia [25, 59] however AD pathology including neurofibrillary tangles were also abundant in some patients. The neuropathology of late stage vascular dementia and FTD has not been defined although advance stage FTD patients typically demonstrate high densities of tau-based pathology such as Pick bodies as well as neuronal loss and gliosis. White matter loss is described in all advanced stage dementias however the neuropathology has not been defined.

Clinicopathological Correlates of Capacity and Competency

Many decisions related to hospice care depend on the ability of family or patient to give informed consent or of family to accurately predict a person's wishes. Cognitive impairment, severe mental illness, neuropsychiatric complications and severe sensory disability may impact ability to give informed consent. Different types of dementia can selectively damage regions involved with judgment early in the disease, such as Frontotemporal dementia. The development of psychiatric complications such as depression or psychosis can also impair judgment. Individuals with advanced directives or durable powers of attorney are more likely to get the care they directed and less likely to die in hospital [60]. However, even clearly defined wishes may be ignored by physicians as surveys show that a large number of internists may be unwilling to adhere to patients' instructions to withhold or withdraw life saving interventions [61]. Surrogates may make errors in 12–22 % of decision situations and can be unclear in 11–16 % [62]. Surrogate decision makers accurately predict the patient's wishes in 68 % of the cases [63]. The best option is defining wishes while the patient retains capacity to give informed consent and explain those decisions to the family who will execute the directions.

The precise neuroanatomy of consent is unknown. The cognitive tasks for consent and capacity must involve multiple brain regions and networks including the saliency and default mode systems. The neuropathology of advanced dementia may include severe damage to mesial and lateral temporal brain regions as well as atrophy of the frontal lobes. The neurobiology of capacity is unknown as few scientists have attempted to define the functional neuroanatomy of capacity and develop biomarkers that correlate to risk for loss of this function. Capacity requires that a patient have the ability to understand the verbal or written information about the consequences of their decisions and also the ability to reflect on those decisions by remembering the conversation and facts. The patient must weigh the benefits and consequences of those decisions in the context of their value and belief systems. The patient must have sufficient motivation to consider these difficult issues.

The patient with moderate or severe Alzheimer's disease usually has significant damage to the hippocampus and the lateral temporal cortices (Fig. 2). An intact hippocampus is required to acquire and retain new information. Damage to the lateral temporal cortices is most intense in the auditory association cortices with relative sparing of the transverse temporal gyrus that contains the primary auditory cortex. These patients may be able to hear but not understand or interpret. The frontal lobes and the orbitofrontal cortices are involved with sophisticated decision making and risk-benefit assessment. Functional imaging studies of moral judgments indicate two distinct pathways. The first person judgment of "how I perceive an issue' is distinct from the third person judgment of "What is he doing". Preliminary studies suggests that first person decisions activate the medial prefrontal cortex while third person decisions activate hippocampus and visual cortex [64].

The frontal lobes are usually damaged in Alzheimer's disease and Lewy body dementia. FTD specifically damages these brain regions early in the disease producing the combination of personality change and impaired judgment. Patients with alcohol related dementia often have damage to the frontal lobe. Individuals with post concussive dementia may have significant damage to the orbitofrontal cortices. Components of the default mode system and the saliency network such as the anterior cingulate gyrus, temporal pole; temporal-parietal junction and the insula cortex are damaged in Alzheimer's disease, Lewy body dementia and FTD [65]. These systems are critical to insight and "moral reasoning" where risk-benefit and contextual information is processed. These systems would help process information about life choices, reflect on those choices and weigh the moral value of the decision [66]. Dysfunction of these systems is identified with impaired insight such as the continued use of cocaine in humans. In summary, most common dementias produce damage to the brain regions that are used in weighing decisions and providing informed consent. The multifocal damage associated with most common dementia impacts brain regions that acquire, remember and process information as well as regions that reflect on information and weigh the information against the internalized set of moral standards.

Management of the Patient with Dementia in Hospice Care

The hospice team may assume management of medical problems for the patient with dementia or the team may work with other physicians such as the primary care provider or the nursing home physician. Specific common clinical concerns arise such as managing medications, nutrition, hydration, pain control and the decision to hospitalize for common end-of-life medical problems such as pneumonia.

Avoiding Hospitalization

Individuals with multiple medical morbidities are more likely to be hospitalized and they are more likely to deteriorate rapidly [67]. Hospitals can be fraught with danger, even for a relatively healthy person. For older adults, especially those with dementia, the situation is often even more dire. The hospital is an unfamiliar environment and the change in routine, including the lack of adherence to usual sleep-wake cycles, can be particularly disruptive, increasing the risk of delirium. Medications frequently change and new "poisons" are added, which may worsen cognition thorough anticholinergic, sedating or other mechanisms. Patients are routinely held as "NPO" as they await procedures, leading to a more compromised nutritional status; anesthesia or sedating medications associated with these procedures can often worsen cognition. Patients are often placed on bed rest, out of fear of falls, but the enforced bed rest only further weakens the patient, thus increasing fall risk. Bed rest can also be associated with deep venous thrombosis, pulmonary embolism, pressure ulcers, placement

of bladder catheters which may then lead to urinary infections, etc. Most nursing home residents who are transferred from nursing home to inpatient hospital care have infections (59 %) while the majority of emergency room visits are caused by issues about PEG tubes (43 %) [68].

The hospital experience for dementia patients is often more difficult than the experience for cognitively intact individuals [69]. Hospital environments are rarely dementia friendly except perhaps in the setting of specialized programs such as Acute Care for Elderly (ACE) units. The negative hospital experience for the patient with dementia may begin in the admissions area where demented patients may wait longer for admission. The negative experience may extend into the inpatient unit where the patients may experience fear, overstimulation, excessive thirst and pain. The physical structure of the care environment, philosophical approach of the staff, and quality measures are not focused on the needs of persons with dementia. This reality is important to communicate to caregivers as they determine the level and intensity of medical care and weigh the risk benefit ratio for each hospitalization.

Because of these inherent issues, it is often difficult to know when the burdens of hospitalization outweigh the benefits for a person with worsening dementia. At end of life, the risks of hospitalization more frequently outweigh the benefits, but treatment should always be guided by the person's prognosis and goals of care. A person with mild dementia, who happens to be on hospice for a recent diagnosis of metastatic lung cancer but is otherwise well, may have a fairly prolonged hospice course. If this person should fall and suffer a hip fracture early on, hospitalization and repair of the fracture may be the best course of action if the patient is well enough to withstand the surgery and recovery/rehabilitation process. In persons with more advanced dementia, treatment in place is often more appropriate for other medical problems, whether it be antibiotics for infection, intravenous fluids for dehydration, diuretics for volume overload, or other issues. In contrast, many people with advanced dementia are inappropriately hospitalized at end of life, so it is imperative to discuss the option of

"Do Not Hospitalize" (DNH) orders beforehand, with their family and caregivers.

The decision to forego hospitalization at the end of life often occurs following admission to the nursing home. Although there is scant evidence for the value of hospitalization for most dying patients, the majority of nursing home patients do not have an order to forego hospitalization. The utilization of the DNH order to reduce disruptive transitions of care varies by geographical region ranging from 0.7 % in Oklahoma to 25.9 % in Rhode Island based on a year 2000 study of nursing home residents with advanced dementia. Older individuals with severe disability or those with a person as a designated durable power of attorney were most likely to have a DNH order [8]. Advanced directives are critical to avoiding unhelpful hospitalizations. Surveys of family caregivers suggest that family members often overestimate the presence of an advanced directive for their loved one. Individuals with higher education, older age, a recent significant change in health status and residents of assisted living are more likely to have proper documentation of their wishes [70]. In one European study of nursing home residents in the last month of life 19.5 % of patients were hospitalized and 4.6 % went to the ICU [40]. None of the hospitalizations occurred at the request of the patient with 37 % occurring at the request of family who were seeking extension of life or curative interventions [71]. The cost effectiveness studies of hospitalization for patients with end stage dementia show an incremental increase in Medicare expenditure of $5,972 with a quality adjusted survival or 3.7 days demonstrating the low effectiveness of this treatment decision [72]. Medicare data comparisons between 2000 and 2007 of ICU admissions of nursing home residents with advanced dementia in the last 30 days of life show increased ICU utilization with regional variation from 0.82 % for Montana to 22 % in the District of Columbia. Hospitalized patients with dementia hadsignificantly increased risk of developing organ failure and sepsis during the course of hospitalization as compared to matched non-demented elders [73].

Hospitalization can occur during the dying process for a variety of reasons. Older demented patients are more likely to have multiple medical comorbidities such as hypertension, diabetes, Parkinson's disease, congestive heart failure and others that may increase the possibility of acute care hospitalization [74]. Post mortem studies on individuals with dementia define common health problems in deceased patients to include pneumonia 66.3 % as cause of death, 16.3 % with cardiovascular disease, 20.9 % with lung disease, and 18.6 % with evidence of recent or old myocardial infarction [75].

Post mortem studies on cause of death in elderly patients with dementia as compared to similar groups without dementia identify pneumonia (45 % vs. 28 %) and cardiovascular disease (46 % vs. 31 %) as major causes [76]. Pulmonary thromboembolism (17.3 %) has been identified in some reports [77] however available studies show a low rate of easily reversible diseases in persons who die with dementia. The low frequency of treatable illness or missed diagnosis in post mortem studies suggests that end of life hospitalization would not identify and reverse simple medical problems.

Decisions Regarding Life-Sustaining Medical Treatment

Families, patients and clinicians may be confronted by difficult decisions about the wisdom of employing heroic health measures including dialysis, surgical procedures, mechanical ventilation, pacing devices and implanted defibrillators. Treatment of people with dementia and other terminal illness should always be guided by the person's prognosis and goals of care. While earlier in the course of illness, a person with dementia may have elected to undergo aggressive life-sustaining medical treatments such as dialysis, operations, mechanical ventilation or defibrillators, these treatments become less appropriate as patients progress to more advanced stages of disease. Clinicians and family are often confronted with decisions to continue life sustaining treatment such as dialysis or discontinue the care with the understanding that the patient will deteriorate and eventually die. Treatments like dialysis are complicated and painful for the patient with dementia and the team should consider discontinuing this care as a measure to assure comfort.

Hopefully, the person with mild dementia and end stage renal disease who initiates dialysis will discuss with powers of attorney (POA) and health care proxies (HCP) his or her wishes about when to discontinue dialysis as dementia progresses. Describing specific scenarios to help guide decision-making at various stages of dementia can be helpful in advance care planning. For example, the person with dementia and end stage renal disease who initiates dialysis may feel that it would be acceptable to continue dialysis after he or she has lost decision-making capacity, but that same person may say that he or she would want to have dialysis discontinued if unable to recognize his or her own family members. A 2009 study found that after older people viewed videos depicting patients with advanced dementia, they were more likely to choose comfort as a goal of care [78].

Another question that may arise is whether to perform an operation on a person with dementia. Regardless of diagnosis or prognosis, operations on people who are not expected to survive the procedure, recover from it and later benefit from it in at least some small way should be considered very carefully. This is particularly true for people with more advanced dementia, who will not understand for what potential benefit they are suffering. Ideally, the only surgeries performed on hospice patients with advanced dementia would be palliative procedures, deemed to significantly improve the person's quality of life at end of life.

The use of mechanical ventilators and pacing devices would not likely fall under this "palliative" category for hospice patients with advanced dementia. Mechanical ventilation often requires careful sedation and analgesia, which would limit a person's ability to interact with and communicate with loved ones at end of life; even if the person is still awake, sedating and analgesic medications will likely worsen already poor cognition. If a person with advanced dementia requires mechanical ventilation, discussions regarding initiation of therapy should always include expected duration of therapy and a plan for compassionate discontinuation if the therapy is not successful. In the case of emergent intubations

these discussions may happen after the fact, in which case discussion of a reasonable "time trial" of mechanical ventilation is appropriate.

While a standard pacemaker is not likely to significantly prolong death or interfere with quality of life in a dying person, more advanced devices such as an implantable cardioverter-defibrillator (ICD) certainly can have untoward effects at end of life. As with other life-sustaining treatments, the discussion about initiation of therapy should include a discussion of circumstances in which the therapy should be discontinued. Unfortunately, this part of the discussion is frequently lacking or not performed at all [79]. As these devices become more common, it is important to ask patients and family if these devices are in place and if so, if they are still active. People with active ICDs (or their family, if the person lacks decision-making capacity) who enroll in hospice should be counseled on the likelihood of shocks at end of life unless these devices are deactivated beforehand [80].

Again, discussion should reference the person's prognosis and goals of care, and discussion of various scenarios at advancing stage of illness may help the person/family decide at what point they feel it is appropriate to discontinue the device. In a planned situation, the cardiologist or electrophysiologist who placed the device may be involved, otherwise the hospice attending physician should consult with a representative from the device manufacturing company regarding device deactivation. In an emergency situation, a cardiac device magnet placed over the ICD can prevent the device from delivering shocks. The magnet must be left in place; if removed, the ICD will be able to deliver shocks [81].

Nutritional Issues

Malnutrition is a common problem for people with advanced dementia [82].

Appetite often decreases near the end of life as part of the natural history of dying from many different diseases or illnesses, and dementia is no exception. Cessation of eating is common in the last week of life. Even early in their disease, people with dementia may forget to eat at regular mealtimes, and may only eventually be prompted to eat by an uncomfortable sensation of hunger. As their disease progresses, people with dementia may "unlearn" how to feed themselves, chew and swallow, and they may have dyscordination of the swallowing mechanism. Mechanical difficulty with proper swallowing is common in older adults with dementia, and it is estimated that 13–57 % of patients have dysphagia [83]. Other issues such as poor dentition, dry oral and pharyngeal mucosa and esophageal reflux can contribute to swallowing problems. A Cochrane review [84] did not find a survival benefit to enteral tube feeding for people with advanced dementia, and the American Geriatrics Society published a position paper [85] endorsing careful hand-feeding as preferable to artificial nutrition via gastrostomy feeding tube (commonly referred to as PEG tube) for many reasons including increased risk of agitation leading to restraint use, increased risk of pressure ulcers and other complications related to the feeding tube itself. The benefits of hand-feeding include enjoyment of the taste of food and increased social interaction from having another person feed or assist with meals. The American Society of Parenteral and Enteral Nutrition concluded that enteral therapy was not obligatory in patients with malnutrition and the use of nasogastric tubes should be avoided.

Unfortunately, people with advanced dementia frequently receive feeding tubes despite this information. In our medicalized society, it can be almost reflexive to place a feeding tube for a patient who cannot or will not swallow food. The idea that people with dementia are "starving" if they are not eating is a very difficult topic for most of us. In most cultures, sharing food is an expression of caring and love. It is very natural for us to eat, and can seem so un-natural when we do not. In addition, particularly in nursing homes with limited staffing, there may be multiple financial incentives to send the person who is no longer swallowing properly to the hospital for a tube (this saves nursing home staff time when the person is actually in the hospital, saves time from not having to hand-feed the person several times daily, the nursing home may charge an increased billing rate in the post-acute hospitalization period, etc).

Caregivers, family and hospice staff benefit from education to help them understand the risks of and lack of benefit from artificial nutrition via feeding tube. Countering the thought of "starvation" with the negative ramifications of of "force-feeding" through a feeding tube, emphasizing the benefits of careful hand-feeding and describing the natural history of dementia, can all help alleviate the understandable anxiety surrounding this sensitive issue. The insertion of a PEG tube into a hospice patient with dementia is rarely indicated, rarely beneficial and sometimes harmful. The reinsertion of a displaced or blocked tube should be carefully discussed with the family; especially given the likelihood of a trip to the emergency room or the hospital. The discontinuation of tube feedings may be indicated for specific reasons such as stasis or vomiting. The team should consider removing a tube that was inserted with disregard for the expressed wishes of the patient or the presence of an advanced directive that prohibits this type of life support.

Treatment of Infections

Antimicrobial therapy, though relatively benign compared to other aggressive life-sustaining treatments, is often the topic of end of life discussions for people with dementia. Infections such as pneumonia and urinary tract infections are frequently recurrent in this population. Treatment with antibiotics can temporarily bring a person "back from the brink of death", only to have them live to aspirate another day. The cycle of acute illness followed by recovery, followed by recurrent acute illness, is stressful for patients and families alike. Antibiotic treatment is often associated with hospitalization with all of its attendant perils, as well as with side effects of the antibiotic drugs themselves-antibiotic associated diarrhea/colitis, drug reactions, renal failure, development of multi-drug resistant organisms, site issues, hypernatremia or volume overload from fluids, etc. Half of treated pneumonia patients with advanced dementia were dead in 6 months and most 92 % died in the hospital [86] producing an unwanted outcome for most dying patients. Do antibiotics help with symptom management in people with advanced dementia pneumonia? A 2010 study evaluated the effect of antibiotic use on comfort in people with advanced dementia and pneumonia [87]. The study found that although antibiotics prolong survival in people with advanced dementia and pneumonia, they do not improve overall comfort. Again, decision-making should be guided by the person's prognosis and goals of care, so oral antibiotics should be considered in the person who values prolonged survival, while people at end of life who are focusing solely on comfort may choose to opt out of treatment.

Medication Management

Medications are frequently added or changed in people with advanced illness, especially as new symptoms develop or as a person moves from one location of care to another. Increasing the overall number of medications a person takes will increase the risk of drug–drug or drug–disease interactions. Many of the medications commonly prescribed to hospice patients can worsen cognition thorough anticholinergic, sedating or other mechanisms [88]. The effects of these medications are often amplified in people with underlying dementia. The result is that people with advanced dementia are often on multiple medications of questionable benefit, some of which can negatively impact their quality of life. A recent study found that over half of people with advanced dementia in nursing homes; over half were prescribed at least one medication of questionable benefit [89].

Medications should be closely evaluated in all patients, but particularly in people with advanced illnesses such as dementia, to assess for potentially harmful side effects. Any medications which are clearly harmful should be stopped; medications which are of questionable benefit should be examined closely and discontinued if risks outweigh benefits. Of course, medications of clear benefit may be continued if the patient is willing and able to tolerate them. The Beers Criteria offers a helpful tool to identify potentially inappropriate medication use in older adults, including those with dementia [90]. All

psychotropic medications can be stopped in the actively dying patient to reduce stress caused by administration except those that might cause intolerable abstinence syndromes such as alprazolam or other unacceptable complications such as anticonvulsants in patient with active seizures.

Pain Management

Pain management is extremely important in people with dementia. One key issue for people with advanced dementia is the need for careful attention to non-verbal pain behaviors. A demented person may not have a typical expression or report of pain. Localization, articulation and emotional processing of pain is primarily controlled at the cortical level of the brain where there is extensive damage in end stage dementia. The thalamic processing of pain remains unclear although the emotional component to pain may be reduced in dementia given the severity of limbic neuropathology. Patients may suffer from hyperalgesia or increased sensitivity to a stimulus as well as allodynia or a painful response to a non-noxious stimulus [91]. The expectation and placebo effect of analgesic medications are probably diminished or eliminated in advanced stage dementia. The loss of placebo effect suggests that patients might require higher doses to achieve the same relief as individuals who can anticipate the benefit via mechanisms in the prefrontal cortex [92]. However, these patients may be highly susceptible to adverse effects of the medication. Demented patients with hip fracture are shown to receive less opioid in both the pre and post-operative period and at doses of one third of the standard dose. Patients with vascular dementia or mixed Alzheimer's-vascular dementia may be more vulnerable to problems with pain management but others common types of dementia have little data to guide the clinician [92]. Untreated pain is common and obviously quite distressing to the person with dementia, and can lead to delirium or worsened behavioral disturbances. It is necessary to closely attend to non-verbal expressions of pain in people with dementia, who often will not have typical pain behaviors or reports of pain. Multiple clinical tools are available to assess for non-verbal expressions of pain in people with dementia, with no clear consensus as to which is best [91]. In patients with a fracture or other painful injury who cannot adequately communicate their experience of pain, it is particularly important to premedicate with pain medications as needed prior to repositioning and bathing, for wound debridement or dressing changes. Effective pain management requires clear communication between staff, family and prescribers.

Initial treatment of mild-moderate pain may start with non-opioid analgesics such as acetaminophen; these medications may be scheduled as needed. Avoid potential acetaminophen toxicity by limiting total daily doses to 3,000 mg or less per 24 h period. Though low doses of NSAIDS can be acceptable for very short periods of time, it is important to recognize the risk of gastrointestinal irritation and bleeding, worsening renal function and worsening heart failure with these medications. If pain is not controlled with these medications or low doses of other adjuvant analgesics, it is reasonable to add low-dose opioid analgesics such as short-acting morphine or oxycodone 2.5 mg to 5 mg orally every 3–4 h as needed. Because patients with more advanced dementia may not consistently report pain, it is important to assess for and treat pain on a regular (every hour or two) basis. If constant pain is expected, a dosing schedule of "offer-may-refuse, while awake, hold for sedation" may be most appropriate. Titrate up short-acting medications slowly as needed for appropriate analgesia, and monitor closely for adverse side effects. Almost all patients will require a laxative when taking opioids, so make sure to prescribe one at the time that opioids are initiated. Family education and effective communication between the caregivers and hospice team is important for patients managed at home. Individuals residing in nursing homes may depend on staff assessments and reports. The hospice team may need to determine the familiarity of the nursing home staff with the patient and their ability to monitor for pain behaviors. Many non-pain behaviors need to be tolerated by the staff rather than medicated. Analgesic medications should reduce suffering rather than sedating a "problem" patient.

People with dementia may be less mobile for many years before death, unlike other illnesses in which people reach the debilitated state more rapidly. These individuals are often nutritionally depleted and at risk for decubiti. Pressure ulcers and contractures will develop without careful, scheduled repositioning, appropriate skin care and range of motion exercises. Family and other caregivers will benefit from education on range of motion exercises, with a physical therapist who is knowledgeable regarding care of people with dementia. Wound care is generally not significantly different in hospice patients with advanced dementia than it is in other populations, though a focus on comfort in line with appropriate goals of care should be of primary concern in any person with advanced illness.

Management of Neuropsychiatric Complications and Behavioral Manifestations of Dementia

Psychiatric and behavioral manifestations of dementia are common in all clinical stages of dementia from mild cognitive impairment through advanced stage dementia and in all causes of dementia. These symptoms can be psychiatric, behavioral or both. The symptoms usually develop slowly and often spontaneously remit over the course of the disease as well as fluctuate on a daily or weekly basis. The most common neuropsychiatric complication in hospice-eligible nursing home residents with advanced dementia were agitation or aggression (50.4 %) depression (45 %) and withdrawal/lethargy (43.1 %) [93]. Behavioral and psychiatric complications during the final stages of dementia can be present with any underlying neuropathology such as Alzheimer's disease, vascular dementia, Lewy body dementia, etc. Disease-specific behavioral features that are common in the early stages of the dementia such as visual hallucinations in Lewy body disease or personality changes in FTD may no longer be present in the later stages of dementia (Behavioral manifestations of dementia are extensively discussed in Chapter "Treatment of Dementia: Non-pharmacological Approaches"). Relatively few dementia patients will receive inpatient psychiatric care in the last 90 days of life and few were referred to a hospice service either at home (1.6 %) or as part of nursing home care (7.1 %) [94]. Many (43 %) dementia patients who are transferred to a hospital have some neuropsychiatric symptoms with aggression (57 %), sleep disturbance (42 %) or anxiety (35 %) (Sampson et al.).

Excessive medication is common in advanced stage dementia with 53.9 % of nursing home residents receiving at-least one medication of questionable benefit [89]. Polypharmacy is linked to increased mortality among nursing home residents with advanced dementia [95]. Studies show that enhanced psychosocial care for residents with severe dementia can reduce the use of neuroleptics from 42 to 23 % [96]. Most (85 %) hospice eligible nursing home resident exhibit some neuropsychiatric symptoms related to dementia [93]. Most (70 %) patients in the "final phase" of dementia had clinically relevant neuropsychiatric symptoms and most (87 %) had multiple symptoms [97]. Nursing home residents with dementia and psychosis pose a challenge to staff because they are at-risk for adverse events including accidental injury, anorexia, infections, weight change and death [98]. Psychotic symptoms are associated with accelerated cognitive decline, institutionalization, and higher mortality which may place psychotic patients in the group at higher risk for using end-of-life services [99].

The management strategy for neuropsyciatric symptoms and behavioral problems should emphasize non-pharmacological interventions. Physicians are more likely to use medication in contrast to psychologists or nurse practitioners who are more likely to use behavioral management [100]. The plan of care should define target behaviors, behavioral approaches and treatment. The intervention should be preceded by an evaluation to identify possible causes. For example, screaming can be an expression of pain, hunger, thirst, wetness, position, need to toilet, boredom and fear. The team should consider these causes prior to using PRN medications as behavioral interventions avoid sedation and allow the patient to interact with the family.

A transitional patient, such as a person moving from home to the nursing home may need several days to several weeks for adjustment to the new environment regardless of the stage of dementia. Psychotropic medications may be required on a PRN basis during this adjustment phase but the decision to initiate routine medication should occur after the patient becomes familiar with their new surroundings. For example, a patient may fight during the first few days after discharge home from the hospital or transfer to a nursing home but that patient may stop fighting when the staff learns to communicate using non-verbal methods and the patient becomes familiar with the sounds and the scent of the nursing home.

The management of neuropsychiatric problems begins with a proper assessment of each symptom. The family caregiver will often have detailed information about the nature of problems, the cause of the behavior and methods to reduce the behavior or circumvent the functional consequences of the behavior. Patients with dementia often develop a schedule despite severe cognitive deficits. For example, a patient may struggle if bathed in the morning rather than the afternoon. Specific food preferences are common and hospice patients can be offered what they are willing to eat regardless of whether the nutritional content is optimal. The family caregiver or the direct care staff is often familiar with such nuances and their input is invaluable in assessing the behavior. Psychiatric and behavioral symptoms are dynamic over time and symptoms such as delusions may remit in a matter of months. Often, clinicians are hesitant to simultaneously stop multiple psychotropic medications for fear that dangerous symptoms may re-emerge and the team will not know which medication was critical to patient safety.

Delirium Medications that were prescribed to manage the behavioral manifestations of delirium can be rapidly stopped if the cause of delirium has been corrected. For instance, the new hospice admission who was combative as a result of a urinary tract infection can have the antipsychotic medication stopped following resolution of the infection. Individuals transferred from the ICU may have been combative from the intense environmental and sensory stimulation while the calm of a home environment or an inpatient hospice unit may be sufficient to reduce the agitation. Profoundly demented hospice patients who are close to death can have rapid discontinuation of multiple medications to improve alertness and reduce the need to swallow pills or liquids. These individuals are typically immobile and minimally responsive. Other patients with some intact function and expected survival of weeks or months may require a more methodical approach for medication reductions to assure comfort and behavioral stability.

Depression Recognition of depression in advanced stage disease with severe communication deficits can be challenging, even though it is a common disorder in mid to late stages of dementia (56 %) [101]. Depression is common in demented nursing home residents [102]. The DSM criteria for depression are not proven valid in patients with advanced dementia and clinicians must diagnose based on clinical judgment. Symptoms such as agitation or distress in a patient with prior depression may signify a depressive relapse. Most patients with advanced dementia lack the ability to recognize and report complex internal emotions such as mood. Intense emotional outbursts can be caused by depression, fear, anxiety and multiple other emotional stressors. A past history of mood disorder increases the chance of recurrent depression. Verbal distressed patients may sometimes make alarming statements such as, "I might as well be dead" and such statements can raise concerns about suicide. Suicidality is associated with poor health in older persons, especially persons with past depression, and functional impairments [103]. Dementia is not identified as a major risk factor for suicidality in older persons although anyone who expresses suicidal thoughts should be evaluated for depression and safety [104, 105]. Many dementia patients will be admitted to hospice with a diagnosis of depression and some will develop symptoms of depression following admission to the program. Some patients may already receive polypharmacy for depression to include two or more antidepressants as well as mood stabilizers such as second generation antipsychotic medications.

The decision to stop, reduce or continue mood stabilizing medications depends on the clinical circumstances of the individual. Patients with very short life expectancies can have rapid dose reductions to reduce the number of medications. Some antidepressants such as venlafaxine must be tapered over several weeks to avoid instability of blood pressure. Others, such as the SSRI medications must be tapered to avoid a discontinuation syndrome.

A risk benefit consideration of using these medications is needed when starting antidepressants for dementia patients in hospice. The clinician should weigh the expected onset of symptom improvement in a 2–6 week period versus the burden of additional medications and potential side effects. The efficacy of antidepressant therapy in advanced stage dementia is unknown. Common major side effects include gastrointestinal symptoms, prolongation of the QTc interval and hyponatremia. Bupropion carries the risk of lowering seizure threshold in patients who are already at risk for seizures and this medication may also worsen vascular headaches [106]. Venlafaxine can increase blood pressure. Antidepressant treatment of a bipolar patient can provoke a manic episode with additional behavioral problems.

Adjunctive therapy for depression involves prescribing two antidepressant medications or one antidepressant with other medications such as second generation antipsychotics like quetiapine, or anticonvulsants like lamotrigine. Polypharmacy is common, especially in patients with severe or therapy resistant depression. Available data does not support the use of two antidepressants in persons with dementia or the use of super-therapeutic doses of any medication. Older patients tend to be more sensitive to the side effects of medications and more at risk for drug-drug interactions. Individuals on large doses of medications such at 80 mg/day of fluoxetine may benefit from dose reduction into the geriatric normal range even in the presence of depressive symptoms. The older antidepressant medications such as amitriptyline should be used with care as urinary retention and confusion are possible. The selective serotonin reuptake inhibitors and the norepinephrine serotonin reuptake inhibitors are the medications of choice for depression in elderly patients and those with dementia. Duloxetine improves mood and neuropathic pain but this medication has limited data in patients with dementia. Mirtazapine in low dose such as 7.5 mg at bed time can assist with sleep and enhance appetite while in higher doses produce the antidepressant effect.

Anxiety The symptoms of anxiety are common in mid to late stage dementia (42 %) [101]. The treatment of anxiety in advanced stage dementia requires an accurate diagnosis and therapeutic endpoints that are consistent with the patient's clinical status. There are no established behavioral correlates for anxiety in patients with advanced stage dementia who are usually nonverbal. Pain, thirst, rectal impaction and fear can produce agitation, restlessness and distress that mimic anxiety. The prevalence of anxiety in advanced stage patients is unknown. Patients with pre-morbid panic disorder or generalized anxiety disorder may continue to have symptoms into later stage disease. Veterans with post-traumatic stress disorder may have a reoccurrence of some symptoms with dementia. The treatment of anxiety in dementia can include SSRI therapy and benzodiazepines. The use of benzodiazepines in persons with dementia is fraught with risks. Addiction is not the major concern but delirium, disinhibition, dysphagia and falls are potential problems. Other serotonergic agents such as buspirone have not been shown effective in demented patients with anxiety disorders [105].

A verbal patient with mild to moderate dementia can report typical symptoms of anxiety or panic. Anxiety in a verbal patient can be treated with a SSRI like sertraline or an NSRI like mirtazapine. Starting dose should be low such as 25 mg of sertraline and a careful titration should target symptom relief and side effect monitoring [107]. A very low dose of lorazepam, e.g., 25 mg every 6 h as needed can be used for severe distressing anxiety. Long half-life benzodiazepine such as clonazepam should be used with caution. Alprazolam should be avoided in patients with dementia as the medication has no injectable preparation and high risk for rapid dependence.

Psychotic Symptoms Hallucinations and/or delusions are common in mid to late stage dementia and occur in 22 % of nursing home residents [101, 102]. Psychotic symptoms in dementia are associated with a worse outcome as defined by increased mortality, faster functional decline and increased risk of institutionalization [99]. Psychotic symptoms can be caused by depression, dementia or delirium and symptoms can include a variable mixture of hallucinations or delusions but none are distinctive for end stage dementia. Tactile hallucinations are not common and suggest delirium. Advanced stage patients usually lack the capacity to describe complex internal events such as hearing voices and the clinicians may need to depend on behavioral clues to these symptoms and behavioral endpoints to assess efficacy of the medications. The presence of psychotic symptoms does not warrant treatment unless the patient has distress, adverse behavioral responses or dangerous behavior. For instance, a patient may be delusional about caregivers but the person is happy to follow instructions versus the delusional patient who is combative out of fear of the caregivers. The use of antipsychotic medications in dementia is highly controversial due to concerns about increased risk for death, stroke, DVT and other serious health problems [108]. Neurological complications from all antipsychotic medications include tardive dyskinesia, dystonic reactions, drug induced Parkinsonism and others. Both older medications like haloperidol and newer antipsychotic medications like risperidone have a potential role in treatment of neuropsychiatric symptoms of patients with end stage dementia. Older medications like haloperidol have higher affinity for the dopamine receptor and may cause more Parkinsonism however these medications are safe, effective and available in a variety of preparations to include liquid. Newer medications such as risperidone can be administered as sol-tabs and other preparations. Both medications can produce sedation or calming and both can augment the sedation caused by narcotics or other medications commonly prescribed in older adults. Long acting depot preparations like Haldol deaconate should be avoided in advanced stage dementia patients and patients who were receiving the shots for pre-existing mental illness such as schizophrenia can have cessation of injections. Doses of anti-psychotic medications should be slowly titrated to define the therapeutic dosing parameters for each individual. For example, the clinician can start 0.5 mg haloperidol or 0.25 mg risperidone to determine level of sedation and the slowly titrating to minimal effective dose. Acute agitation can be managed with IM haloperidol in the 1–2 mg range. Newer medications such as injectable olanzapine or ziprasidone are expensive and neither has good published data in advanced stage dementia [105].

The type and frequency of behavioral or psychiatric symptoms seen in a hospice patient can depend on severity of dementia, type of dementia, associated medical problems, environmental cues and the medications already prescribed for the patient as they enter the hospice service. The goal of hospice care is to reduce the number and dosage of psychotropic medications while maintaining the comfort of the patient and assuring the safety of both the caregivers and the patient.

Behavioral Manifestations of Distress in Late Stage Dementia Many late stage dementia patients are nursing home residents and these individuals commonly exhibit behavioral manifestations that are distinct from psychiatric complications. Behavioral management is discussed elsewhere in the book (see Chapter "Treatment of Dementia: Non-pharmacological Approaches"). A meta-analysis of 28 studies showed that 82 % of demented residents had at least one neuropsychiatric or behavioral problem. The mean range for the frequency of aggression was 32 % of all residents. Residents in late stage disease demonstrated a moderate severity of apathy and agitation as well as vocalization 44 %, grabbing 33 %, spitting 15 %, hitting 13 % and screaming [97]. The management of these behavioral problems begins with a review of the patient's cognitive deficits and past patterns of behavior. Common basic human needs such as hunger, thirst, pain, fear, boredom and loneliness may increase the frequency of such behaviors. For example, a patient who fights during skin care may have pain from the repositioning or fear from being disrobed. The staff can address those symptoms

through pain medications or verbal reassurances and keeping the patient covered as much as possible. The family caregiver can often explain the causes of the behavior and the best behavioral approaches to reduce the frequency of the behavior. Some behaviors such as" grabbing" may result from frontal lobe damage causing frontal release signs such as the grasp response. Spitting may result from chewing or swallowing dyspraxia. Medications should be reserved for patients who have failed behavioral interventions and who engage in dangerous activity.

Discontinuation or Dose Reduction of Psychotropic Medications in Advanced Stage Dementia

A patient may be admitted to hospice receiving multiple psychotropic medications and multiple non-psychiatric medications that are used for psychotropic purposes. Polypharmacy is used in over half of nursing home residents with advanced dementia and excess polypharmacy is present in 10–20 % of these residents [109]. For example diphenhydramine is commonly used as a sedative hypnotic and such medications are designated as "potentially inappropriate" for long term care according to the Beers criteria [90]. The team should establish the indication and target symptoms for each medication to determine the risk of dose reduction. For example, a SSRI may be prescribed for depression or irritability. Dose reduction or discontinuation can be guided by peer reviewed literature about the efficacy of specific classes of medications and their potential side effects in patients with dementia. Considerable data exists on the efficacy of cholinesterase inhibitors, antipsychotic medications, antidepressants, sedative hypnotics, benzodiazepines, mood stabilizing agents and other medications. Some patients receive polypharmacy with little data to support either interclass or cross class polypharmacy [110]. The pharmacist and the medical director for the hospice organization should carefully review medications with the greatest potential for toxicity and work backwards to review all medications that treat psychiatric or behavioral symptoms.

Most advanced-stage patients can have reduction or elimination of psychotropic medications but patients who are mildly or moderately demented may require continued therapy or adjustment of medications to address new behavioral symptoms. The efficacy of psychotropic medications prescribed in the final stages of dementia in unknown. A reasonable strategy is to first withdraw the medications with the least robust efficacy data followed by reduction of evidence-based medications that might no longer be required; such as stopping the benzodiazepine but continuing the cholinesterase inhibitor. Medications with significant anticholinergic toxicity should be discontinued as quickly as is reasonable. The anti-epileptic medications have little data to support their efficacy in reducing behavioral symptoms. Medications like valproic acid and lamotrigine can produce significant sedation. The cessation of antiepileptic medications may reduce global sedation however seizures are more common in patients with dementia than the general age matched population. Antiepileptic medications prescribed for either seizures or behavior can be tapered and patients should be monitored to detect new onset seizures [106].

Benzodiazepines are not effective for the sustained treatment of behavioral problems in patients with end-stage dementia, merely sedating the patient. Medications like lorazepam can be administered to achieve short term sedation. Long term prescription of these medications is tightly controlled in the nursing home setting by federal regulations and survey standards. Some patients with pre-existing anxiety disorders may be taking long term high dose benzodiazepine therapy. Long half-life medications like diazepam or clonazepam, can accumulate over time, especially in the dehydrated patient [105]. Shorter half life benzodiazepines such as lorazepam or alprazolam can produce a significant abstinence syndrome if abruptly discontinued. Alprazolam is noteworthy for its potential to produce a complicated withdrawal state. Patients receiving stable long term therapy for psychiatric diagnoses should have very gradual back titrations of benzodiazepine's to the lowest dose that assures symptom control for anxiety or panic. Patients who received these medications for control of behavioral complica-

tions caused by dementia can have a more rapid dose reduction. Anyone receiving high dose alprazolam should either continue the medication or undergo a very slow, gradual dose reduction. The chronic use of benzodiazepines as sedative hypnotic agents is not supported by published evidence and these medications can produce side effects as well as rebound insomnia if stopped. Hypnotic medications such as zolpidem add to the net burden of sedation produced by other medications such as benzodiazepines and antipsychotic medications. This class of medication should be used with care and discontinued early in the medication simplification phase of the management strategy. Benzodiazepine therapy should be initiated with great care in the demented, dying patient. Although these medications are routinely used for distress, anxiety and dyspnea in dying cognitively intact patients, the prescription of these medications or inclusion in the emergency medication kit requires careful monitoring and family education.

Antidepressant medications can be tapered in dying patients. Abrupt cessation is not recommended to avoid a rebound effect. Patients treated for depression in the past should be monitored for behavioral manifestations that suggest re-occurrence of depression. Dose reductions can be done in several weeks for patients with some level of alertness and more rapidly in obtunded patients. Antidepressant may have benefit for agitation in demented patients and discontinuation may cause a re-emergence of symptoms over several weeks [107].

Antipsychotic medications should be tapered or discontinued based on the patient's level of alertness, swallowing competency and ongoing psychiatric or behavioral symptoms [111]. Antipsychotic medications can be synergistic to narcotics and produce excess sedation as well as problems with swallowing. However, data shows that antipsychotic medications may be beneficial for selected psychiatric and behavioral symptoms in late stage dementia [110]. Some (20 %) patients with dementia entering hospice care are receiving cholinesterase inhibitors. Clinicians may recommend cessation to families but the caregivers may be hesitant to stop treatment [16]. Donepezil may have a beneficial effect on life expectancy after onset of symptoms where studies report 7.9 years for treated versus 5.3 years in untreated but there is no evidence that cessation of therapy will hasten death [112]. Cholinsterase therapy may be beneficial for reducing behavioral symptoms in persons with advanced disease. A dose taper is the safest approach to avoid symptom relapse. Both donepezil and memantine are shown to have some benefits from continued therapy [113, 114]. Acute withdrawal of cholinesterase inhibitors from patients with Lewy body dementia or Parkinsonism can cause abrupt increase in hallucinations and decrease of cognitive function [115] Individuals who have failed dose tapers should restart medications for at least 2 months to determine whether the loss can be corrected.

Memantine, a NMDA antagonist may be beneficial for Alzheimer's disease when used with a choline esterase inhibitor as determined by slowing progression in the late phase of the disease [113, 114]. Memantine can be tapered over a 2–4 week period or rapidly discontinued in the actively dying patient. Cholinesterase inhibitors and memantine should be discontinued in actively dying patients. Clinicians can employ a dose reduction for individuals with a longer life expectancy such as several months.

Optimal hospice care for behavioral and psychiatric symptoms is to treat first with behavioral interventions. Psychotropic medications should be reduced or eliminated whenever possible. New psychotropic medications should be initiated for specific symptoms that defy behavioral management. The impact on the quality of life for the patient and the caregivers should be weighed against the benefit offered by the medication. Sedation, reduced responsiveness to family and reduced oral intake can occur with many psychotropic medications. Low dosages of short half-life medications are preferable.

Home Hospice Management for the Patient with Dementia

Older patients from many cultural backgrounds choose to die at home. Studies show that one half to three quarters of all elders identify home care as their best option in the event they develop a terminal illness [14, 15]. Critical elements to home hospice care for persons with dementia are: (1) the availability of caregivers in the home; (2) expertise and knowledge of dementia care; (3) communication between the staff and the caregivers; and (4) organizational procedures that accommodate the needs of dementia patients residing at home with complex medical and psychiatric problems. The home care of a patient dying with dementia differs from the care of a terminal cancer at many levels. The team must address the need for behavioral and the long term stress on the family caregiver.

The organizational structure of a home hospice agency needs to be flexible and capable of accommodating patients who are dying with dementia at home. The admission process must include sufficient information to capture the cognitive and psychiatric needs of the patient. The transmission of critical information such as whether the patient has aphasia or has aggressive behaviors is critical to treating the patient. Printed materials should include information about persons with dementia. Each "on-call" nurse must be capable of distinguishing symptoms that require behavioral support from symptoms that require use on medications from the home emergency kit. Chaplains and other professionals who will assist the family at the time of death or assist during the period after death need to understand the unique dementia-related issues for caregivers and their families. Hospice clinical leadership should be familiar with obtaining autopsies on persons who need definitive diagnosis. Older individuals with the typical history of Alzheimer's disease are infrequently examined however younger individuals such as those below the age of 60 may be candidates for post mortem examinations. Early onset Alzheimer's disease and frontotemporal dementia both have genetic components that may impact risk assessments in future generations. In general, funeral directors are comfortable providing services for individuals dying with dementia however prion diseases can present a unique challenge. Most funeral directors are familiar with prion diseases and many are hesitant to embalm such individuals.

The family may need to identify a willing service provider prior to death to avoid delays in the funeral.

Dementia may account for the second largest number of hospice referrals (17.7 %) but cancer remains the most common disease and attracts the greatest attention (34.6 %) [88]. Lorazepam, morphine, atropine and haloperidol were among the five most commonly prescribed medications. For persons with dementia, these medications were more likely prescribed for symptomatic relief rather than on a chronic basis. Home emergency kits are utilized in up to two thirds of all cases with morphine, lorazepam and haloperidol topping the list of medications that are commonly used at home [116]. Home hospice nurses report that the kit was used in half the cases and helped to prevent emergency room visits. The kits cost less than $50. Families may need assistance with using the medications and 22 % of home family hospice caregivers for all patients reported formal support from the hospice team while 31 % reported informal support such as a friend with medical training [117]. The administration of benzodiazepines to demented patients may produce delirium as will medications that have anticholinergic side effects. The team should be monitoring the use of such medications to avoid new behavioral problems caused by delirium. Haloperidol is an old, first generation antipsychotic medication that is effective in psychotic or severely agitated persons with dementia. Haloperidol can sometimes produce sedation when administered along with other medications in the emergency kit such as lorazepam or morphine. Initial reduced dosages are advisable until the patient's medication tolerance is determined.

The administration of medications for pain, psychiatric distress, nausea and other common conditions is complicated with a non-verbal patient. The experienced family caregiver may recognizes behaviors that indicate thirst, pain, dampness or distress but the inexperienced caregiver or the paid health provider may lack that knowledge. Studies show that many (40 %) caregivers reported no additional support for administering medications in the home setting. Caregivers who live at home and come from minority or lower socioeconomic backgrounds were more likely to lack home support [118].

Excellent home care involves staff with knowledge about dementia communicating in a regular, dependable manner with direct care staff in the home and utilizing the caregiver's knowledge to optimize the behavioral approaches.

Adaptation of the home environment for a dying patient with dementia is similar to that of any other cause of death. The usual equipment to include hospital bed, oxygen, suction, and other devices are usually required for the patients comfort. The training of the family caregiver depends on the needs of the patient for issues such as interpretation of pain behaviors, vocalization, misidentifications etc. Restraints are a poor option in any setting. The caregiver may need encouragement in asking for assistance from other members of the family to avoid exhaustion or health problems.

Supporting and Working with Caregivers

Caregiver stress and burn out are discussed elsewhere in the text (see Chapter "Experiences and Perspectives of Family Caregivers of the Person with Dementia") but most caregivers of end stage patients have engaged in caregiving for over 5 years and may themselves have health problems. The caregiver network may include other family members, friends and paid staff. All individuals who will provide direct services to the patient need basic knowledge about dementia and the dying process to maximize their contribution to the care of the individual. Some distant or disconnected family members may visit or interact with the team for the first time creating a situation where misunderstanding or lack of caregiver knowledge may cause stressful discussions between the distant relatives and the caregiver family and the hospice team. The quality of hospice care has been related to the strength of the relationship between the family and the hospice professionals, the family's emotional commitment to caring and the family's ability to think about dying and death [119]. Lack of support from the health care team is consistent concern for caregivers at the end of life [120].

Dementia usually causes death through a protracted process for the patient that can produce increased frailty for the caregiver. Dementia caregiving may increase the risk for cognitive loss and produce 40.5 % higher odds of increased frailty for the primary caregiver by time of death [121]. Many caregivers who choose hospice may not have received the psychoeducational interventions that can reduce stress in some individuals [122]. These caregivers have been shown to struggle with multiple issues at the hospice stage of care including the struggle to navigate the medical system to get hospice care, "reaching the boiling point" with a complex and difficult system and welcoming death for the patient [123]. The hospice team can assess the level of caregiver distress by looking at the health of caregiver and the burden of caregiving for the patient. Understanding the mental and physical health of the caregiver can be helpful in predicting the impact of the dying process, the features of bereavement and the quality of recovery following the death of the patient. Each caregiver or caregiver family is unique and the strategy to help during the dying process must accommodate those unique features [124].

The family caregiver usually experience physical, psychological, social and financial stress over the course of the illness [125] and the caregiver may view impending death of a patient with a mixture of sadness and relief. Caregivers showed high levels of depressive symptoms while caregiving but the depression diminished in 3 months following the death of the patient. Most (72 %) reported that death was a relief to them and even more (92 %) believed that death was a relief to the patient [124]. Risk factors for increased caregiver burden include female gender, lower socioeconomic status, and residence with the care recipient, and higher numbers of hours of care per week, depression, social isolation, financial hardship and lack of choice in assuming the role as caregiver [126]. Caregiver strain at the end of the patient's life is increased in patients with more behavioral problems, higher levels functional needs and situations wherein the caregiver perceives a lack of support from the clinical

team [120]. Pharmacological and psychosocial interventions that assist the patient with dementia may reduce caregiver burden. Even minor reductions of burden may improve the symptoms endorsed by the caregiver. The cumulative impact on the caregiver then reflects the severity of symptoms for the hospice patient and the efforts to mitigate those symptoms by the treatment team. The transition of a patient into hospice care requires a review and/or change of the previous plan of care that met palliative care goals. In some instances, the admission to hospice may be the first effort at constructing a plan for the family. The care plan or goals of care should identify of primary and secondary caregivers, incorporate the preferences of the patient and the caregiver in all care planning, provide education and skills for the caregiver and finally, be adjusted over time.

The hospice team can best assist with this process by providing information and guidance to the proximate family and educational materials to the distant relatives or friends. Studies that examine the value of simple informational booklets like "Family Booklets about Comfort Care in Advanced Dementia" show that almost all (94 %) viewed the material as helpful and most wanted the information early in the process rather than later. Families are experts about their patients and staff must be mindful and respectful of that knowledge. Family's members are often not health care professionals and require information in a non-technical format. The nursing staff and any other staff that interacts with the family needs to speak in appropriate terminology and the staff must send a consistent, accurate message about the nature of this disease.

Members of the Hospice team should be prepared to manage the stress experienced by the family and the possible ventilation of that stress onto the front line team members. Staff should employ a patient thoughtful approach when dealing with family who are perceived as angry, demanding or difficult to please. Aging family members may be cognitively impaired and require frequent reminders. Aging individuals who have rarely had outsiders in their home may find home services as intrusive and unsettling. Older persons are encouraged by law enforcement to be wary of unknown outsiders to prevent exploitation and the presence of unknown strangers in the home can cause anxiety. The hospice team can address issues with an empathic, careful approach that begins with validation of the caregivers fatigue and stress. The team members should focus on the accomplishments of the family and remind the caregivers of the support that the family members have provided. Some families may view the need for institutional help such as a nursing home or "outside help" such as home hospice as a failure. Team leadership should listen to each concern expressed by the family and attempt to address those issues in a calm, empathic manner. Intense emotional responses from caregivers to non-critical issues such as small details of personal grooming or placement of objects in the room can signify distress in the caregiver. All direct care workers or office staff that handles caregiver calls should understand caregiver stress and demonstrate the ability to communicate in a therapeutic manner.

Physicians can also play a critical role in managing caregiver stress during the dying process. Physicians can promote excellent communications with the family, support home care when appropriate, facilitate advanced care planning, demonstrate empathy to the family and recognize bereavement during the dying process and after death [127]. Physicians are sometimes challenged by end-of-life situations as the discussions are often stressful, time consuming, and may not be reimbursable.

The type and features of dementia can influence caregiver coping. Younger onset dementia such as familial early onset AD, FTD and Huntington's disease may impact both the spouse and the children of the patient. The spouse or child of a younger patient who may engage in bizarre behaviors may cause embarrassment and social discomfort for the family. This may lead to guilt and remorse later. This behavior may isolate the family from friends and the faith community [128]. The family, particularly children of early onset dementia, may need counseling and support over time.

Hospice services may be initiated in conjunction with placement from home or independent living into a nursing home setting. While some caregivers experience an improvement in stress-related symptoms following transition to a nursing home, some continue to experience depression and burdens; especially for patients with greater behavioral symptomology or intense functional needs [129]. Simple interventions can help reduce this stress during the transition such as conducting a discussion about advanced directives, exploring issues that help patient comfort, depicting the specialized understanding of dementia and avoiding feeding tubes [130]. Available published data describing caregiver views of helping persons dying with dementia is limited. A common theme focused on" the family's belief of death and their choice of treatment" [119]. These reviews seemed to share common themes such as (1) The relationship with professionals is a core component to care quality. (2) Caring is physically and emotionally demanding. (3) The caregivers' ability to consider death is an important factor in making decisions.

Managing Bereavement Issues Experienced by Family Caregivers

The caregiver grief reaction produced by supporting a patient with dementia over a period of years can be complex and prolonged. Despite years of caregiving, many (23 %) report that they are not prepared for death [131]. Many caregivers experience anticipatory grief as well as the bereavement following death. The grieving process for both the patient and the caregivers may begin at the time of diagnosis or recognition of symptoms.

Anticipatory grief is mourning the loss of the person who remains alive but manifests evidence of psychological decline. Anticipatory grief can occur in family caregivers of patients with mild cognitive impairment (MCI) or dementia especially among individuals who live with the patient. Different themes may be present with families of persons with MCI "missing the person" while caregivers of individuals with dementia mourn the loss of function [132]. Anticipatory grief can be predicted in 47–71 % of caregivers and complicated grief can occur in about 20 % of caregivers following death [133, 134]. Complicated grief may occur more often in caregivers with more pre-loss depression, caregiving for more severely impaired patients and experiencing more positive aspects of caregiving. Caregivers participating in psychosocial support activities were less likely to develop complicated grief [134]. The treatment of complicated grief may include referral to a psychiatrist.

Although epidemiology studies are limited, there is a consensus that grief is common in caregivers in all stages of the disease. At the end, many caregivers (23 %) report that they were not prepared for the death of their loved one and these individuals are at higher risk for depression and anxiety following the loss [131]. Anticipatory grief has not been shown to reduce the intensity of post-death grief [135]. Caregivers who provided daily support to patients may exhibit increased risk for symptoms of depression and anxiety which may increase during the dying process but many caregivers show significant resiliency and return to baseline after 1 year.

Among those who needed assistance post death, many used the family support group (65.5 %) or individual counseling (53.3 %). In some instances, the caregiver spouse may resume a life style as a single person with the limitations of marriage and some caregivers may have new intimate relationships to fill the void of companionship despite the presence of the spouse. The patient and the caregiver may not have the opportunity to resolve issues as the patient loses cognitive abilities. Patients and adult children may not have the ability to reminisce or engage in discussions that often occur with individuals capable of reflecting back over their lives and resolving old conflicts.

Bereavement Support

Bereavement counseling before or after death can be a critical element of hospice care. Alzheimer's disease is identified as a disorder that increased the need for psychological bereavement services. Caregivers are at increased risk for depression following the death of the patient and post death studies indicate that dementia caregivers who use hospice experience less depression than those who employ aggressive medical measures for the patient [136].

The caregiver experience during the dying phase, including their perception of the patient's suffering, may impact post death psychiatric morbidity. Caregivers report choking and pain as particularly distressing; symptoms that are specifically targeted for treatment during hospice care [68]. Grief may be more common in dementia than in other chronic diseases such as cardiac disease where twice as many dementia caregivers are reported to have symptoms of bereavement. Some caregivers may continue to grieve at 1 year following the death and clinicians should be vigilant to detect these conditions given the adverse physical and mental health consequences of complicated grief [133]. Patients with complicated grief demonstrate persistent, intense feelings of "missing the person." Some individuals may describe a sense that the deceased patient is still in the home or the caregiver may report hearing the deceased patient's voice. While this does not imply psychotic features, these symptoms do warrant further evaluation by a mental health professional [137]. Prophylactic antidepressant therapy is not indicated for grieving caregivers and clinicians should avoid benzodiazepines for anxiety or sleep in older persons. Suicidality has not been shown to increase in bereaved caregivers but older, frail individuals with depression are always at greater risk for self-harm, especially individuals with chronic pain or substance abuse. Grief counseling, grief support groups, continued participation in dementia support groups and other psychological interventions are preferable for the caregiver. The grief counselor should be familiar with dementia and caregiving. Caregivers may have disruption of sleep cycle from the chronic caregiver role and clinicians should avoid benzodiazepines for sleep but rather suggested behavioral interventions such as sleep hygiene, avoiding naps and resuming regular activities.

The caregiving family may have lost the support of the faith community over the years of service. The family may be disconnected from their church when the patient is no longer able to attend worship services and the family is not able to identify respite support to allow participation. Child care during worship service is frequent in faith communities but adult day care is less common. Pastors may not continue home visits as the patient loses memory of the church and ability to communicate. Spiritual isolation can be painful and stressful, especially in rural communities.

The therapist or chaplain who treats grief in dementia caregivers should understand dementia and the impact of caregiving. Depression is common in the post death phase and chaplains should be alert to signs that the caregiver has transitioned from bereavement to depression. The role of the chaplain or pastor in hospice care for patients with dementia may differ from their role in patients with other diseases. Patients may no longer attend church regularly due to functional or behavioral problems. Pastors can sometimes struggle to cope with the demented patient and the distressed caregiver. Families may sometimes feel abandoned by the faith community in settings where the community has not attempted to accommodate the needs of cognitively impaired individuals.

The chaplain and the faith community can be emotionally and spiritually supportive to the family and the patient. The chaplain's role is not bound by faith belief system but rather by a spirit-to spirit relationship. While many elements of chaplain-patient relationship are not available in dementia, others such as" focusing on the presence or journeying together" are possible" [138]. Spiritual care can be beneficial at many levels in cognitively intact persons although this support may be underutilized with persons suffering from all terminal diseases. Chaplains may not understand the complex neuropsychiatric manifestations of dementia and they may feel uncomfortable spending time with these individuals who may appear unresponsive. Ministering to such patients may seem unrewarding but clergy should be advised that they may be making spiritual connections that are not readily apparent. The interest by clergy in patients with dementia can send a powerful message to the staff that cares for the individual. The attention of the clergy may validate the human value of the person. Clergy should know that their presence in activities such as spiritual readings or a spiritual musical expression may touch the patient but more importantly affirm the humanity of the patient to the staff. From the spiritual perspective, the distinction between brain, mind and soul is critical. A possible teaching model is the conceptualization of spiritual music appreciation. A powerful hymn will be heard by the auditory cortex of the brain. The mind will process the information and place the music in context but the soul is moved in a way that cannot readily be defined by neuroscience. The clergy can be advised that while the brain and mind of the dementia patient may have significant deficits, the state of the soul is not known and should be assumed to be intact until the time of death.

Managing Bereavement in Patients with Dementia

An individual with dementia may mourn the loss of function and independence, especially in cases where only selective function is impaired such as the ability to communicate in progressive nonfluent aphasia. The sense of loss and fear may continue until the patient loses insight. Patient grieving is less common in persons with late stage dementia however individuals with early stage dementia and other lethal disease such as cancer need bereavement services that match their cognitive abilities. A mild or moderately demented patient with cancer may understand that they are gravely ill and they deserve an informed discussion at least once to alert them to the prognosis. Repeated explanations about their condition that are promptly forgotten due to amnesia may provoke intense emotional response for the patient and not help with their care [139]. While any patient questions should be answered honestly by the clinicians (e.g., Do I have a serious illness?—Yes), the team should move to other subjects or activities that sustain quality of life. For example, an appropriate response might be, "Yes, you are seriously ill but today will be a good day because your grandchildren are coming."

Mild to moderately demented patients may experience other losses such as the death of caregivers or adult children during the course of their illness. In some instanced, individuals may ask for deceased family or friends. Individuals with dementia deserve to know about a recent loss but the subject does not need to be revisited except in response to a direct question from the patient. Repeated reminders of the loss may be forgotten and the patient may re-experience the grief as a new event when reminded. Redirection and distraction may be employed to avoid patient distress. The treatment team may experience difficulties when family insists that the patient not be informed. The team can discuss the ethical issues for informing the patient with the family unless a guardian is in place as a surrogate decision maker. There is no specific rule or guideline on the merits of informing versus withholding information from individuals with impaired capacity. Studies of grief among demented elders suggest that some individuals can process the information about the loss while others will react with confusion or bewilderment. Patients may react by seeking the dead, emotional outbursts and the need for comfort that may last for months [139]. Reassurance and behavioral interventions are the first line treatment for such symptoms and staff should avoid psychotropic medications. Patients may make alarming statements such as, "I wish I were dead too." Such statements may not reflect suicidality; however recurrent statements warrant a psychiatric assessment. There are no specific guidelines for distinguishing normal grief from pathological grief in demented patients and clinicians must use their best judgment based on the patients past psychiatric history, intensity of symptoms, duration from the actual event and behavioral impact.

The decision about whether a demented person can attend a funeral is complicated. The presence of the individual may comfort the family but some patients may be overwhelmed by the emotion and the stimulation. The decision whether to attend a wake or funeral must be made on a case by case basis. Severely demented patients rarely comprehend such events and these individuals may be traumatized by the environmental stressors. Mildly demented patients may be able to attend the service but these individuals may need constant attendance

by a person with detailed knowledge about their needs and the team needs a strategy to manage a behavioral problem if the patient experiences distress. For instance, if there is concern the patient will become very upset, the family can identify a quiet area to help with de-escalation, they can have a driver ready to return to the facility. Two caregivers should accompany a mobile patient to assure safety while driving.

Management of Special Hospice Populations with Cognitive Deficits

Special populations for hospice care with cognitive impairment and unique behavioral challenges include older individuals with serious mental illness and those with intellectual disability. Excluding dementia as a psychiatric diagnosis, over a half million persons with mental illness are thought to reside in American nursing homes [140]. Most (89 %) residents admitted to nursing homes have some psychiatric diagnosis with 89 % having depression, 5.6 % schizophrenia and 5.2 % having bipolar disorder. As compared to the general older population, both groups have higher risks for age-related dementia with aging, are more likely to receive psychotropic medications and are more likely to have unrecognized health problems that might contribute to the patient's symptoms and suffering [140]. Individuals with severe mental illness or substance abuse in middle life have increase risk of dementia in later life [141].

Little is written about hospice care for persons with schizophrenia or bipolar disorder who are at greater risk for cognitive decline than other elders [142]. The overall life expectancy for persons with serious mental illness is 10–20 years shorter than the general population. Access to health care is often limited and many patients may have untreated or undertreated health problems. Schizophrenia is a neurodevelopmental disorder that impacts both the frontal and temporal lobes of the brain and psychotic symptoms persist in many patients throughout life. The need for continued antipsychotic therapy in later life must be determined on a case by case basis. Hallucinations and delusions can be quite distressing to persons with schizophrenia. The impact of dementia on the manifestation of psychotic symptoms can vary by individual however some patients with dementia may have worsening of psychotic symptoms. Older patients with schizophrenia have a greater risk for adverse events from antipsychotic medications and have higher levels of frailty that mandate the use of lower doses of antipsychotic drugs [143].

Cognitive symptoms are often overlooked in the hospice patient with serious mental illness and the staff should be particularly alert to assessing their cognition with appropriate instruments. Few cognitive screening instruments have been normed in the mentally ill however the Folstein Mini Mental Status Examination is simple and valid in these populations [105]. The mental status examination on admission should identify hallucinations and delusions as older patients may not volunteer that information because past endorsement of symptoms may have resulted in hospitalization or escalation of doses of antipsychotic medications. Patients with schizophrenia and more severe negative symptoms such as apathy are most likely to have cognitive symptoms [144]. The combination of mental illness, unrecognized cognitive deficits and unrecognized age-related sensory deficits may predispose the patient to delirium. These individuals may have silent psychotic symptoms that can re-emerge with stress or illness as manifest by behavioral problems. Many patients with schizophrenia have limited ties with their families and surrogate decision-making can become a major challenge.

Demented patients with bipolar disorder or psychotic depression can pose unique challenges to the hospice team. Frail, elderly, cognitively impaired patients may have unstable symptoms of mania or depression as well as symptoms that may become unstable as a result of their illness. Patients may be inclined to discuss issues such as suicide that can become alarming to the hospice team. Some patients may seem hostile or threatening as a baseline. The withdrawal of mood stabilizing medications in patients with mood disorders and cognitive impairment should be conducted with the assistance of the treating psychiatrist. Specific medications such as second generation antipsychotic medications, lithium

and anticonvulsants such as valproic acid used to stabilize mood can be systematically tapered. Lithium has a very narrow therapeutic range in older adults and great care is needed to avoid drug-drug interactions with other medications such as NSAIDs that can increase serum lithium levels. Reduced oral intake and dehydration may likely increase the lithium level. The mood stabilizers can be reduced in the dying patient as the first step followed by the antipsychotic medications which are less likely to cause delirium and which also stabilize mood. Patients with psychotic depression can sometimes develop somatic delusions where they are convinced that they cannot swallow or they can become paranoid about the food and stop eating. Antipsychotic medications are indicated in these patients to reduce the psychological suffering associated with their delusion and maintain optimal nutrition during the dying process. Severe depression can cause catatonia or cognitive symptoms that resemble dementia and patients with severe depression should receive aggressive therapy if other lethal diseases are not present such as cancer of end stage heart failure.

Suicidality is a major issue in both demented patients and those with mental illness. There is no evidence that persons with dementia are at increased risk for suicide at any point in their illness as compared to other older, chronically medically ill individuals. Patients may express morbid thoughts, especially if depressed. A psychiatrist with expertise in older patients should be consulted in cases where demented patients begin to express suicidal thoughts. Patients may become tearful or catastrophic in any phase of dementia and express thoughts of self-harm during periods of intense, transient emotions. For example the severely confused older adult who states "I have been left here by my family, I might as well be dead" but 2 h later is having a pleasant conversation with the chaplain.

Patients with intellectual disability are living longer than 50 years ago and this group is at increased risk for developing dementia. All-cause mortality is increased almost three fold in persons with intellectual disability [145]. Some groups, such as patients with Down's syndrome or fragile X, are at high risk for dementia and age related care-giver burden [146]. Most individuals with intellectual disability are in the mild range with IQ's above 60 but dementia can occur in groups across the IQ spectrum. Commonly used cognitive screening instruments such as the SLUMS or the MMSE are not valid in this group. Patients often develop loss of previously acquired functions as the manifestation of the dementia. For example, a 60 year old individual with mild intellectual disability who can no longer self-toilet but who has been continent of urine for the last 40 years and the individual has no medical explanation for the loss of function. Many persons with intellectual disability are managed by very aged parents and the loss of the caregiver can produce bereavement or depression that looks like dementia in the middle aged care recipient. Patients with intellectual disability are at higher risk for serious mental illness than the general population and persons with moderate to severe impairment may have specific behaviors such as self-injurious behavior. Many clinical skills that are helpful in caring for dementia patients are also valuable in caring for persons with intellectual disability. Loss of caregivers, physical health problems, relocation to new home or residential program and a range of other stressors can induce behaviors such as head slapping, biting and others. The hospice team should consult with developmental behavioral specialists to assess these new behaviors and treat appropriately [147].

Frailty is common in all older persons with intellectual disability; 11 % of individuals age 50–65 and 18 % over age 65 are frail. Risks for frailty include Down's syndrome, dementia, motor impairments and lower baseline intellectual function [148]. Premature deaths are increased in persons with intellectual disability and this increased mortality is associated with problems with health care [149, 150]. Determination of a terminal illness in a person with intellectual disability should include a defined cause such as metastatic carcinoma or documentation of a thorough evaluation to identify a cause for the patient's decline. Most individuals with intellectual disability do not have accelerated aging and do not spontaneously die at an early age.

The access of hospice services may be limited for the older frail intellectually disabled patient who is dying. A large survey in New Jersey found that few group homes (22 %) and developmental centers 60 % reported a familiarity with hospice services [147].

Ethical Challenges for Hospice Care in Persons with Dementia

Dementia presents a unique challenge to the legal and ethical constructs for society and healthcare. Dementia can be a relentless, expensive, demoralizing disease to both patient and caregiver. The patients may not wish to be a burden to their family and the demented person may not wish to live without their mental abilities. There is no guidance to define when cognitive loss is sufficiently progressed to diminish personhood or indicate that a treatment represents medical futility [151].

Assisted dying remains a controversial issue for many reasons. Based on guidance from the European Association of Palliative Care, assisted dying encompasses both voluntary euthanasia and physician assisted suicide. Physicians may be more comfortable with physician assisted suicide as the doctor merely provides the medication so the patient can voluntarily take the lethal dose. Euthanasia requires a more active role for the doctor. (Some) European countries have offered patients with dementia the right to choose assisted suicide as long as the patient made the choice while they were cognitively intact [152]. The choice of assisted suicide involves many factors for the patient including: (1) the suffering, dependency and loss of self caused by dementia; (2) potential for pain and suffering; (3) the desire for a dignified, good quality of death; and (4) the desire to exert self determination. Several concerns exist about assisted suicide including: (1) the need for safeguards against financial or social pressures; (2) moral and religious objections; and (3) the possibility that a decisions made years before to use assisted suicide may no longer be chosen by the patient. Depression is common in both caregivers and patients. The mental health status of the decision makers can impact the capacity to make truly informed decisions.

Surveys conducted with patients and families show great variation of attitude based on the study sample. Anywhere between 14 % and 65 % of patients, and 15–77 % if caregivers may consider assisted suicide [153]. The attitudes of both groups were impacted by age, gender and faith background. Individuals with greater cognitive impairment but retained insight were more likely to favor access to this option. Health care professionals are generally against any form of assisted dying for many reasons and this attitude is unlikely to change in the immediate future. Likewise, the medical community is not likely to develop specific criteria of medical futility for patients with dementia and aggressive care for some severely demented patients will continue.

References

1. Alzheimer's Association. Alzheimer's disease facts and figures. Alzheimers Dement. 2014;10(2):e47–92.
2. Johnson KS, Elbert-Avila K, Kuchibhatla M, Tulsky JA. Characteristics and outcomes of hospice enrollees with dementia discharged alive. J Am Geriatr Soc. 2012;60(9):1638–44.
3. Li Q, Zheng NT, Temkin-Greener H. Quality of end-of-life care of long-term nursing home residents with and without dementia. J Am Geriatr Soc. 2013;61(7):1066–73.
4. Wachterman MW, Marcantonio ER, Davis RB, McCarthy EP. Association of hospice agency profit status with patient diagnosis, location of care, and length of stay. JAMA. 2011;305(5):472–9.
5. Irwin SA, Zurhellen CH, Diamond LC, Dunn LB, Palmer BW, Jeste DV, Twamley EW. Unrecognised cognitive impairment in hospice patients: a pilot study. Palliat Med. 2008;22(7):842–7.
6. Aminoff BZ, Adunsky A. Their last 6 months: suffering and survival of end-stage dementia patients. Age Ageing. 2006;35(6):597–601.
7. Aragon K, Covinsky K, Miao Y, Boscardin WJ, Flint L, Smith AK. Use of the Medicare posthospitalization skilled nursing benefit in the last 6 months of life. Arch Intern Med. 2012;172(20):1573–9.
8. Mitchell SL, Teno JM, Intrator O, Feng Z, Mor V. Decisions to forgo hospitalization in advanced dementia: a nationwide study. J Am Geriatr Soc. 2007;55(3):432–8.
9. Teno JM, Gozalo PL, Bynum JP, Leland NE, Miller SC, Morden NE, Scupp T, Goodman DC, Mor V. Change in end-of-life care for Medicare beneficiaries: site of death, place of care, and health care transitions in 2000, 2005, and 2009. JAMA. 2013; 303(5):470–7.
10. Dobbs D, Meng H, Hyer K, Volicer L. The influence of hospice use on nursing home and hospital use in assisted living among dual-eligible enrollees. J Am Med Dir Assoc. 2012;13(2):189.e9–13.
11. Perrels AJ, Fleming J, Zhao J, Barclay S, Farquhar M, Buiting HM, Brayne C, Collaboration Cambridge City over-75s Cohort Study. Place of death and end-of-life transitions experienced by very old people with differing cognitive status: retrospective analysis of a prospective population-based cohort aged 85 and over. Palliat Med. 2014;28(3):220–33.
12. Hales S, Zimmermann C, Rodin G. The quality of dying and death. Arch Intern Med. 2008;168(9): 912–8.
13. Lawrence V, Samsi K, Murray J, Harari D, Banerjee S. Dying well with dementia: qualitative examination of end-of-life care. Br J Psychiatry. 2011;199(5): 417–22.
14. Kulkarni P, Kulkarni P, Anavkar V, Ghooi R. Preference of the place of death among people of Pune. Indian J Palliat Care. 2014;20(2):101–6.
15. Fukui S, Yoshiuchi K, Fujita J, Sawai M, Watanabe M. Japanese people's preference for place of end-of-life care and death: a population-based nationwide survey. J Pain Symptom Manag. 2011;42(6):882–92.
16. Shega JW, Hougham GW, Stocking CB, Cox-Hayley D, Sachs GA. Patients dying with dementia: experience at the end of life and impact of hospice care. J Pain Symptom Manag. 2008;35(5):499–507.
17. Shemie SD, Hornby L, Baker A, Teitelbaum J, Torrance S, Young K, Capron AM, Bernat JL, Noel L, The International Guidelines for Determination of Death Phase 1 Participants, in Collaboration with the World Health Organization. International guideline development for the determination of death. Intensive Care Med. 2014;40(6):788–97.
18. Burkle CM, Sharp RR, Wijdicks EF. Why brain death is considered death and why there should be no confusion. Neurology. 2014;83(16):1464–9.
19. Koppitz A, Bosshard G, Schuster DH, Hediger H, Imhof L. Type and course of symptoms demonstrated in the terminal and dying phases by people with dementia in nursing homes. Z Gerontol Geriatr. 2015;48(2):176–83.
20. Pinzon LC, Claus M, Perrar KM, Zepf KI, Letzel S, Weber M. Dying with dementia: symptom burden, quality of care, and place of death. Dtsch Arztebl Int. 2013;110(12):195–202.
21. Vandervoort A, Houttekier D, Vander Stichele R, van der Steen JT, Van den Block L. Quality of dying in nursing home residents dying with dementia: does advanced care planning matter? A nationwide postmortem study. PLoS One. 2014;9(3):e91130.
22. Klapwijk MS, Caljouw MA, van Soest-Poortvliet MC, van der Steen JT, Achterberg WP. Symptoms and treatment when death is expected in dementia patients in long-term care facilities. BMC Geriatr. 2014;14:99.

23. Macleod AD, Taylor KS, Counsell CE. Mortality in Parkinson's disease: a systematic review and meta-analysis. Mov Disord. 2014;29(13):1615–22.

24. Miyasaki JM, Long J, Mancini D, Moro E, Fox SH, Lang AE, Marras C, Chen R, Strafella A, Arshinoff R, Ghoche R, Hui J. Palliative care for advanced Parkinson disease: an interdisciplinary clinic and new scale, the ESAS-PD. Parkinsonism Relat Disord. 2012;18 Suppl 3:S6–9.

25. Kempster PA, O'Sullivan SS, Holton JL, Revesz T, Lees AJ. Relationships between age and late progression of Parkinson's disease: a clinico-pathological study. Brain. 2010;133(Pt 6):1755–62.

26. Carter JH, Lyons KS, Lindauer A, Malcom J. Predeath grief in Parkinson's caregivers: a pilot survey-based study. Parkinsonism Relat Disord. 2012;18 Suppl 3:S15–8.

27. Garcia-Ptacek S, Farahmand B, Kareholt I, Religa D, Cuadrado ML, Eriksdotter M. Mortality risk after dementia diagnosis by dementia type and underlying factors: a cohort of 15,209 patients based on the Swedish Dementia Registry. J Alzheimers Dis. 2014;41(2):467–77.

28. Gill DP, Hubbard RA, Koepsell TD, Borrie MJ, Petrella RJ, Knopman DS, Kukull WA. Differences in rate of functional decline across three dementia types. Alzheimers Dement. 2013;9(5 Suppl):S63–71.

29. van der Steen JT, van Soest-Poortvliet MC, Hallie-Heierman M, Onwuteaka-Philipsen BD, Deliens L, de Boer ME, Van den Block L, van Uden N, Hertogh CM, de Vet HC. Factors associated with initiation of advance care planning in dementia: a systematic review. J Alzheimers Dis. 2014;40(3):743–57.

30. Mitchell SL, Black BS, Ersek M, Hanson LC, Miller SC, Sachs GA, Teno JM, Morrison RS. Advanced dementia: state of the art and priorities for the next decade. Ann Intern Med. 2012;156(1 Pt 1):45–51.

31. Teno JM, Gozalo PL, Lee IC, Kuo S, Spence C, Connor SR, Casarett DJ. Does hospice improve quality of care for persons dying from dementia? J Am Geriatr Soc. 2011;59(8):1531–6.

32. Robinson L, Dickinson C, Rousseau N, Beyer F, Clark A, Hughes J, Howel D, Exley C. A systematic review of the effectiveness of advance care planning interventions for people with cognitive impairment and dementia. Age Ageing. 2012;41(2):263–9.

33. Badrakalimuthu V, Barclay S. Do people with dementia die at their preferred location of death? A systematic literature review and narrative synthesis. Age Ageing. 2014;43(1):13–9.

34. Penders YW, Albers G, Deliens L, Vander Stichele R, Van den Block L, Euro Impact on behalf of. Awareness of dementia by family carers of nursing home residents dying with dementia: a post-death study. Palliat Med. 2015;29(1):38-47.

35. van der Steen JT, Onwuteaka-Philipsen BD, Knol DL, Ribbe MW, Deliens L. Caregivers' understanding of dementia predicts patients' comfort at death: a prospective observational study. BMC Med. 2013;11:105.

36. Brody AA, Galvin JE. A review of interprofessional dissemination and education interventions for recognizing and managing dementia. Gerontol Geriatr Educ. 2013;34(3):225–56.

37. Albrecht JS, Gruber-Baldini AL, Fromme EK, McGregor JC, Lee DS, Furuno JP. Quality of hospice care for individuals with dementia. J Am Geriatr Soc. 2013;61(7):1060–5.

38. Vandervoort A, Houttekier D, Van den Block L, van der Steen JT, Vander Stichele R, Deliens L. Advance care planning and physician orders in nursing home residents with dementia: a nationwide retrospective study among professional caregivers and relatives. J Pain Symptom Manag. 2014;47(2):245–56.

39. Temkin-Greener H, Zheng NT, Xing J, Mukamel DB. Site of death among nursing home residents in the united states: changing patterns, 2003-2007. J Am Med Dir Assoc. 2013;14(10):741–8.

40. Fulton AT, Gozalo P, Mitchell SL, Mor V, Teno JM. Intensive care utilization among nursing home residents with advanced cognitive and severe functional impairment. J Palliat Med. 2014;17(3):313–7.

41. Gozalo P, Teno JM, Mitchell SL, Skinner J, Bynum J, Tyler D, Mor V. End-of-life transitions among nursing home residents with cognitive issues. N Engl J Med. 2011;365(13):1212–21.

42. Sleeman KE, Ho YK, Verne J, Gao W, Higginson IJ, GUIDE Care Project. Reversal of English trend towards hospital death in dementia: a population-based study of place of death and associated individual and regional factors, 2001-2010. BMC Neurol. 2014;14:59.

43. Poppe M, Burleigh S, Banerjee S. Qualitative evaluation of advanced care planning in early dementia (ACP-ED). PLoS One. 2013;8(4):e60412.

44. Edwards R, Voss S. Education about dementia in primary care: is person-centredness the key? Dementia. 2014;13(1):111–9.

45. McCarty CE, Volicer L. Hospice access for individuals with dementia. Am J Alzheimers Dis Other Demen. 2009;24(6):476–85.

46. Jayes RL, Arnold RM, Fromme EK. Does this dementia patient meet the prognosis eligibility requirements for hospice enrollment? J Pain Symptom Manag. 2012;44(5):750–6.

47. Brown MA, Sampson EL, Jones L, Barron AM. Prognostic indicators of 6-month mortality in elderly people with advanced dementia: a systematic review. Palliat Med. 2013;27(5):389–400.

48. Morrison RS, Siu AL. Survival in end-stage dementia following acute illness. JAMA. 2000;284(1):47–52.

49. Modi S, Moore C, Shah K, Organization National Hospice. Which late-stage Alzheimer's patients should be referred for hospice care? J Fam Pract. 2005;54(11):984–6.

50. Coleman AM. End-of-life issues in caring for patients with dementia: the case for palliative care in management of terminal dementia. Am J Hosp Palliat Care. 2012;29(1):9–12.

51. Razlighi QR, Stallard E, Brandt J, Blacker D, Albert M, Scarmeas N, Kinosian B, Yashin AI, Stern Y. A new algorithm for predicting time to disease endpoints in Alzheimer's disease patients. J Alzheimers Dis. 2014;38(3):661–8.

52. Mitchell SL, Miller SC, Teno JM, Kiely DK, Davis RB, Shaffer ML. Prediction of 6-month survival of nursing home residents with advanced dementia using adept vs hospice eligibility guidelines. JAMA. 2010;304(17):1929–35.

53. Casarett DJ, Farrington S, Craig T, Slattery J, Harrold J, Oldanie B, Roy J, Biehl R, Teno J. The art versus science of predicting prognosis: can a prognostic index predict short-term mortality better than experienced nurses do? J Palliat Med. 2012;15(6): 703–8.

54. Kaffashian S, Dugravot A, Elbaz A, Shipley MJ, Sabia S, Kivimaki M, Singh-Manoux A. Predicting cognitive decline: a dementia risk score vs. the Framingham vascular risk scores. Neurology. 2013;80(14):1300–6.

55. Huskamp HA, Stevenson DG, Grabowski DC, Brennan E, Keating NL. Long and short hospice stays among nursing home residents at the end of life. J Palliat Med. 2010;13(8):957–64.

56. Rothenberg LR, Doberman D, Simon LE, Gryczynski J, Cordts G. Patients surviving six months in hospice care: who are they? J Palliat Med. 2014;17(8):899–905.

57. Toledo JB, Weiner MW, Wolk DA, Da X, Chen K, Arnold SE, Jagust W, Jack C, Reiman EM, Davatzikos C, Shaw LM, Trojanowski JQ, Initiative Alzheimer's Disease Neuroimaging. Neuronal injury biomarkers and prognosis in ADNI subjects with normal cognition. Acta Neuropathol Commun. 2014;2:26.

58. Andrade-Moraes CH, Oliveira-Pinto AV, Castro-Fonseca E, da Silva CG, Guimaraes DM, Szczupak D, Parente-Bruno DR, Carvalho LR, Polichiso L, Gomes BV, Oliveira LM, Rodriguez RD, Leite RE, Ferretti-Rebustini RE, Jacob-Filho W, Pasqualucci CA, Grinberg LT, Lent R. Cell number changes in Alzheimer's disease relate to dementia, not to plaques and tangles. Brain. 2013;136(Pt 12): 3738–52.

59. Irwin DJ, White MT, Toledo JB, Xie SX, Robinson JL, Van Deerlin V, Lee VM, Leverenz JB, Montine TJ, Duda JE, Hurtig HI, Trojanowski JQ. Neuropathologic substrates of Parkinson's disease dementia. Ann Neurol. 2012;72(4):587–98.

60. Silveira MJ, Kim SY, Langa KM. Advance directives and outcomes of surrogate decision making before death. N Engl J Med. 2010;362(13):1211–8.

61. Farber NJ, Simpson P, Salam T, Collier VU, Weiner J, Boyer EG. Physicians' decisions to withhold and withdraw life-sustaining treatment. Arch Intern Med. 2006;166(5):560–4.

62. Moorman SM, Carr D. Spouses' effectiveness as end-of-life health care surrogates: accuracy, uncertainty, and errors of overtreatment or undertreatment. Gerontologist. 2008;48(6):811–9.

63. Shalowitz DI, Garrett-Mayer E, Wendler D. The accuracy of surrogate decision makers: a systematic review. Arch Intern Med. 2006;166(5):493–7.

64. Avram M, Hennig-Fast K, Bao Y, Poppel E, Reiser M, Blautzik J, Giordano J, Gutyrchik E. Neural correlates of moral judgments in first- and third-person perspectives: implications for neuroethics and beyond. BMC Neurosci. 2014;15:39.

65. Sevinc G, Spreng RN. Contextual and perceptual brain processes underlying moral cognition: a quantitative meta-analysis of moral reasoning and moral emotions. PLoS One. 2014;9(2):e87427.

66. Moeller SJ, Konova AB, Parvaz MA, Tomasi D, Lane RD, Fort C, Goldstein RZ. Functional, structural, and emotional correlates of impaired insight in cocaine addiction. JAMA Psychiatry. 2014;71(1): 61–70.

67. Melis RJ, Marengoni A, Rizzuto D, Teerenstra S, Kivipelto M, Angleman SB, Fratiglioni L. The influence of multimorbidity on clinical progression of dementia in a population-based cohort. PLoS One. 2013;8(12), e84014.

68. Givens JL, Selby K, Goldfeld KS, Mitchell SL. Hospital transfers among nursing home residents with advanced dementia. J Am Geriatr Soc. 2012;60(5):905–9.

69. Dewing J, Dijk S. What is the current state of care for older people with dementia in general hospitals? A literature review. Dementia. 2014.

70. Hirschman KB, Abbott KM, Hanlon AL, Prvu Bettger J, Naylor MD. What factors are associated with having an advance directive among older adults who are new to long term care services? J Am Med Dir Assoc. 2012;13(1):82.e7–11.

71. Houttekier D, Vandervoort A, Van den Block L, van der Steen JT, Vander Stichele R, Deliens L. Hospitalizations of nursing home residents with dementia in the last month of life: results from a nationwide survey. Palliat Med. 2014;28(9):1110–7.

72. Goldfeld KS, Hamel MB, Mitchell SL. The cost-effectiveness of the decision to hospitalize nursing home residents with advanced dementia. J Pain Symptom Manag. 2013;46(5):640–51.

73. Shen HN, Lu CL, Li CY. Dementia increases the risks of acute organ dysfunction, severe sepsis and mortality in hospitalized older patients: a national population-based study. PLoS One. 2012;7(8): e42751.

74. Poblador-Plou B, Calderon-Larranaga A, Marta-Moreno J, Hancco-Saavedra J, Sicras-Mainar A, Soljak M, Prados-Torres A. Comorbidity of dementia: a cross-sectional study of primary care older patients. BMC Psychiatry. 2014;14:84.

75. Magaki S, Yong WH, Khanlou N, Tung S, Vinters HV. Comorbidity in dementia: update of an ongoing autopsy study. J Am Geriatr Soc. 2014;62(9): 1722–8.

76. Attems J, Konig C, Huber M, Lintner F, Jellinger KA. Cause of death in demented and non-demented elderly inpatients; an autopsy study of 308 cases. J Alzheimers Dis. 2005;8(1):57–62.

77. Fu C, Chute DJ, Farag ES, Garakian J, Cummings JL, Vinters HV. Comorbidity in dementia: an autopsy study. Arch Pathol Lab Med. 2004;128(1):32–8.

78. Volandes AE, Paasche-Orlow MK, Barry MJ, Gillick MR, Minaker KL, Chang Y, Cook EF, Abbo ED, El-Jawahri A, Mitchell SL. Video decision support tool for advance care planning in dementia: randomised controlled trial. BMJ. 2009;338:b2159.

79. Buchhalter LC, Ottenberg AL, Webster TL, Swetz KM, Hayes DL, Mueller PS. Features and outcomes of patients who underwent cardiac device deactivation. JAMA Intern Med. 2014;174(1):80–5.

80. Thanavaro JL. ICD deactivation: review of literature and clinical recommendations. Clin Nurs Res. 2013;22(1):36–50.

81. Goldstein N, Carlson M, Livote E, Kutner JS. Brief communication: management of implantable cardioverter-defibrillators in hospice: a nationwide survey. Ann Intern Med. 2010;152(5):296–9.

82. Pivi GA, Bertolucci PH, Schultz RR. Nutrition in severe dementia. Curr Gerontol Geriatr Res. 2012;2012:983056.

83. Alagiakrishnan K, Bhanji RA, Kurian M. Evaluation and management of oropharyngeal dysphagia in different types of dementia: a systematic review. Arch Gerontol Geriatr. 2013;56(1):1–9.

84. Sampson EL, White N, Leurent B, Scott S, Lord K, Round J, Jones L. Behavioural and psychiatric symptoms in people with dementia admitted to the acute hospital: prospective cohort study. Br J Psychiatry. 2014;205(3):189–96.

85. American Geriatrics Society Ethics Committee, Practice Clinical and Committee Models of Care. American Geriatrics Society feeding tubes in advanced dementia position statement. J Am Geriatr Soc. 2014;62(8):1590–3.

86. Rozzini R, Sleiman I, Ranhoff A, Maggi S, Trabucchi M. Decision making in elderly patients with severe dementia and pneumonia. Int J Geriatr Psychiatry. 2010;25(3):325–6.

87. Givens JL, Jones RN, Shaffer ML, Kiely DK, Mitchell SL. Survival and comfort after treatment of pneumonia in advanced dementia. Arch Intern Med. 2010;170(13):1102–7.

88. Sera L, McPherson ML, Holmes HM. Commonly prescribed medications in a population of hospice patients. Am J Hosp Palliat Care. 2014;31(2):126–31.

89. Tjia J, Briesacher BA, Peterson D, Liu Q, Andrade SE, Mitchell SL. Use of medications of questionable benefit in advanced dementia. JAMA Intern Med. 2014;174:1763–71.

90. Fick DM, Cooper JW, Wade WE, Waller JL, Maclean JR, Beers MH. Updating the beers criteria for potentially inappropriate medication use in older adults: results of a US Consensus Panel of experts. Arch Intern Med. 2003;163(22):2716–24.

91. Corbett A, Husebo B, Malcangio M, Staniland A, Cohen-Mansfield J, Aarsland D, Ballard C. Assessment and treatment of pain in people with dementia. Nat Rev Neurol. 2012;8(5):264–74.

92. Achterberg WP, Pieper MJ, van Dalen-Kok AH, de Waal MW, Husebo BS, Lautenbacher S, Kunz M, Scherder EJ, Corbett A. Pain management in patients with dementia. Clin Interv Aging. 2013;8:1471–82.

93. Kverno KS, Black BS, Blass DM, Geiger-Brown J, Rabins PV. Neuropsychiatric symptom patterns in hospice-eligible nursing home residents with advanced dementia. J Am Med Dir Assoc. 2008;9(7):509–15.

94. Epstein-Lubow G, Fulton AT, Marino LJ, Teno J. Hospice referral after inpatient psychiatric treatment of individuals with advanced dementia from a nursing home. Am J Hosp Palliat Care. 2014. doi:10.1177/1049909114531160.

95. Onder G, Liperoti R, Foebel A, Fialova D, Topinkova E, van der Roest HG, Gindin J, Cruz-Jentoft AJ, Fini M, Gambassi G, Bernabei R, Shelter Project. Polypharmacy and mortality among nursing home residents with advanced cognitive impairment: results from the Shelter Study. J Am Med Dir Assoc. 2013;14(6):450.e7–12.

96. Fossey J, Ballard C, Juszczak E, James I, Alder N, Jacoby R, Howard R. Effect of enhanced psychosocial care on antipsychotic use in nursing home residents with severe dementia: cluster randomised trial. BMJ. 2006;332(7544):756–61.

97. Koopmans RT, van der Molen M, Raats M, Ettema TP. Neuropsychiatric symptoms and quality of life in patients in the final phase of dementia. Int J Geriatr Psychiatry. 2009;24(1):25–32.

98. Oliveria SA, Liperoti R, Italien GL, Pugner K, Safferman A, Carson W, Lapane K. Adverse events among nursing home residents with Alzheimer's disease and psychosis. Pharmacoepidemiol Drug Saf. 2006;15:763–74.

99. Scarmeas N, Brandt J, Albert M, Hadjigeorgiou G, Papadimitriou A, Dubois B, Sarazin M, Devanand D, Honig L, Marder K, Bell K, Wegesin D, Blacker D, Stern Y. Delusions and hallucinations are associated with worse outcome in Alzheimer disease. Arch Neurol. 2005;62(10):1601–8.

100. Cohen-Mansfield J, Jensen B, Resnick B, Norris M. Knowledge of and attitudes toward nonpharmacological interventions for treatment of behavior symptoms associated with dementia: a comparison of physicians, psychologists, and nurse practitioners. Gerontologist. 2012;52(1):34–45.

101. Hart DJ, Craig D, Compton SA, Critchlow S, Kerrigan BM, McIlroy SP, Passmore AP. A retrospective study of the behavioural and psychological symptoms of mid and late phase Alzheimer's disease. Int J Geriatr Psychiatry. 2003;18(11):1037–42.

102. Selbaek G, Engedal K, Bergh S. The prevalence and course of neuropsychiatric symptoms in nursing home patients with dementia: a systematic review. J Am Med Dir Assoc. 2013;14(3):161–9.

103. Conwell Y, Duberstein PR, Hirsch JK, Conner KR, Eberly S, Caine ED. Health status and suicide in the

second half of life. Int J Geriatr Psychiatry. 2010;25(4):371–9.

104. Chan J, Draper B, Banerjee S. Deliberate self-harm in older adults: a review of the literature from 1995 to 2004. Int J Geriatr Psychiatry. 1995;22(8):720–32.

105. Coffey CE, Cummings JL. The American Psychiatric Publishing textbook of geriatric neuropsychiatry. 3rd ed. Arlington: American Psychiatric Publishing; 2011.

106. Imfeld P, Bodmer M, Schuerch M, Jick SS, Meier CR. Seizures in patients with Alzheimer's disease or vascular dementia: a population-based nested case-control analysis. Epilepsia. 2013;54(4):700–7.

107. Seitz DP, Adunuri N, Gill SS, Gruneir A, Herrmann N, Rochon P. Antidepressants for agitation and psychosis in dementia. Cochrane Database Syst Rev. 2011;(2):CD008191.

108. O'Brien J. Antipsychotics for people with dementia. BMJ. 2008;337:64–5.

109. Vetrano DL, Tosato M, Colloca G, Topinkova E, Fialova D, Gindin J, van der Roest HG, Landi F, Liperoti R, Bernabei R, Onder G. Polypharmacy in nursing home residents with sever cognitive impairment: results from the SHELTER Study. Alzheimers Dement. 2013;9:587–93.

110. Wang J, Yu JT, Wang HF, Meng XF, Wang C, Tan CC, Tan L. Pharmacological treatment of neuropsychiatric symptoms in Alzheimer's disease: a systematic review and meta-analysis. J Neurol Neurosurg Psychiatry. 2015;86(1):101–9.

111. Declercq T, Petrovic M, Azermai M, Vander Stichele R, De Sutter AI, van Driel ML, Christiaens T. Withdrawal versus continuation of chronic antipsychotic drugs for behavioural and psychological symptoms in older people with dementia. Cochrane Database Syst Rev. 2013;3, CD007726.

112. Meguro K, Kasai M, Akanuma K, Meguro M, Ishii H, Yamaguchi S. Donepezil and life expectancy in Alzheimer's disease: a retrospective analysis in the Tajiri project. BMC Neurol. 2014;14:83.

113. Howard R, McShane R, Lindesay J, Ritchie C, Baldwin A, Barber R, Burns A, Dening T, Findlay D, Holmes C, Hughes A, Jacoby R, Jones R, Jones R, McKeith I, Macharouthu A, O'Brien J, Passmore P, Sheehan B, Juszczak E, Katona C, Hills R, Knapp M, Ballard C, Brown R, Banerjee S, Onions C, Griffin M, Adams J, Gray R, Johnson T, Bentham P, Phillips P. Donepezil and memantine for moderate-to-severe Alzheimer's disease. N Engl J Med. 2012;366(10):893–903.

114. Wilkinson D, Wirth Y, Goebel C. Memantine in patients with moderate to severe Alzheimer's disease: meta-analyses using realistic definitions of response. Dement Geriatr Cogn Disord. 2014;37(1–2):71–85.

115. Minett TS, Thomas A, Wilkinson LM, Daniel SL, Sanders J, Richardson J, Littlewood E, Myint P, Newby J, McKeith IG. What happens when donepezil is suddenly withdrawn? An open label trial in

dementia with Lewy bodies and Parkinson's disease with dementia. Int J Geriatr Psychiatry. 2003;18(11):988–93.

116. Leigh AEK, Burgio L, Williams BR, Kvale E, Bailey FA. Hospice emergency kit for veterans: a pilot study. J Palliat Med. 2013;16(4):356–61.

117. Bishop MF, Stephens L, Goodrich M, Byock I. Medication kits for managing symptomatic emergencies in the home: a survey of common hospice practice. J Palliat Med. 2009;12(1):37–44.

118. Joyce BT, Berman R, Lau DT. Formal and informal support of family caregivers managing medications for patients who receive end-of-life care at home: a cross-sectional survey of caregivers. Palliat Med. 2014;28(9):1146–55.

119. Davies N, Maio L, Rait G, Iliffe S. Quality end-of-life care for dementia: what have family carers told us so far? A narrative synthesis. Palliat Med. 2014;28(7):919–30.

120. Diwan S, Hougham GW, Sachs GA. Strain experienced by caregivers of dementia patients receiving palliative care: findings from the palliative excellence in Alzheimer care efforts (PEACE) program. J Palliat Med. 2004;7(6):797–807.

121. Dassel KB, Carr DC. Does dementia caregiving accelerate Frailty? Findings from the Health and Retirement Study. Gerontologist. 2014.

122. Beinart N, Weinman J, Wade D, Brady R. Caregiver burden and psychoeducational interventions in Alzheimer's disease: a review. Dement Geriatr Cogn Dis Extra. 2012;2(1):638–48.

123. Lewis LF. Caregivers' experiences seeking hospice care for loved ones with dementia. Qual Health Res. 2014;24(9):1221–31.

124. Schulz R, Mendelsohn AB, Haley WE, Mahoney D, Allen RS, Zhang S, Thompson L, Belle SH, Resources for Enhancing Alzheimer's Caregiver Health Investigators. End-of-life care and the effects of bereavement on family caregivers of persons with dementia. N Engl J Med. 2003;349(20):1936–42.

125. Thompson GN, Roger K. Understanding the needs of family caregivers of older adults dying with dementia. Palliat Support Care. 2014;12(3):223–31.

126. Adelman RD, Tmanova LL, Delgado D, Dion S, Lachs MS. Caregiver burden: a clinical review. JAMA. 2014;311(10):1052–60.

127. Rabow MW, Hauser JM, Adams J. Supporting family caregivers at the end of life: "they don't know what they don't know". JAMA. 2004;291(4):483–91.

128. Massimo L, Evans LK, Benner P. Caring for loved ones with frontotemporal degeneration: the lived experiences of spouses. Geriatr Nurs. 2013;34(4):302–6.

129. Gaugler JE, Mittelman MS, Hepburn K, Newcomer R. Clinically significant changes in burden and depression among dementia caregivers following nursing home admission. BMC Med. 2010;8:85.

130. Engel SE, Kiely DK, Mitchell SL. Satisfaction with end-of-life care for nursing home residents with advanced dementia. J Am Geriatr Soc. 2006;54(10):1567–72.

131. Hebert RS, Dang Q, Schulz R. Preparedness for the death of a loved one and mental health in bereaved caregivers of patients with dementia: findings from the reach study. J Palliat Med. 2006;9(3):683–93.

132. Garand L, Lingler JH, Deardorf KE, DeKosky ST, Schulz R, Reynolds 3rd CF, Dew MA. Anticipatory grief in new family caregivers of persons with mild cognitive impairment and dementia. Alzheimer Dis Assoc Disord. 2012;26(2):159–65.

133. Chan D, Livingston G, Jones L, Sampson EL. Grief reactions in dementia carers: a systematic review. Int J Geriatr Psychiatry. 2013;28(1):1–17.

134. Schulz R, Boerner K, Shear K, Zhang S, Gitlin LN. Predictors of complicated grief among dementia caregivers: a prospective study of bereavement. Am J Geriatr Psychiatry. 2006;14(8):650–8.

135. Peacock SC. The experience of providing end-of-life care to a relative with advanced dementia: an integrative literature review. Palliat Support Care. 2013;11(2):155–68.

136. Irwin SA, Mausbach BT, Koo D, Fairman N, Roepke-Buehler SK, Chattillion EA, Dimsdale JE, Patterson TL, Ancoli-Israel S, Mills PJ, von Kanel R, Ziegler MG, Grant I. Association between hospice care and psychological outcomes in Alzheimer's spousal caregivers. J Palliat Med. 2013;16(11):1450–4.

137. Simon NM. Treating complicated grief. JAMA. 2013;310(4):416–23.

138. Edwards A, Pang N, Shiu V, Chan C. The understanding of spirituality and the potential role of spiritual care in end-of-life and palliative care: a meta-study of qualitative research. Palliat Med. 2010;24(8):753–70.

139. Johansson AK, Grimby A. Anticipatory grief among close relatives of patients in hospice and palliative wards. Am J Hosp Palliat Care. 2012;29(2):134–8.

140. Aschbrenner KA, Cai S, Grabowski DC, Bartels SJ, Mor V. Medical comorbidity and functional status among adults with major mental illness newly admitted to nursing homes. Psychiatr Serv. 2011;62(9):1098–100.

141. Zilkens RR, Bruce DG, Duke J, Spilsbury K, Semmens JB. Severe psychiatric disorders in mid-life and risk of dementia in late-life (age 65-84 years): a population based case-control study. Curr Alzheimer Res. 2014;11(7):681–93.

142. Vohringer PA, Barroilhet SA, Amerio A, Reale ML, Alvear K, Vergne D, Ghaemi SN. Cognitive impairment in bipolar disorder and schizophrenia: a systematic review. Front Psychiatry. 2013;4:87.

143. Jeste DV, Maglione JE. Treating older adults with schizophrenia: challenges and opportunities. Schizophr Bull. 2013;39(5):966–8.

144. Lewandowski KE, Cohen BM, Keshavan MS, Ongur D. Relationship of neurocognitive deficits to diagnosis and symptoms across affective and non-affective psychoses. Schizophr Res. 2011;133(1–3):212–7.

145. Chesney E, Goodwin GM, Fazel S. Risks of all-cause and suicide mortality in mental disorders: a meta-review. World Psychiatry. 2014;13(2):153–60.

146. Iosif AM, Sciolla AF, Brahmbhatt K, Seritan AL. Caregiver burden in fragile X families. Curr Psychiatry Rev. 2013;9(1).

147. Stein GL. Providing palliative care to people with intellectual disabilities: services, staff knowledge, and challenges. J Palliat Med. 2008;11(9):1241–8.

148. Evenhuis HM, Hermans H, Hilgenkamp TI, Bastiaanse LP, Echteld MA. Frailty and disability in older adults with intellectual disabilities: results from the healthy ageing and intellectual disability study. J Am Geriatr Soc. 2012;60(5):934–8.

149. Heslop P, Blair PS, Fleming P, Hoghton M, Marriott A, Russ L. The confidential inquiry into premature deaths of people with intellectual disabilities in the UK: a population-based study. Lancet. 2014;383(9920):889–95.

150. Tyrer F, McGrother C. Cause-specific mortality and death certificate reporting in adults with moderate to profound intellectual disability. J Intellect Disabil Res. 2009;53(11):898–904.

151. Congedo M, Causarano RI, Alberti F, Bonito V, Borghi L, Colombi L, Defanti CA, Marcello N, Porteri C, Pucci E, Tarquini D, Tettamanti M, Tiezzi A, Tiraboschi P, Gasparini M, Bioethics and Neurology Palliative Care in Neurology Study Group of Italian Society of Neurology. Ethical issues in end of life treatments for patients with dementia. Eur J Neurol. 2010;17(6):774–9.

152. Hendry M, Pasterfield D, Lewis R, Carter B, Hodgson D, Wilkinson C. Why do we want the right to die? A systematic review of the international literature on the views of patients, carers and the public on assisted dying. Palliat Med. 2013;27(1):13–26.

153. Tomlinson E, Stott J. Assisted dying in dementia: a systematic review of the international literature on the attitudes of health professionals, patients, carers and the public, and the factors associated with these. Int J Geriatr Psychiatry. 2015;30(1):10–20.

Challenges in Dementia Care Policy

Jane Tilly and Kate Gordon

Introduction

Dementia is a word that describes brain diseases, like Alzheimer's, that cause people to be more dependent on others over time because of increasing problems with communication, thinking, behavior, or physical function. We fear developing dementia, have it, care for a loved one who has it, or interact with people with disabilities resulting from dementia. The symptoms of dementia as well as its progression have profound implications for all of us and the service systems we depend upon. Model health and community care systems recognize the special nature of dementia through their policies and practices, ranging from eligibility for program services and how to manage them to quality assurance. Dementia care policy challenges involve ensuring that programs' policies and practices meet the needs of this very vulnerable population and their family caregivers.

Getting an accurate diagnosis of dementia is critical. Some researchers estimate that only about half of people with dementia actually have a diagnosis [1]. In addition, a few causes of dementia may be reversible and other diseases can resemble dementia. For example, normal pressure hydrocephalus often can be resolved with a shunt in the brain that drains excess fluid [2]. Symptoms of other conditions, such as depression, thyroid disease, vitamin deficiencies, excessive use of alcohol, and brain tumors can resemble dementia. So can the effects of certain drugs and medication interactions. For example, over the counter sleep aids and antihistamines can harm memory and cognition [3]. Even people who have problems with their hearing that affect their communication may receive an inaccurate diagnosis of dementia. An accurate diagnosis enables practitioners to effectively treat dementia, and those conditions that are reversible or resemble dementia.

Once a person has a definitive diagnosis of dementia, he/she or the caregiver should begin to plan for future health and community care, as well as make arrangements for managing finances. When diagnosis occurs late in the disease process, people with dementia may have declined to the point where it is difficult for them to understand their options and communicate their wishes about health and community care.

People with dementia generally depend on family and friends for help in living their lives. These caregivers provide assistance with activities ranging from managing finances to help with the most intimate tasks like eating, bathing, and dressing. Caregivers generally help without receiving payment out of a feeling of love or duty to the person who has the disease. Eventually, the demands of caring for someone with dementia

J. Tilly, DrPH (✉)
U.S. Administration for Community Living,
Washington, DC, USA
e-mail: jane.tilly@acl.hhs.gov

K. Gordon, MSW
Splaine Consulting, Columbia, MD, USA

© Springer International Publishing Switzerland 2016
M. Boltz, J.E. Galvin (eds.), *Dementia Care*, DOI 10.1007/978-3-319-18377-0_17

may become more than caregivers can manage on their own. Then, people with dementia and their families rely on paid workers in the home, community, or in institutions. Caregivers need education about their loved one's disease, its progression, and how to handle symptoms. Workers who help or interact with those who have dementia need to be able to identify them and their caregivers, understand how the condition progresses and be able to communicate with them appropriately. Caregivers and workers need to understand how to care for their own health when they are providing physically and emotionally demanding care to those with dementia.

Dementia policy requires consideration of a number of issues, ranging from research priorities to dementia-friendly communities. Research that targets prevention, cure, or stabilization of the disease is critical. For example, prevention is important because those who do not get dementia will not experience the decline in independence that results from it, nor will their caregivers experience the stresses of helping their loved ones cope. While we wait for effective prevention or treatment of dementia, many people have dementia with or without an accurate diagnosis, so detecting who has it and what type of dementia they have is vital to helping ensure that those with dementia receive good care. As the diseases progress, management of an individual's health and long-term services and supports becomes more complicated and requires teamwork as well as education of caregivers and service providers. Finally, some populations are more likely to acquire dementia and have special needs as a result.

Discussion of dementia policy requires a full understanding of its impact on people with the condition, their caregivers, workers, and public and private programs. We start by exploring the impacts and then move on to their policy implications.

The Impact of Dementia

The number of people with dementia and their caregivers is large and growing, as are the costs of dementia care in the U.S. and across the world.

The best estimates of the number of people with dementia come from studies of those who have Alzheimer's disease. About five million Americans may have Alzheimer's disease. Estimates vary from about three million people over age 65 from 1999 through 2001 [4] to about 5.2 million in 2014 [5]. Since age is a major risk factor for dementia, the number of people with the condition likely will grow as the U.S. population ages. There are some people who acquire dementia before age 65, including people with Down syndrome.

World-wide, in 2013, researchers estimated that 44.4 million people 60 years or older had dementia. Assuming no changes in current therapies for the disease, they projected that this number will reach 75.6 million in 2030 [6]. In most countries, the prevalence of dementia among those 60 years and older ranges from 5–7 % [6]. Over time, the percentage of the world's population with dementia in low and middle income countries is likely to grow from 62 % in 2013 to 71 % in 2050 [6]. This is due to population growth and aging in these countries.

Estimates of the number of caregivers for people with dementia in the U.S. vary. The Alzheimer's Association estimates that at least 15 million people provide unpaid care for those with dementia in the U.S [1]. An analysis of the 2011 National Health and Aging Trends Survey of Medicare beneficiaries aged 65 and over shows that 5.8 million caregivers were helping people who probably have dementia [7]. The number of caregivers of people with dementia is likely to grow with the aging of the population.

People with dementia and their caregivers deal with a disease that makes daily living and management of finances, medical care, and social lives more and more difficult as time passes. Behavioral or physical symptoms may eventually cause many people with dementia to pay for care at home, in adult day centers, or in nursing homes. In the end stages of the dementia, people have difficulty communicating in any way, they fail to recognize family, and need round-the-clock care.

As dementia progresses, caregivers experience more stress as they provide more services and supports, such as supervision and personal care [8]. Caring for people with dementia is particularly difficult because of the way it affects abilities and behavior. Caregivers of people with dementia are more likely than caregivers of other older people to help with all daily activities [8]. In addition, caregivers of people with dementia are more likely to help them with the most demanding daily activities—getting out of bed, bathing, using the toilet, and eating. The resulting strain causes many caregivers to have high levels of stress, become depressed, and have financial worries [9–11].

If peolpe with dementia live alone, their lives and those of any caregivers they may have are even more complicated. Researchers estimate that 25 % of American aged 71 and older with moderate dementia and 17 % of those with severe dementia live alone [12]. People living alone with dementia are especially vulnerable to self-neglect, emotional and physical abuse, and financial exploitation because they can be socially isolated and left on their own much of the time. Older adults with cognitive impairments are likely to be at greater risk of abuse and exploitation, leading to negative effects on their health [13]. In addition, two US-based studies have found that people with dementia who live alone are placed into nursing homes earlier, on average, than otherwise similar people with dementia who do not live alone [10, 14].

Use of Medical and Long Term Services and Supports

As compared to those without dementia, people with dementia are more likely to have other chronic conditions, such as heart disease, diabetes, and arthritis [15, 16] Cognitive problems can lead to poor management of these other diseases [17, 18] because people with dementia have difficulty managing complex tasks in the early stages of the disease and have much more difficulty as dementia progresses. Symptoms of dementia and poor management can lead to such things as greater use of health care services. For example, on average, people with dementia have

three times as many hospital stays and three times the average Medicare expenditure as other older people [15]. Recent demonstrations of care that help people with a cognitive disability and their caregivers move from medical settings to home appear to better meet their needs than usual care [19].

Many people who need long-term services and supports (LTSS) have cognitive problems, which often come from dementia. In the U.S., 15 % of older adults, who do not live in institutions like nursing homes and have at least one limitation in a daily activity, have a cognitive disability and the percentage increases with severity of disability [20]. People with these disabilities represent a large percentage of people using LTSS and many of them have a dementia diagnosis. In the U.S., approximately 24 % of people of all ages who receive Medicare or Medicaid-funded home health care have moderate to severe cognitive impairment [21]. Similarly, more than a quarter of people eligible for Medicare and Medicaid who receive home and community-based services through Medicaid waiver programs have Alzheimer's disease or other dementias [22]. Over 40 % of nursing home residents in the U.S. have a diagnosis of dementia, most often a result of Alzheimer's disease [4], and the proportion is higher among nursing home residents who are dually eligible for Medicare and Medicaid. The percentage of people with dementia in institutions varies across the world, depending upon the family and care system structures.

The large number of people with dementia makes it a costly condition. Researchers estimate that dementia care for people 70 years and older in the U.S. cost between $159 billion and $215 billion in 2010, depending on how family caregivers' care costs are calculated [23]. Costs stem from supports and services, and from loss of paid employment for caregivers, among other causes. Costs would be even higher if people with dementia under age 70 were included in these estimates. A similar world-wide cost estimate for dementia care for people of all ages was $610 billion in 2010 [24].

Dementia's effects on persons with dementia and their caregivers highlight the need for effective public policy. So does the estimated economic impact of the disease. Countries around the world face similar issues, although those in developing countries where the population is rapidly aging have a particularly difficult future related to dementia.

Dementia Policy and Planning

Since the early 1980s, state and national governments have recognized the special needs of people with dementia and their caregivers through development and implementation of "Alzheimer's Plans." These plans started in response to the public's recognition of the scope of Alzheimer's disease on the people who have it and their families. In the U.S., the 1980s saw passage of 23 plans and 2 more in the 1990s. For the most part, these plans remained on the shelf with little implementation [25]. However, a few states did address narrow issues, such as impoverishment of one spouse when the other became eligible for Medicaid and the coordination of services for those with dementia.

Starting in the mid-2000s, advocates successfully pushed for a new wave of state plans, culminating in the existence of 36 state plans, plus the District of Columbia in 2014, with more on the way [26]. These plans' policy recommendations fall into 16 categories. The most frequently mentioned are: care management, worker training and quality of care, caregiver support, and public awareness of Alzheimer's. When discussing services, the more recent plans primarily address community services, not those in institutions. Implementation of those plans focuses on caregiver support, care management, worker training. In addition, many U.S. states have implemented the cognitive impairment component of the Behavioral Risk Factor Surveillance System, which the Centers for Disease Control and Prevention (CDC) sponsor, to estimate the proportion of their population who report this type of disability. This gives states information about how cognitive disability affects their residents, which can be very useful for planning purposes.

In the late 2000s, U.S. advocates started their push for the National Alzheimer's Project Act, which became law created in 2012 and 2011. Among other provisions, the Act called for creation of a national plan. The U.S. Secretary of Health and Human Services (HHS) leads the ***National Plan to Address Alzheimer's Disease Research, Care, and Services***. The U.S. plan updated annually, contains actions that federal agencies, states, and communities can use to address the unique needs of people with dementia, and their families and caregivers. The Plan has five goals:

1. Prevent and effectively treat Alzheimer's disease by 2025.
2. Optimize care quality and efficiency.
3. Expand supports for people with Alzheimer's disease and their families.
4. Enhance public awareness and engagement.
5. Track progress and drive improvement.

Other countries have developed and are implementing their own plans. According to Alzheimer's Disease International, 15 mostly European countries now have governmental plans to address the disease [27]. The non-European countries are Israel, Republic of Korea, and the United States. Australia, Canada, Switzerland, and the U.S. have state or provincial Alzheimer's plans. Costa Rica, Cuba, and Mexico are releasing plans in 2014.

The European Union, under the leadership of France, began joint work to address Alzheimer's disease as a major public health challenge in 2008 and to develop international and national plans. In 2013, the United Kingdom led another international effort to address Alzheimer's disease, resulting in several international meetings of the G-7 countries (Canada, France, Germany, Italy, Japan, UK, and U.S.) to promote cooperative developmental work on research, health, and community care.

Most recent national governmental Alzheimer's plans call out a number of policy issues needing attention:

- Funding research into effective treatments for dementia
- Increasing public awareness of dementia and reducing stigma associated with the condition

- Identification of those with possible dementia and the need for an accurate diagnosis
- Effective management of health and community care and expansion of supports for family caregivers
- Delivery of quality services that are able to meet the needs of those with the disease and their caregivers

Using these policy issues to guide the remainder of this chapter, we will discuss how those who interact with and provide services to people with dementia and their caregivers can help support them, that is be—*dementia-capable*. We discuss how a model dementia-capable system would address the issues that national and state plans raise. We provide examples of dementia capability from around the U.S. and other countries. We begin by explaining why dementia-capability is so important for people with the condition and their families, communities, states, and nations.

Importance of Dementia-Capability

Many people are at risk of having dementia or are already living with it. They live alone or with family and they use many public and private service systems. People with dementia rely on their families and faith communities, grocery stores and banks, as well as health, community, and institutional care. Given the long, slow progress of the dementia, their needs and those of their caregivers become more intense with time.

Service systems that wish to be dementia-capable could consider adopting policies that support key aspects of a model dementia-capable service system. The following list of key aspects of a model system comes from two sets of information: dementia-related research, and an evaluation of dementia program experience. A model, dementia-capable system would:

1. Educate the public about risk factors associated with dementia and the diseases that cause it, indicators of cognitive problems, symptom management, evidence-based support programs, and opportunities to participate in research.
2. Identify people with possible dementia and recommend that they see a physician for a timely, accurate diagnosis and to rule out reversible causes of dementia or conditions that resemble dementia.
3. Ensure that program eligibility and resource allocation take into account the impact of cognitive disabilities.
4. Ensure that staff communicate effectively with people with dementia and their caregivers and provide services that:
   - Are person and family-centered
   - Offer self-direction of services
   - Are culturally appropriate
5. Educate workers to identify possible dementia, and understand the symptoms of dementia and appropriate communication and services.
6. Implement quality assurance systems that measure how effectively providers serve people with dementia and their caregivers.
7. Encourage development of dementia-friendly communities, which incorporate key aspects of dementia-capability.

Key Aspects of Model Dementia-Capable Systems

Below we elaborate on how various public and private agencies might approach developing those aspects of a model system that apply to their mission, work, and communities. These aspects are for discussion purposes and could be adapted to an organization or community's individual situation.

Educate the Public

While no one now knows how to prevent Alzheimer's disease, nations, states and communities have a role in educating the public about research findings and opportunities to help that can affect their lives. There are four general educational categories and free U.S. resources are available on each.

a) The general public needs to know about **risk factors associated with dementia**. The risk factors include many of those related to heart health, such as hypertension and smoking—as well as poor sleeping and eating habits. Physical exercise and social and mental engagement can promote brain health. HHS' *Brain Health Resource* provides current, evidence-based information and resources related to brain health. Using this information, states and communities can educate people about how to promote their own brain health. The *Brain Health Resource*, which is available at http://www.acl.gov/Get_Help/BrainHealth/Index.aspx, contains a consumer fact sheet, presentation slides, educator guide, and list of resources that people can consult as they consider changes in their life style. Other countries have educational efforts underway too, either through government, or national advocacy organizations. Examples include the United Kingdom's National Health Services *Dementia Guide*, available at http://www.nhs.uk/Conditions/dementia-guide/Pages/dementia-prevention.aspx and Alzheimer's Australia's *Your Brain Matters* program at http://www.yourbrainmatters.org.au/.

b) People with dementia, their families and providers need to know about **management of physical, cognitive, emotional, and behavioral symptoms of dementia**. As dementia progresses families may find that their loved ones have many difficult symptoms. Consumer-friendly information about how to cope with symptoms can be found at the Alzheimer's Disease Education and Referral Center's website—http://www.nia.nih.gov/alzheimers. It offers current, evidence-based information for consumers and professionals on a wide range of dementia issues. In addition, the HHS' Administration for Community Living (ACL) helps support the Alzheimer's Association's 24 h/7 day a week call center for people who have questions and need advice about dementia. The National Alzheimer's Call Center's phone number is 1.800.272.3900.

c) Staff who serve people with dementia can find out about **evidence-based programs to serve people with dementia and their caregivers** by consulting a white paper—*Translating Innovation to Impact: Evidence-based interventions to support people with Alzheimer's disease and their Caregivers at home and in their communities*. This paper and its related webinar describe successful interventions that help people in the early stages of dementia, family caregivers, and those who coordinate health and long term services and supports for them. These resources are available at: http://www.aoa.acl.gov/AoA_Programs/HPW/Alz_Grants/index.aspx.

d) The public needs to know about **opportunities to participate in research**. The U.S. National Institute on Aging (NIA) sponsors Alzheimer's Disease Research and Education Centers, which conduct research on various dementia topics. Connections to them and opportunities to participate in research are available at http://www.nia.nih.gov/alzheimers. Another resource is the Alzheimer's Association TrialMatch located at http://www.alz.org/research/clinical_trials/find_clinical_trials_trialmatch.asp?type = alzchptfooter. This website lists opportunities to participate in research that come from publicly available sources such as the National Institutes of Health, and a wide variety of research facilities and trial sites across the country.

Identify People with Possible Dementia

Providing appropriate services to people with dementia and their caregivers will not happen unless agencies and health care providers identify people with the condition. Individuals or caregivers may contact programs or service providers to discuss memory problems, trouble managing finances or medical care or behavior changes. Agency workers and health care providers can learn to recognize whether a person may be showing signs of cognitive impairment and refer them for an accurate diagnosis.

Local agencies in the U.S. have adopted several types of strategies for identifying people who may have dementia. These agencies are called Aging and Disability Resource Centers (ADRCs) and Area Agencies on Aging (AAAs); they are the agencies that people with disabilities in the U.S. often contact for help. These strategies include:

a. Information gathering and assessment forms include dementia-specific questions. Minnesota's adds this type of question to its assessment forms [28]. In Missouri, AAA staff use the AD8 assessment to screen for dementia and to refer people who appear to have problems to the Alzheimer's Association (G. Meachum-Cain, Aging Program Specialist, Missouri Department of Health and Senior Services, personal communication, June 15, 2011). In Washington State, AAAs use the TCARE® tool in their Family Caregiver Support Program to provide reliable screening and assessment, identify high-risk caregivers, ensure that available resources go to those most in need, and to determine whether services make a measurable difference to caregivers [29].
b. Staff at local agencies receive training to recognize possible cognitive impairment in their conversations with callers and in other interactions and about how various ethnic groups regard dementia [30].
c. Agencies create processes for referral of people with possible cognitive impairment for professional assessment.
d. Agencies partner with organizations specializing in dementia. For example, staff of the local chapter of the Alzheimer's Association spend one day per month at the ADRC in Racine, Wisconsin, providing training for ADRC staff and information and referral for callers and walk-in ADRC clients (K. Scheel, Program Director, Alzheimer's Association, Southeastern WI chapter, personal communication, October 4, 2011).

Serving people with concerns about dementia requires that physicians and other practitioners understand the possible signs of dementia, which

can be found at the following website: http://www.nia.nih.gov/research/dn/alzheimers-diagnostic-guidelines. If necessary, practitioners must be able to assess a person's cognition or refer them for appropriate evaluation. The U.S. NIA provides a searchable database of brief screening tools available to identify cognitive problems, available at http://www.nia.nih.gov/research/cognitive-instrument. The Alzheimer's Association also offers recommendations for screening tools for use in primary care, available at www.alz.org/documents_custom/jalz_1528.pdf.

If an assessment shows that a person has cognitive problems, it is important to find out the cause. A few causes of dementia may be reversible and some other conditions can resemble it. In addition, while Alzheimer's disease is responsible for 60–80 % of dementia, there other diseases that cause dementia, like Parkinson's disease, Lewy body disease, and fronto-temporal dementia, among others. The HHS offers a free educational program on this topic for practitioners available through Medscape, which provides continuing education units for those who complete it. This program is called *Case Challenges in Early Alzheimer's Disease*, which is available after a free registration at www.medscape.com. The World Health Organization published the Mental Health Gap Action Programme Intervention Guide for mental, neurological and substance use disorders in non-specialized health settings" to address the lack of care, especially in low- and middle-income countries, for people suffering from disorders, including dementia. The Intervention Guide, available from: http://whqlibdoc.who.int/publications/2010/9789241548069_eng.pdf?ua=1, includes an assessment and management guide for dementia.

Ensure Appropriate Eligibility Criteria and Resource Allocation

Most public programs offering home and community services have criteria for deciding whether a person can receive them. Those programs with eligibility criteria based on a person's ability to carry out daily activities sometimes do not take into account cognition. People with dementia may be physically able to carry out daily activities, but still need prompting to complete them. And, the behavioral symptoms that most people with dementia experience may mean that they need supervision to avoid being a danger to themselves or others.

A 2006 examination of Medicaid nursing home level-of-care criteria in six states found that some states weighted "hands-on" assistance more heavily than prompting even if the service time exceeded that for people with physical disabilities only [31]. In addition, state eligibility criteria sometimes do not include the need for supervision due to behavioral symptoms or poor judgment. Medicaid eligibility criteria that accurately measure the needs of people with dementia can promote equitable access to publicly-funded home and community services.

Measuring cognitive disability is more difficult and less standardized than measuring a person's physical ability to carry out daily activities. There are dozens of measures of cognitive impairment. Studies find that one of the most widely used measures—the Mini-Mental Status Examination (MMSE)—has scores that are unrelated to the disability or service needs of people with dementia [32]. One approach that states use is to recognize that if a person needs prompting or supervision when carrying out daily activities, that person has a disability. For example, the Virginia Department of Health, Office of Licensure and Certification has guidelines on assessing activities of daily living. They can be found at: http://www.vdh.state.va.us/ OLC/Laws/documents/HomeCare/ADLs%20 for%20HCOs.pdf.

Model dementia-capable service systems recognize that people with dementia: (1) use more and different services than people with physical disabilities and, (2) rely on their caregivers in order to remain in their communities. Research using the Health and Retirement Study found that older people with cognitive disabilities who needed help with daily activities used twice as many hours of paid care on average as people who had physical disabilities only [20]. People with dementia often need constant supervision

and special services due to behavioral and memory symptoms. Some states have accommodated these needs. For example, in Tennessee, a program found that partnering with adult day care centers enabled caregivers to participate in training because respite was available [33]. Massachusetts' Home Care program staff identified four services as being of particular value for people with Alzheimer's disease and related disorders: Alzheimer's Day Care, Supportive Home Care Aides, habilitation therapy, and occupational therapy (J. Quirk, Director of Home and Community-Based Programs, Massachusetts Executive Office of Elder Affairs, personal communication, August 11, 2011).

Ensure Effective Communication and Person and Family-Centered Services

Model systems offer information, person-centered planning and opportunities for self-direction of services and address cultural differences. Information about services and supports helps people with dementia and their caregivers choose what they need. Information can be made available in several ways. People with dementia and their caregivers can get help in choosing services from a variety of public and private agencies. These local agencies can offer information, assistance, help with managing services, and access to publicly-funded programs like Medicaid and the National Family Caregiver Support Program. Some states host websites with relevant information. For example, the Alabama Department of Mental Health and Mental Retardation sponsors a website (http://alzbrain.org) that provides information for caregivers, professionals, and people with memory loss (J. Miller, Programs Chief, Alabama Department of Senior Services, personal communication, July 8, 2011). Virginia's Alzheimer's Disease and Related Disorders Commission has a virtual Alzheimer's disease center (http://www.alzpossible.org) that offers information about the disease (J. Hoyle, Policy Analyst, Virginia Department on Aging, personal communication, May 31, 2011).

Person and family-centered planning enables people with dementia and their caregivers to choose services that will best meet their unique needs. Person-centered planning is a process that the person with dementia directs. This approach identifies the person's strengths, goals, preferences, service needs, and desired outcomes. Staff, family, and other multidisciplinary team members help the person to identify and access a unique mix of paid and unpaid services to meet their needs. The best person-centered planning helps people live better lives, with support to do the things most important to them.

Section 2402(a) of the Affordable Care Act requires the U.S. Secretary of HHS to ensure all states develop home and community care systems that respond to the changing needs of program beneficiaries, maximize independence, and support self-direction. The Secretary recently offered guidance on person-centered planning and self-direction, which can be found at: http://www.acl.gov/Programs/CDAP/OIP/docs/2402-a-Guidance.pdf. The Secretary's guidance also has standards for self-direction. Self-direction allows the people to control their services and choose providers, which may include family or friends. It may allow people to purchase goods and supports that traditional systems fail to offer.

People with dementia may participate in self-directed programs with the support of representatives. Despite the challenges people with dementia face, people with mild to moderate dementia are able to show preferences for their care. A study of 51 pairs of older adults with their caregivers living in the community found that individuals with mild to moderate cognitive disability were able to respond to questions about preferences for care and their involvement in making decisions consistently over time [34]. Almost all people with mild to moderate cognitive disability were able to identify someone they wished to make health and personal care decisions for them [35]. Almost three quarters of these individuals named their primary family caregiver as the person who should be making these decisions and most individuals preferred help from family and friends. Although people

who do not have severe dementia can express preferences, they may not able to manage care on their own because of losses in decision-making ability. As a result, having the assistance of a representative who can act on behalf of the person with dementia is important [36].

Model dementia-capable systems recognize and support the important role that caregivers play in helping people with dementia remain in the community by helping with decision-making about services and providing them with support. States may offer caregiver training and education as a distinct service under a Medicaid home and community-based services waiver. Covered services may include home-based training, special classes and workshops, and arranging for substitute services when caregivers are learning outside the home. Medicaid rehabilitation services may cover caregiver training. In Kentucky, for example, rehabilitation covers home visits to assist family members and beneficiaries with serious mental health conditions to practice effective communication to cope better with stressful situations that occur at home [37]. Self-directed service budgets generally permit expenditures for caregiver training and education. Sixteen states have a local Medicare coverage policy that provides guidance on Medicare payment for home health nurses to provide teaching and training for families and other caregivers of Medicare beneficiaries with Alzheimer's disease and behavioral symptoms [38].

Model dementia-capable systems also recognize and accommodate the cultural aspects of care, particularly since certain racial and ethnic groups have a higher risk of getting dementia and cultural aspects of dementia vary. For example, older African-Americans are about twice as likely to have Alzheimer's and other dementias as older whites [39] and Hispanics are about 1.5 times as likely to have Alzheimer's and other dementias as older whites [40]. These groups tend to have different symptoms of dementia than whites [41]. In addition, African Americans and Hispanics often have more than one generation living together [42, 43] and faith communities are particularly important to them [30, 44]. Cultural attitudes toward dementia also vary. Hispanics tend to see dementia as a natural part of aging [45] and many Asian communities tend to view dementia as something to hide from others [46]. Finally, lesbian, gay, bisexual, and transgender groups may experience poor treatment from families, faith communities, and certain parts of society and may have limitations on their ability to marry. Poor treatment and isolation from family can complicate dementia care [47].

Resources are available related to help meet the varying needs of diverse groups. *Serving Diverse Communities: A Self-Assessment of Alzheimer's Disease Services Provided by the Aging Network and Its Partners*, available at www.adrc-tae.acl.gov/tiki-download_file. php?fileId=33539, provides information about dementia capability related to cultural issues and a tool to assess an organization's cultural dementia capability related to the communities it serves. There is a companion document that provides resources for those interested in improving their services to diverse communities—*Serving Diverse Populations with Alzheimer's Disease and Related Dementias: A Resource List* at http:// www.adrc-tae.acl.gov/tiki-download_file. php?fileId=33540.

People with certain intellectual disabilities, like Down syndrome, have higher rates of dementia. Six percent of adults with an intellectual disability will have dementia after the age of 60. At least 50–70 % of those with Down syndrome will have it after the age of 60 [48]. Two U.S.-based advocacy groups have addressed the special concerns of adults with intellectual disabilities who have acquired community living skills but find their skills deteriorate as dementia progresses. Resources, like the Caregiver's Guide to Down syndrome and Alzheimer's Disease, from the National Down Syndrome Society can be found at http://www.ndss.org/Resources/Aging-Matters/ Alzheimers-Disease/A-Caregivers-Guide-to-Down-Syndrome-and-Alzheimers-Disease. The National Task Group on Intellectual Disabilities and Dementia Practice has a number of resources ranging from recommendations for assessment to opportunities to join workgroups on health care practice available at http://aadmd.org/ntg.

Worker Training

Staff who work with people with dementia need special training due to the unique needs of this group and their caregivers. Dementia training is uncommon among direct care workers. Federal regulations require 75 h of overall training for home health aides and certified nursing assistants. States vary widely in their requirements for personal care aides [49].

Several sections of the Affordable Care Act address training direct care workers to serve people with dementia. Section 5305 of the Affordable Care Act authorizes $10.8 million in supplemental grants to Geriatric Education Centers (established under Titles VII of the Public Health Service Act) to develop and offer training courses to family caregivers and direct care providers at no charge or minimal cost and incorporate mental health and dementia "best practices" training into their courses. Section 6121 of the Affordable Care Act requires the U.S. Centers for Medicare & Medicaid Services (CMS) to ensure that nurse aides receive regular training on how to care for residents with dementia and on preventing abuse. CMS and its team of experts created the Hand-in-Hand training, which is based on person-centered care, to address this requirement. The training is offered free to all nursing homes, regional offices and state survey agencies and is available at https:// www.cms.gov/Medicare/Provider-Enrollment-and-Certification/SurveyCertificationGenInfo/ Downloads/Survey-and-Cert-Letter-12-44.pdf. However, nursing homes are not required to use the Hand-in-Hand training; other tools and resources are also available.

Sweden undertook a similar effort in 2010 by issuing guidance about person-centered dementia care in residential care facilities. One facility successfully implemented the guidelines using an interactive staff education program. A pre-post design study showed increases in delivery of person-centered dementia care and decreases in staff stress related to delivery of care [50]. These positive results lasted at least one year after the training occurred.

Several U.S. states have developed dementia training programs for direct care workers. For example, Washington developed a comprehensive training program on dementia for service providers, which covers the basics of dementia, communication, behaviors, and providing assistance with daily activities. Massachusetts developed standards for provider training and qualifications, hired a dementia trainer, and provides special training for Supportive Home Care Aides who specialize in serving people with dementia (J. Quirk, Director of Home and Community-Based Programs, Massachusetts Executive Office of Elder Affairs, personal communication, August 11, 2011). In Alabama, the Dementia Education and Training Act provides for training of caregivers and agencies about dementia (J. Miller, Programs Chief, Alabama Department of Senior Services, personal communication, July 8, 2011). Because of the high turnover among LTSS workers, training needs are ongoing and many of the workers who are trained this year may leave the field in a few years.

State grantees, in collaboration with ACL and its National Resource Center on dementia, crafted a toolkit that includes links to trainings, knowledge tests, staff competencies, and information on state dementia training policies and state Alzheimer's disease plan recommendations. The toolkit can be found at: http://www.aoa.acl.gov/AoA_Programs/HPW/Alz_Grants/index.aspx.

Quality Assurance

Improvements in dementia-capability could result in better quality care because staff become knowledgeable about the special needs of people with dementia and their caregivers. Effective quality assurance policies would have at least three components. First, quality measures would assess whether the health and community care system is dementia-capable. Second, systematic and regular measurement of the experience of people with dementia and their caregivers would provide an assessment of how the service system is working from their perspectives. Third, a process of continuous quality improvement would

provide feedback information about dementia service quality which could be used to improve services. This implies that the measures are tracked over time so that comparisons in performance can be made. So far, very little attention has been given to developing these measures and implementing them on an ongoing basis. A special learning collaborative with ACL grantees participating in the Alzheimer's Disease Supportive Services Program developed a set of measures of a system's dementia-capability related to community care. Systems using this set of measures will be able to track their progress in improving dementia-capability. The measures can be found at: http://www.aoa.acl.gov/AoA_Programs/HPW/Alz_Grants/index.aspx.

Dementia-Friendly Communities

A small number of communities in Europe and the U.S. are becoming dementia-friendly. They are implementing policies and practices designed to create communities that are sensitive to the needs of those with dementia. These communities are learning about dementia through education and awareness efforts, providing various types of support to caregivers, and accommodating the needs of racially and ethnically diverse communities. Dementia-friendly services promote meaningful participation in community life for those with the disease, while promoting good quality of life for them and their caregivers.

These efforts go beyond developing dementia-capable health and long term services and supports. Dementia-friendly communities involve improved customer service at participating agencies and businesses, supportive faith or spiritual communities, emergency services that understand dementia, and suitable transportation and public spaces. One of the leading organizations promoting dementia-friendly communities in the U.S. is *ACT on Alzheimer's*. Their website—www.ACTonALZ.org has a number of tools to help communities explore how they might become dementia-friendly. In the UK, a similar website can be found at: http://www.alzheimers.org.uk/dementiafriendlycommunities.

Conclusions

Ensuring that state and local service systems are dementia-capable and friendly is critical to address the policy challenges in dementia care. Many people who seek assistance from these systems have dementia and likely have cognitive disabilities as a result. In addition, caregivers of people with dementia regularly contact these systems seeking assistance in coping with their loved ones' special needs. These needs relate to ever more dependence on others for help with daily activities, short-term memory loss, impaired decision-making capacity, and behavioral and physical symptoms. The types of supports that people with dementia and their caregivers use include assistance with planning for service needs, identifying dementia-capable services, options counseling, and home and community services providers who understand dementia.

In dementia-capable and dementia-friendly systems, information and assistance services identify those with dementia who contact them, staff have training and special communication skills they use with people with dementia and their families, and public and private services programs offer services tailored to the unique needs of this population through the use of person and family-centered planning. To promote optimum quality of services, self-direction is a viable option for those with dementia and their caregivers, workers at all levels have dementia training, and the quality assurance system incorporates some measures of progress toward dementia-capability. A number of states in the U.S. have begun working toward dementia-capability, and others are well along the path. Many communities are becoming dementia-friendly through incorporation of key aspects of dementia-capability in public and private sector agencies and businesses. By taking these actions, states and communities can work to improve care and quality of life for people with dementia and their caregivers, who are among our most vulnerable groups.

References

1. Alzheimer's Association. 2014 Alzheimer's disease facts and figures. Chicago: The Association; 2014. 75 p.
2. National Institutes of Health. The dementias hope through research. Bethesda, MD: The Institutes; 2013. 40 p.
3. Rueben D. Presentation at Easter Seals Webinar: the real scoop on brain health; 2014.
4. Bernstein A, Remsburg R. Estimated prevalence of people with cognitive impairment: results from nationally representative community and institutional surveys. Gerontologist. 2007;47(3):350–4.
5. Herbert L, Weuve J, Scherr P, Evans D. Alzheimer disease in the United States (2010–2050) estimated using the 2010 census. Neurology. 2013;80(19):1178–83.
6. Alzheimer's Disease International. Policy brief for heads of government: the global impact of dementia 2013–2050. London: The International Federation; c2013 [cited 2014 Aug 12]. Available from: http://www.alz.co.uk/research/GlobalImpact-Dementia2013.pdf
7. Spillman B, Kasper J. Dementia and informal caregiving analyses of the national study of caregiving. Presentation before the National Advisory Council on Alzheimer's Disease, Care and Services; 2014 Jul 21.
8. Alzheimer's Association. 2011 Alzheimer's disease facts and figures. Chicago: The Association; 2011. 68 p.
9. The Shriver Report and the Alzheimer's Association. A woman's nation takes on Alzheimer's. Chicago: The Report and the Association; 2010. 320 p.
10. Yaffe K, Fox P, Newcomer R, Sands L, Lindquist K. Patient and caregiver characteristics and nursing home placement in patients with dementia. J Am Med Assoc. 2002;287(16):2090–7.
11. Taylor D, Ezell M, Kuchibhatia M, Ostbye T, Clipp E. Identifying the trajectories of depressive symptoms for women caring for their husbands with dementia. J Am Geriatr Soc. 2008;56(2):322–7.
12. Okura T, Plassman B, Steffens D, Llewellyn D, Potter G, Langa K. Neuropsychiatric symptoms and the risk of institutionalization and death: the aging, demographics, and memory study. J Am Geriatr Soc. 2011; 59(3):473–81.
13. Government Accountability Office. Elder justice: stronger federal leadership could enhance national response to elder abuse highlights of GAO-11-208, a report to the Chairman, Senate Special Committee on Aging, U.S. Senate. Washington, DC: The Office; 2011. 60 p.
14. Freedman VA. Family structure and the risk of nursing home admission. J Gerontol B Psychol Sci Soc Sci. 1996;51(2):S61–9.
15. Bynum J. Characteristics, costs and health service use for Medicare beneficiaries with a dementia diagnosis:

report 1: medicare current beneficiary survey. Dartmouth: Dartmouth Institute for Health Policy and Clinical Care, Center for Health Policy Research; 2009.

16. Hill J, Futterman R, Duttagupta S, Mastey V, Lloyd J, Fillit H. Alzheimer's disease and related dementias increase costs of comorbidities in managed Medicare. Neurology. 2002;58(1):62–70.

17. Doraiswamy P, Leon J, Cummings J, Marin D, Neumann P. Prevalence and impact of medical comorbidity in Alzheimer's disease. J Gerontol A Biol Sci Med Sci. 2002;57(3):M173–7.

18. Tilly J, Riggs J, Maslow K, Brown K. Medicaid managed long-term care for people with Alzheimer's disease and other dementias. Washington, DC: The Alzheimer's Association; 2006.

19. Naylor M, Hirschman K, Bowles K, Bixby M, Konick-McMahan J, Stephens C. Care coordination for cognitively impaired older adults and their caregivers. Home Health Care Serv Q. 2007;26(4): 57–78.

20. Johnson R, Wiener J. A profile of frail older Americans and their caregivers. Washington, DC: The Urban Institute; 2006. 78 p.

21. U.S. Department of Health and Human Services, Centers for Medicare, Medicaid Services (n.d.). Unpublished data from rollup summary reports, case mix means and episode counts, national values for the 12-month period from March 2003–February 2004, Baltimore, MD.

22. Walsh E, Freiman M, Haber S, Bragg A, Ouslander J, Wiener J. Cost drivers for dually eligible beneficiaries: potentially avoidable hospitalizations from nursing facility, skilled nursing facility, and home and community-based services waiver programs: draft task 2 report. Waltham, MA: RTI International; 2010. 262 p.

23. Hurd M, Martorell P, Delavande A, Mullen K, Langa K. Monetary costs of dementia in the United States. N Engl J Med. 2013;368(14):1326–34.

24. Wimo A, Jonsson L, Bond J, Prince M, Winblad B. The worldwide economic impact of dementia 2010. Alzheimers Dement. 2013;9(1):1–11.

25. Baumgart M. Presentation before the Advisory Council on Alzheimer's Research, Care and Services; 2014 April 29. Accessed 27 Aug 2014.

26. Alzheimer's Association [Internet]. Chicago: The Alzheimer's Association; c2014 [cited 2014 Sept 6] State Alzheimer's Disease Plans. Available from: http://act.alz.org/site/DocServer/STATE_AD_PLANS.pdf?docID=4641accessed

27. Alzheimer's Disease International [Internet]. London: Alzheimer's Disease International; c2014 [cited 2014 Aug 27]; [about 33 screens]. Available from http://www.alz.co.uk/alzheimer-plans

28. Brown D, Wiener J. Alzheimer's disease demonstration grants to states: Minnesota prepared for the administration on aging. Research Triangle Park, NC: RTI International; 2007.

29. Korte L. Washington state dementia partnerships project: final report. Olympia, WA: Washington Department of Social and Health Services; 2011.

30. Grey H, Jimenez D, Cucciare M, Tong H-Q, Gallagher-Thompson D. Ethnic differences in beliefs regarding Alzheimer disease among dementia family caregivers. Am J Geriatr Psychiatry. 2009;17(11): 925–33.

31. O'Keeffe J, Tilly J, Lucas C. Medicaid eligibility criteria for long-term care services: access for people with Alzheimer's disease and other dementias. Chicago, IL: Alzheimer's Association; 2006. 20 p.

32. Royall D. Use of the mini-mental status examination to categorize dementia. Nurs Home Med. 1997;5(11): 11A–3.

33. Gould E, Hughes S, O'Keeffe C, Wiener J. The Alzheimer's disease supportive services program: report on completed grants. Alzheimer's Disease Supportive Services Program National Resource Center for the U.S. Administration on Aging at the Administration for Community Living; 2014 Sept.

34. Friss Feinberg L, Whitlatch C. Are people with cognitive impairment able to state consistent choices? Gerontologist. 2001;41(3):374–82.

35. Friss Feinberg L, Whitlach C. Decision-making for people with cognitive impairment and their family caregivers. Am J Alzheimers Dis Other Dement. 2002;17(4):237–44.

36. O'Keeffe J, Saucier P, Jackson B, Cooper R, McKenney E, Crisp S, Moseley C. Understanding home and community-based services: a primer. Research Triangle Park, NC: RTI International; 2010. 253 p.

37. The Alzheimer's Association. Medicare home health benefit for caregiver training in 16 states. Chicago, IL: The Association; 2014. 2p.

38. Potter G, Plassman B, Burke J, Kabeto M, Langa K, Llewellyn D. Cognitive performance and informant reports in the diagnosis of cognitive impairment and dementia in African Americans and whites. Alzheimers Dement. 2009;5(6):445–53.

39. Gurland B, Wilder D, Lantigua R, Stern Y, Chen J, Killeffer E. Rates of dementia in three ethnoracial groups. Int J Geriatr Psychiatry. 1999;14(6):481–93.

40. Sink K, Covinsky K, Newcomer R, Yaffe K. Ethnic differences in the prevalence and pattern of dementia-related behaviors. J Am Geriatr Soc. 2004;52(8): 1277–83.

41. Alzheimer's Association. Lighting the path for people with Alzheimer's: a guide for African American clergy. Chicago, IL: The Association; 2006.

42. Napoles A, Chadiha L, Eversley R, Moreno-John G. Developing culturally sensitive dementia caregiver interventions: are we there yet? Am J Alzheimers Dis Other Dement. 2010;25(5):389–406.

43. Eiser A, Ellis G. Cultural competence and the African American experience with health care: the case for specific content in cross-cultural education. Acad Med. 2010;82(2):176–83.

44. National Alliance for Hispanic Health. Alzheimer's disease: outreach to the Hispanic community. Washington, DC: The Alliance; 2006.

45. Ethnic Elders Care Network. Chinese Americans and dementia. Washington, DC: The Network; 2013.

46. National Resource Center on LGBT Aging. Inclusive questions for older adults a practical guide to collecting data on sexual orientation and gender identity. New York: The Center; 2013. 28 p.

47. National Task Group on Intellectual Disabilities and Dementia. My thinker's not working a national strategy for enabling adults with intellectual disabilities to remain in their community and receive quality supports. Chicago, IL: The Group; 2012. 48 p.

48. Institute of Medicine. Retooling for an aging America: building the health care workforce. Washington, DC: National Academy of Sciences; 2010. 316 p.

49. Edvardsson D, Sandman P, Borell L. Implementing national guidelines for person-centered care of people with dementia in residential aged care: effects on perceived person-centeredness, staff strain, and stress of conscience. Int Psychogeriatr. 2014;26(7):1171–9.

50. Konrad T, Morgan J, Green-Royster T. North Carolina long-term care workforce turnover survey: descriptive results, 2010. Chapel Hill, NC: North Carolina Institute on Aging, University of North Carolina at Chapel Hill; 2011. 7 p.

Index

A

Aβ. *See* Amyloid beta (Aβ)
Acetaminophen, 278
Acetylcholinesterase inhibitors (AChEIs), 160, 252
    donepezil, 75
    galantamine, 76
    ginkgo biloba, 84
    memantine, 77
    rivastigmine, 75
AChEIs. *See* Acetylcholinesterase inhibitors (AChEIs)
Activities of daily living (ADL), 197, 269
AD. *See* Alzheimer's disease (AD)
ADACs. *See* Alzheimer's Disease Assistance Centers (ADACs)
ADCs. *See* Alzheimer's Disease Centers (ADCs)
ADEPT. *See* Advanced dementia prognostic tool (ADEPT)
ADL. *See* Activities of daily living (ADL)
Adler, G., 128
ADRCs. *See* Aging and Disability Resource Centers (ADRCs)
Adult Day Service (ADS), 206
Advanced care planning (ACP)
    cognitive function, 250
    CPR/intubation, 250
    family/proxy, 251
    healthcare proxy, 249
    medical interventions, 250
    POLST, 250
    primary care providers, 249
Advanced dementia prognostic tool (ADEPT), 269
Advanced practice nurses (APNs), 237
Aging and Disability Resource Centers (ADRCs), 305
Aging, Demographics, and Memory Study (ADAMS), 192
Agitation
    psychomotor, 98
    psychotic symptoms, 98
    resistance, 99
Alcohol, 13, 265, 271, 299
Alder, C.A., 113–120
ALF. *See* Assisted living facility (ALF)
Alzheimer's disease (AD). *See also* Dementia prevention
    AD8, 41

anti-inflammatory approaches, 80
anti-neuroinflammatory, 80
aspirin-generated lipoxin A4 (LXA4), 80
biomarkers, 35–36
dementia policy, 299–310
dementias diagnosis, 154
despair experiences, 154
diagnosis and treatments, 191
DS, 194
early stage, 61–68
emotional care, 200
ethnic diversity factors, 196
hospitalization, 208
insulin receptors, 79–80
and MCI, 33
MoCA, 39
pharmacologic approaches, 77, 78
physical care, 197
prevalence, 1
resilience, 156
sandwich generation caregiver, 193
SBT, 38
symptoms, 1, 2
Tau/Phospho-tau, 79
Alzheimer's Disease Assistance Centers (ADACs), 46
Alzheimer's Disease Centers (ADCs), 46, 306
Ambulatory care-sensitive conditions (ACSCs), 235
American Automobile Association (AAA), 133
AMPS. *See* Assessment of motor and process skills (AMPS)
Amyloid beta (Aβ), 73, 81
    accumulation, 77, 79
    alcohol consumption, 13
    atorvastatin, 80
    berries, 18
    caffeine, 14
    caspase-enzymes, 13
    curcumin, 18
    folate, 16
    hypoinsulinemia, 17
Amyloid precursor protein (APP), 16, 77, 79
Aniracetam, 25
Anstey, K.J., 21
Anticonvulsants, 87

Antidepressants
    adverse effects, 87
    citalopram, 86
    depression, 86
    SSRIs, 86
    trazodone, 87
Anti-inflammatory approaches, 80
Antimicrobial therapy, 276
Antipsychotics, 85–86
Anxiolytics, 87
Apolipoprotein E ε4 allele (ApoE4), 11, 12, 21
APP. *See* Amyloid precursor protein (APP)
Area Agencies on Aging (AAAs), 305
Artificial nutrition and hydration, 250, 252–253
Art therapy, 67
Assessment, BPSD, 100–101, 106
Assessment of motor and process skills (AMPS), 137–138
Assisted living facility (ALF)
    cognitive impairment, 206
    memory care settings, 207
    physical care interventions, 207
    relocation decision, 207
    residential care setting, 207
Austrom, M.G., 113–120
Avila, R., 173

B
Bass, D.M., 173, 184
Baum, L., 19
B12 deficiency, 81, 82
Behavioral and psychological symptoms of dementia
        (BPSD)
    assessment, 100–101
    dementia, 98
    lack confidence, 98
    neuropsychiatric symptoms, 97
    non-pharmacological interventions, 98
Behavioral management
    anticonvulsants, 87
    antidepressants, 86–87
    antipsychotics, 85–86
    anxiolytics, 87
    cholinesterase inhibitors and memantine, 87–88
    limitations, 84
    neuropsychiatric symptoms, 84
    psychopharmacological medications, 84
    resources, 85
Behavioral management strategies, 169, 181
Behavioral Risk Factor Surveillance System
        (BRFSS), 190
Behavioral symptoms
    affective/mood disturbances, 98–99
    agitation/resistance, 99
    BPSD, 99
    caregiver's approach, 100
    environmental factors, 100
    exposure, 100
    psychotic symptoms, 99
    sleep pattern disturbance, 99

Belle, S.H., 173
Bereavement, hospice care
    anticipatory grief, 287
    cardiac disease, 288
    chaplains, 289
    depression, 289
    faith community, 288–289
    life style, caregiver spouse, 288
    management, demented patients, 289–290
    prophylactic antidepressant therapy, 288
Berries, 18
Blom, M.M., 220
Boltz, M., 1–4, 162, 215–222, 233–242
Boustani, M.A., 113–120
BPSD. *See* Behavioral and psychological symptoms of
        dementia (BPSD)
Brain health, 304
Brandt, N.J., 73–89
Brody, A.A., 247–257
Bryan, J., 17
Buddy Program, 66
Budoff, M.J., 13
Buettner, L.L., 174
Burgener, S.C., 173
Burgio, L., 173
Burkhardt, J., 139
B vitamins
    anti-oxidant and anti-inflammatory properties, 15
    B12 deficiency, 81, 82
    cell metabolism, 14
    folate, 16–17
    folic acid supplementation, 81
    serum homocysteine (Hcy), 81
    vitamin B1 (thiamine), 15
    vitamin B2 (riboflavin), 15
    vitamin B6 (pyridoxine), 15–16, 81
    vitamin B12 (cobalamin), 16, 81

C
Caffeine, 13–14
Campbell, J.L., 216, 217
Cardiovascular disease (CVD), 219
Cardiovascular risk factors
    diabetes, 21
    hypercholesterolemia, 20–21
    hypertension, 20–21
    insulin resistance, 21
    physical exercise, 22
    smoking, 21–22
Care collaboration
    care managers, 51
    CMAs, 52
    definition, 51
    neuropsychology, 53
    NPs/PAs, 52
    OTs, 53
    patient evaluation, 50–51
    physicians, 51–52
    psychology, 53

PTs, 53
registered nurse, 52
social work, 53
in Spain, ACE, 51
staffing, 51
Care continuum
AD, 203
ADS, 206
assisted living, 206–208
care management services, 205–206
club sandwich generation, 204
community education, 204–205
diagnostic resources, 203
dying process, 209
home-community care, 205
hospice, 209
hospitalization, 208–209
medical advocacy, 210
neurological diseases, 211
political advocacy, 210
primary care physician, 203
psychological repercussions, 211
social isolation, 210
terminal illness, 204
Caregivers, 100
dementia policy (*see* Policy, dementia care)
hospice team
aging individuals, 286–287
bizarre behaviors, 287
cumulative impact, 286
dying process, 285
family and educational materials, 286
mental and physical health, 286
physicians, 287
psychoeducational interventions, 286
risk factors, 287
stress-related symptoms, 288
Caregiver well-being
coronary heart disease, 215–216
cross-sectional data, 222
ethnic groups, 222
factors, 222
physical health
CVD, 219
electrical stimulation, 219
exercise, 220
home-based, 220
NMS, 220
PEP, 219
psychoeducational interventions, 219
sleep disturbance, 219
technology-based interventions, 220–221
physiologic stress models, 216–217
post-caregiving interventions, 221–222
psychological stress models, 216
psychologic health
CBT, 218
counseling, 217–218
educational programs, 218
group support interventions, 218–219
meditation and mindfulness, 219
PST, 218
PT, 219
web-based training, 218
respite services, 221
TNF-α and C-reactive protein, 215
Caregiving
behavioral management strategies, 169
financial resources, 257
institutionalization, 256
pain, 254
pressure ulcers, 253
PWD, 247
quality of life, 183
supportive interventions, 168
therapeutic agent, 181
Caregiving experiences
abuse, 202
AD, 197
ADL, 197
dementias caregivers, 199
education and resources, 202–203
emotional care, 200–201
ethical dilemmas, 203
family experience, 198
government agencies, 202
informations, 199
male spouses, 197
parent care responsibilities, 200
physical care demands, 197
psychological strains, 200
rehabilitation, 200
relational dynamics, 201–202
teaching resources, 199
time-consuming, 200
Care management, 300. *See also* Case management
Care partners
AD, 209
driving contract, 63
early stage dementia, 61, 65, 68
healthcare professionals, 68
hospitalization, 208
social engagement, 65
Care transitions intervention (CTI), 237
Carr, D., 141
Case management
assessment and prioritization, 56
benefits, patients and caregivers, 58
challenges, case managers, 57
community resources, 56
definition, 56
GCMs, 56
interventions, 57–58
nurses/social workers, 56–57
RCTs, 57
US Department of Health and Human Services, 57
CBT. *See* Cognitive behavioral therapy (CBT)
CCM. *See* Collaborative care model (CCM)
Certified medical assistants (CMAs), 52
Chang, B.L., 174

Chien, W.T., 174
Choi, S.S.W., 167–185
Cholinesterase inhibitors, 87–88
Chromium, 17–18
Clare, L., 62, 174
Cobalamin, 16, 81
Cognition, 299, 305, 306
Cognitive behavioral therapy (CBT)
    "action-oriented" approach, 218
    Cochrane systematic review, 218
    educational program, 221
Cognitive engagement
    cognitive reserve, 22
    cognitive training, 22–23
    depression, 23
    social networks, 23
Cognitive enhancers, 87–88
Cognitive impairment
    agencies, 304, 305
    Behavioral Risk Factor Surveillance System, 302
    Medicare and Medicaid, 301
    older adults, 301
Cognitive rehabilitation (CR), 66–67
Cognitive stimulation and training, 103–104
Collaborative care model (CCM), 234
Collaborative Studies of Long-term care (CS-LTC), 240
Community mobility
    cognitive impairment, 125
    Comfort Zone®, 138
    consumers and health care providers, 143
    driver rehabilitation programs, 143–147
    driving assessment, 141–142
    driving simulator, 142–143
    driving transition, 131–134
    IADL, 136–138
    management, 139
    monitoring, 138
    monitoring instruments, 139
    primary care health provider, 125
    stakeholders, 126
    transportation options, 139
    travel training, 139
Contractures, 250, 253
Coping, early stage dementia, 61–62
Cornus amonis (CA), 16
Cotter, V.T., 61–68
CR. See Cognitive rehabilitation (CR)
Creutzfeldt-Jacob disease, 261
Crucial conversations, 248–249
CTI. See Care transitions intervention (CTI)
Curcumin, 18–19
CVD. See Cardiovascular disease (CVD)

D
Davis, E.S., 125–147
Dehydroepiandrosterone (DHEA), 24–25
Deimling, G.T., 216
Dementia Advocacy and Support Network International (DASNI), 158

Dementia care. See also Memory clinics; Screening tests
    diagnosis, 1
    educational programs, 3
    family caregivers, 3
    health care and social service workers, 3–4
    physical and social environment, 3
    policy, 299–310
    public awareness, 1–2
    quality of life, 3–4
    stages, 1, 2
    support, person, 2
Dementia care models
    cognition and function, 113
    examining, 113
    geriatrics-trained health care, 113
    local response, 119–120
    primary care, 114–117
    purpose, 114
    significant evidence, 113
    specialty care, 117–119
Dementia diagnosis
    assessment, 114
    caregivers, 115
Dementia-friendly communities, 309
Dementia in primary care
    co-morbidities, 115
    dementia screening support, lack, 115–116
    legal requirements, 116–117
    local response, 119–120
    patient and caregiver, 114
    physician attitudes and values, 116
    physician training and diagnostic tools, 114–115
    time, 115
Dementia in specialty care
    communication and care coordination, 118–119
    follow-up services, lack, 118
    lack, resources, 118
    local response, 119–120
    memory care specialists, 117
    patient's acceptance, 117
    reimbursement system, 119
    social support, lack, 117–118
    volume-based incentives, 118
Dementia living, home interventions
    behavioral symptoms, 172, 181
    community interventions, 169–170
    design/random allocation, 170
    disease severity, 171
    dose response, 181
    family caregivers, 170, 181
    institutionalization, 172
    nonpharmacology, 170
    person with dementia, 170–172
    quality of life, 172
    randomized trial design, 171
    therapeutic agent, 181
Dementia management, 117
Dementia prevention
    advancing age, 9
    alcohol, 13

B vitamins, 14–17
caffeine, 13–14
cardiovascular risk factors, 20–22
chromium, 17–18
cognitive decline
   ApoE4, 11
   brain regions, 10
   medial temporal lobes, 10
   mitochondrial dysfunction, 11
   neurodegeneration, 10
   vascular risk factors, 11
cognitive engagement, 22–23
DHA, 19–20
diet, 11–12
economic cost, 9
flavonoids, 18–19
garlic, 12–13
ginkgo biloba, 13
health authorities, 10
hormones, 24–25
learning disabilities, 10
piracetam, 25
recommendations, 25
risk factors, 9–10
vitamins E and C, 17
Desai, A.K., 151–164
Desai, F.G., 151–164
Despair, PwD, 154–156, 160
DHA. *See* Docosahexaenoic acid (DHA)
DHEA. *See* Dehydroepiandrosterone (DHEA)
Diabetes, 21
Dias, A., 174
Dickerson, A.E., 125–147
Dignity experiences
   loss, 154
   resilience, 156
   retrospective, 155
   stress, 154
DNH. *See* Do Not Hospitalize (DNH)
Docosahexaenoic acid (DHA), 19–20, 83
Donepezil (Aricept)®
   adverse reactions, 75
   dosing, 75
Do Not Hospitalize (DNH), 273–274
Down syndrome (DS), 194
Driver rehabilitation specialists (DRS)
   driving evaluation and training, 135
   occupational therapists, 134
   on-road assessment, 134
Driving assessment
   behind-the-wheel (BTW), 134
   "discrete" skills, 141
   DRS, 135
   IADLs, 132–133
   individual screening method, 141
   licensing guidelines and reporting, 130
   medically-at-risk drivers, 141
   MMSE, 141
   mobility and transportation mode, 132
   "motor memory", 142

   on-road performance, 142
   physician, 129
   road test and licensing authority, 134
   Snellgrove Maze test, 141
   Trail Making Test A, 141
   UFOV, 141
Driving cessation
   adult child, 126
   community mobility, 140
   driver to passenger transition, 129
   DRSs, 135
   evidence-based screening tools, 130
   fault crash/acute situation, 131
   fitness-to-drive, 126
   health professionals, 140–141
   IADL, 130
   medically-at-risk drivers, 129
   transportation/medication, 132
Driving screening
   AAA, 133
   Alzheimer's disease, 134
   comprehensive driving evaluation, 134
   evaluator screening, 133
   fitness-to-drive, 133, 134
   FTDS, 133
   functionally-based, 141
   IADLs, 133–134
   motion sickness and symptoms, 143
   obtaining and reviewing data, 133
   Parkinson's Disease, 141
   proxy screening, 133
   screening tools, 130
   self-screening tool, 133
   web-based tool, 133
Driving transition
   Alzheimer's disease, 134
   awareness, 132
   cessation, 132
   educational resources, 132
   evaluator screening, 133
   fault crash/acute situation, 131
   fitness-to-drive, 133
   FTDS, 133
   IADLs, 133–134
   MIT Age Lab, 132
   non-binding agreement, 132
   Proxy screening, 133
   "red flags"/triggers, 131
   Roadwise Review®, 133
   self-screening, 133
   stakeholders, 126
DRS. *See* Drirehabilitation specialists (DRS)
Dyspnea, 248, 254, 255

E
Early stage dementia
   coping, 61–62
   diagnostic disclosure, 62–63
   driving, 63

Early stage dementia (*cont.*)
   healthcare professionals, support, 64–65
   legal and financial planning, 63–64
Early stage resources
   Alzheimer's Association, 65–66
   art therapy, 67
   buddy programs, 66
   cognitive support, 66–67
   physical fitness, 67–68
Eby, D.W., 138, 139
Eloniemi-Sulkava, U., 174
Emotional care
   behavioral symptoms, 201
   denial and confusion, 200
   disease awareness, 200
   early intervention, 201
   frontotemporal dementia, 201
Emotion oriented interventions, 104
Environment, 106
Estrogens, 24
Ethnic diversity factors
   African-Americans, 196
   bisexual respondents, 197
   data collection, 196
   late-onset AD, 196
Exercise and physical activity, 104–105
Experiences, PwD
   negative
      abandonment, 155
      alzheimerization, 155
      care facility, 154
      caregivers, 153
      despair, 154
      excess disability, 154
      HCPs, 153
      loss and grief, 153
      loss of dignity, 154–155
      social rejection, 153
      socio-cultural factors, 156
      supportive resources, 154
   positive
      care practices, 157
      hope, 156
      joy and gratitude, 157
      resilience reflection, 156
      social activities, 156
      social relationships, 158
      spiritual conversion, 157
      vascular dementia, 157

F
Family caregivers
   AD, 189
   care partners, 189
   children caregivers, 192
   decision-making, 189
   employed caregivers, 194–195
   IADL, 189
   long distance caregiver, 195
   male caregivers, 191
   parents
      DS, 194
      early onset, 193
      evidence-based information, 193
      special care environments, 194
   religious communities, 190
   sandwich generation caregiver, 193
   sexual orientation, 190
   spouses, 192
Farias, J., 215–222
Farran, C.J., 220
Fever, 255–256
Fioravanti, M., 16
Fitness-to-drive
   complex medical issues, 136
   occupational therapy, 137
   skilled professional, 136
   stakeholders, 126
   state licensing authority, 134
Fitness to drive screening (FTDS), 133
Fitzsimmons, S., 174
Flavonoids
   berries, 18
   curcumin, 18–19
   ginkgo biloba, 13
   resveratrol, 19
Fletcher, S., 207
Folate, 16–17
Folstein, M.F., 291
Frontotemporal dementia, 1, 265, 272
FTDS. *See* Fitness to drive screening (FTDS)
Functional decline, palliative care
   acetaminophen, 255
   caregiver's pain, 254
   delirium, 255
   dyspnea, 255
   fever, 255–256
   Hospice Dementia Care, 254
   moderate dementia, 254
   psychological symptoms, 254

G
Galantamine (Razadyne)®
   acetylcholinesterase inhibitor, 76
   adverse reactions, 76
   dosing, 76
Galik, E., 97–107
Galvin, J., 1–4, 162
Galvin, J.E., 33–42
Garlic, 12–13
Gaugler, J.E., 221, 238
Gavrilova, S.I., 175
GCMs. *See* Geriatric care managers (GCMs)
Gerdner, L.A., 175
Geriatric care managers (GCMs), 56
Geriatric Resources for Assessment and Care of Elders
      (GRACE), 234
Ginkgo biloba
   antioxidative properties, 83
   benefits, 83

EGb761, 84
   flavonoids and terpenes, 13
   meta-analysis, 84
Gitlin, L.N., 167–185
Godwin, K.M., 15
Gordon, K., 299–310
Gormley, N., 176
Graff, M.J., 176
Grossberg, G., 151–164
Guerra, M., 176
Gu, Y., 12

H
Hamaguchi, T., 18
Haynes, N., 9–25
Healthcare professionals (HCPs).
      See also Community mobility
   AD, 162
   aging, 163
   cognitive impairment, 126
   critical driving skills, 143
   dementia care, 162
   "driver-at-risk", 128
   driver rehabilitation, 134
   DRS, 134, 135
   evaluator screening, 133
   experiences, 160, 161
   inform care decisions, 162
   licensing authority, 130
   physician, 129
   psychiatric consultation, 163
   QOL, 160
   "red flags"/triggers, 132
   renewal policy, 130
   safety risk, 129
   screening tool, 133
   warning signs, 127
Health information technology, 184
Healthy Aging Brain Care Monitor (HAB-C Monitor), 234
Hipoccampal atrophy, 24
Hirano, A., 220
HMG-CoA reductase inhibitors ("statins"), 80
Hodgson, N., 167–185
Home care, 170
Home hospice management
   adaptation, 285
   admission process, 284
   atropine, 285
   critical elements, 284
   emergency kits, 284
   haloperidol, 285
   lorazepam and morphine, 285
   pain, psychiatric distress and nausea, 286
Home interventions. *See* Persons with dementia (PwD)
Hope, 152, 154, 156, 157
Hopkins, J., 163
Hormone replacement therapy (HRT), 24
Horvath, K.J., 176
Hospice dementia care
   agencies, 261

bipolar disorder, 291
causes, 262
centenarians, 263
cognitive symptoms, 262, 291
death and dying process, 263–265
diagnosis, nursing homes, 262
disruptive transitions, 268
education, 267–268
eligibility, 269
environmental consistency, 267–268
ethical challenges, 292–293
expenditures, 261
features, 265, 266
hospice providers, 268–269
intellectual disability, 291–292
interdisciplinary team, 267
Lewy body dementia, 261, 265
in older adults, 261
Parkinson's disease, 265
patient and family
   advanced planning, 266
   aggressive measures, 266
   end-stage dementia, 267
   financial issues, 267
   racial disparities, 266
   recommendations, 266–267
patient management, 273–278
prognostic uncertainty, 270
psychiatric and behavioral manifestations,
   278–284
quality measures, 268
quality of life, 263
referrals, 269
research and ethical issues, 263
schizophrenia, 290
sensory deficits, 262
special populations, 290
suicidality, 291
Hospital avoidance, 256
Hospitalization
   ACSCs, 235
   Alzheimer's Association, 236
   APNs, 237
   cognitive stimulation, 237
   CTI, 237
   decision-making, 235
   delirium, 235
   family caregiver, 235
   Hospice Dementia Care, 238
   medications, 236
   palliative care, 238
   TCM, 237
HRT. *See* Hormone replacement therapy
   (HRT)
Huang, H.L., 176
Huang, Y.C., 239
Humor, 159
Hunt, L.A., 125
Hypercholesterolemia, 20–21
Hypertension, 20–21, 115, 304
Hypoinsulinemia, 17

I

IADL. *See* Instrumental activity of daily living (IADL)
IDE. *See* Insulin-degrading enzyme (IDE)
Implantable cardioverter-defibrillator (ICD), 275
Informant questionnaire on cognitive decline in the
         elderly (IQCODE), 41
Instrumental activity of daily living (IADL)
      AMPS, 138
      driver rehabilitation program, 138
      driving examination, 138
      fitness-to-drive, 138
      gaps and pathways project, 138
      housing and finances planning, 130
      occupational therapy, 130, 136, 137
      on-road evaluation, 137
      physician, 129
      transportation, 128–129
Instrumental ADL (IADL), 189
Insulin-degrading enzyme (IDE), 21
Interventions, caregiver well-being.
         See Caregiwell-being
IQCODE. *See* Informant questionnaire on cognitive
         decline in the elderly (IQCODE)
Isaacson, R.S., 9–25

J

Jansen, A.P.D., 176
Joy, 157

K

Kenny, A.M., 240
Khanassov, V., 57
Kiosses, D.N., 177
Kitwood, T., 2, 151
Koch, T., 57
Krikorian, R., 17
Kruman, I.I., 16
Kurata, T., 78

L

LaMantia, M.A., 113–120
Lam, L.C., 177
Late-onset dementia (LOD), 160
Late stage dementia
      neuropathology, 271
      pathobiology, brain imaging
            atrophy and ventriculomegaly, 271
            biomarkers, 270
            brain death, clinical definition, 270
            capacity, 272
            frontal lobes and orbitofrontal cortices, 272
            hypertensive leukoencephalopathy, 271
            microscopic damage, 270
Lee, H., 15
Lee, I.Y.M., 174
Livingston, G., 177
Long-term care, PwD
      AD, 238
      ADLs, 238
      decision-making, 239
      family caregivers, 238
      hospitalization, 241
      multivariate analysis, 240
      person-centered care, 239–240
      RC/AL facilities, 239
      residences, 240
Long-term services and supports (LTSS), 301–302, 309
LTSS. *See* Long-term services and supports (LTSS)

M

MAB. *See* Medical Advisory Boards (MAB)
Mansour, D.Z., 73–89
Marriott, A., 177
Marsiske, M., 217
Maslow, K., 140
Mavall, L., 221
McCurry, S.M., 177, 178
McFadden, J.T., 163
McFadden, S., 151–164
McFadden, S.H., 157, 163
McGillick, J., 189–211
MCI. *See* Mild cognitive impairment (MCI)
Meador, K., 15
Medical Advisory Boards (MAB), 130–131
Medically-at-risk driving
      automobile *vs.* transit, 128
      community stakeholders, 130
      driving cessation support groups, 129
      family member, 128
      healthcare professionals, 130
      IADL, 128–129
      individual capability, 128
      judicial system, 131
      law enforcement officers, 131
      NHTSA, 130–131
      patient/client, 128
      physician, 129
      screening tools, 130
Medication discontinuation, 251–252
Medication management and safety, 88, 89
Mediterranean diet (MeDi), 11–12
Meeuwsen, E.J., 55
Memantine (Namenda)®, 87–88
      adverse reactions, 77
      dosing, 77
      pivotal study, 77
      stages, 76
Memory care practice, 116, 118
Memory clinic outcomes
      cholinesterase inhibitors, 55
      cognitive complaints, 54
      collaborative care, 55
      community resources, 55
      diagnosis, caregivers, 53
      diagnostic disclosure, 54
      general practitioners (GPs), 54

in Netherlands, physicians, 54
post encounter interviews, 53–54
quality of care, 54
Memory clinics
   ADCs, 46
   assessment and management, 47, 48
   collaborative care, 50–53
   community services, 48
   cost effectiveness, 55–56, 58
   diagnosis, 45
   education and training, 48–49
   funding, 46–47
   health professionals, 48–49
   interdisciplinary team, 47
   NAPA, 46
   NDS, 46
   outcomes, 53–55
   population served, 49
   psychometric testing, 47
   social/ethical issues, 48
   telemedicine, 50
   UK survey, 46, 47
   in US, 45–46
Memory evaluation, 54
Memory Services National Accreditation Programme
      (MSNAP), 47
Mental status examination, screening tests
   cognitive assessment, 36–38
   informant interviews, 36
   neurological, 36
   office setting, 37, 38
   self-rating scales, 36
Mild cognitive impairment (MCI)
   biomarkers, 35
   DHA, 19
   heterogeneous definitions, 20
   hipoccampal atrophy, 24
   HRT, 24
   IQCODE, 41
   Mediterranean diet, 11, 12
   MoCA, 39
   piracetam, 25
   pyridoxine, 16
   SLUMS, 39
Mills, M.A., 159
Mimori, Y., 15
Mini Cognitive Assessment Instrument (Mini-Cog), 38
Mini-mental state exam (MMSE)
   curcumin, 19
   diabetes, 21
   diagnostic tests, 38
   driving assessment, 141
   ginkgo biloba, 84
   insulin, 80
   issues, 38
   Mini-Cog, 38
   MoCA, 39
   omega-3 FA, 83
   riboflavin, 15
   SLUMS, 39

thiamine, 15
vitamin B6, 15
vitamin D, 82
vitamin E and C, 17
Mini mental state examination (MMSE), 269, 292
   category fluency test, 15
   on-road performance, 141
   population-based sample, 21
   riboflavin intake, 15
   vitamin D, 82
   vitamins and carotene, 17
Mitochondrial dysfunction, 11
Mittelman, M.S., 178, 217
Mizrahi, E.H., 15
MMSE. *See* Mini-mental state exam (MMSE)
MoCA. *See* Montreal cognitive assessment (MoCA)
Model dementia-capable systems
   agencies, 304–305
   dementia-friendly communities, 309
   description, 303, 310
   education, public, 303–304
   eligibility criteria and resource allocation, 305–306
   health care providers, 304–305
   person and family-centered services, 306–308
   quality assurance, 309
   worker training, 308–309
Models of care, 46, 51, 55
Mollica, R.F., 205
Moniz-Cook, E., 178
Montreal cognitive assessment (MoCA)
   informant-based tools, 39–41
   MMSE, 39
   neuropsychological testing, 39, 40
   sensitivity, 39
Moore, R.C., 222
Morgan, R.L., 155
Morris, M.C., 16
MSNAP. *See* Memory Services National Accreditation
      Programme (MSNAP)

N
NAPA. *See* National Alzheimer Project Act (NAPA)
National Alzheimer Project Act (NAPA), 33, 46, 97
National dementia strategy (NDS), 46, 58
National Highway Traffic Safety Administration
      (NHTSA)
   evidence-based information, 129
   gaps and pathways project, 138
   law enforcement officers, 131
   MAB, 130–131
   online training developement, 130
NDS. *See* National dementia strategy (NDS)
Neafsey, E.J., 13
New York University Caregiver Intervention (NYUCI)
   caregiver depressive symptoms, 222
   Hispanic caregivers, 222
   multisite program, 217
NHTSA. *See* National Highway Traffic Safety
      Administration (NHTSA)

Nighttime monitoring system (NMS), 220
NMDA receptor. *See* N-methyl-D-aspartate (NMDA)
    receptor
N-methyl-D-aspartate (NMDA) receptor, 74, 76, 284
NMS. *See* Nighttime monitoring system (NMS)
Nobili, A., 178
Non-pharmacological approaches
    behavioral symptoms, 97–100
    BPSD, 100–101
Non-pharmacological interventions
    assessment, environment and caregiver support
        network, 106
    behavioral goals, 106–107
    BPSD, 102
    caregivers, 102
    categorization, 103
    cognition and physical/functional capabilities, 106
    cognitive stimulation and training, 103–104
    education and training, 105–106
    emotion-oriented interventions, 104
    establishment, 106
    mentoring and monitoring, 107
    morbidity and mortality risks, 101
    multi-component interventions, 103
    physical activity and exercise, 104–105
    sensory stimulation, 103
Nonpharmacology
    evidence base support, 168
    family caregivers, 168
    persons with dementia, 168
NPs. *See* Nurse practitioners (NPs)
Nurse practitioners (NPs), 52
Nutraceuticals
    B Vitamins, 81–82
    definition, 81
    Omega-3 fatty acids (FAs), 83–84
    vitamin D deficiency, 82
    vitamin E, 82–83
NYUCI. *See* New York Unisity CaregiIntervention
    (NYUCI)

O
Occupational therapists (OTs), 53
Omega-3 fatty acids (FAs)
    evidence, 83
    Ginkgo biloba, 83–84
    mechanisms, 83
    transgenic mouse model, 83
OTs. *See* Occupational therapists (OTs)
Ouslander, J.G., 241
Oxiracetam, 25

P
PA. *See* Physician assistant (PA)
Palliative care
    ACP, 249
    antipsychotics, 252

    artificial nutrition and hydration, 252–253
    behavioral symptoms, 248
    Caregiver Interventions, 247
    contractures, 253
    functional debility, 252
    Geriatric Depression Scale, 257
    hospitalization, 256
    implementation program, 248
    institutionalization, 256
    non-oncologic settings, 247
    perception and invitation, 249
    pressure ulcers, 253
    prognostication, 248
    psychosocial needs, 247
    serious illness, 247
    specialist vs generalist, 247
    spiritual support, 257
Patient management, hospice care
    antimicrobial therapy, 276
    clinical concerns, 273
    hospitalization, 273–274
    life-sustaining treatments, 276
    mechanical ventilation, 274
    medications, 277
    nutritional issues, 276–277
    pain management, 277–279
PCTs. *See* Primary care trusts (PCTs)
Pearlin, L.I., 216
PEP. *See* Pleasant events program (PEP)
Person-centered dementia care
    African Americans and Hispanics, 307–308
    decision-making, 307
    intellectual disabilities, 308
    Medicaid rehabilitation services, 307
    older adults, 307
    resources, 308
    self-direction, 307
    services and supports, information, 306
Personhood, 160
Persons with dementia (PwD). *See also* Family caregis
    Alzheimer's Society, 152
    behavioral intervention, 168
    bio-measures, 183
    caregivers, 152
    care-partnering, 163
    cognitive functioning, 152, 159
    cognitive impairment, 168
    comorbid processes, 167
    cultural revolution, 151
    dementia interventions, 184
    exercise programs, 169
    family caregiver, 184
    gerontology, 233
    government investments, 168
    growing research, 159
    HCPs, 151, 158
    health care system, 167, 183, 233
    humor sense, 159
    independence, 158

institutionalization, 182
long term sustainability, 184
multi-faceted dementia, 182
neuropsychiatric symptoms, 168, 169
nonpharmacology, 168
persons with dementia, 182
psychometric methods, 183
QOL, 152, 163
quality of life, 167
relocation transitions, 233
reminiscence, 159
research methodology, 152–153
selfhood, 159
severe dementia, 159
social environments, 182
socio-cultural factors, 152
supportive family, 158
supportive interventions, 168
symptomatology, 168
therapeutic agent, 185
Perspectives, PwD. *See* Persons with dementia (PwD)
Pharmacological approaches
AChEIs, 74
AD, 73
donepezil (Aricept)®, 75
galantamine (Razadyne)®, 76
memantine (Namenda)®, 76–77
NMDA, 74
rivastigmine (Exelon)®, 75–76
skin cancers and infections, 73
tacrine (Cognex)®, 74–75
Phelan, E.A., 235
Physical therapists (PTs), 53
Physician assistant (PA), 52
Physicians Orders for Life Sustaining Treatment
        (POLST), 250
Physiologic stress models
cardiovascular response, 216
chronic caregiver stress, 217
cross-sectional studies, 216–217
poor sleep, 217
Piercy, K.W., 217
Pimouguet, C., 56, 57
Piracetam, 25
Pitkala, K.H., 178
Plaques, 79
Pleasant events program (PEP)
CVD biomarkers, 219
IL-6, 219
Polarity therapy (PT), 219
Policy, dementia care
Alzheimer's plans, 302–303
brain diseases, 299
caregivers, 299–300
dementia-capability, 303–309
diagnosis, 299
impact of, 300–301
LTSS, 301–302
prevention, 300

symptoms, 299
Polypharmacy
anticoagulation therapy, 251
antiglycemics, 251
antipsychotics, 252
cardiovascular disease, 251
memantine, 252
severe dementia, 251
statins, 251
Post-acute
behavioral manifestations, 238
Family Caregiver Report, 238
psychoactive medication, 238
unfamiliar environment, 237–238
Post, S., 157
Poulshock, S.W., 216
Powers, B.A., 155
Powers, R.E., 261–293
Pramiracetam, 25
Pressure ulcers, 252, 253, 278
Primary care trusts (PCTs), 47
Problem solving therapy (PST), 218
Prognostication
decision making, 248
life expectancy, 248
onset, 248
PST. *See* Problem solving therapy (PST)
Psychiatric and behavioral manifestations
anxiety, 281
delirium, 279–280
depression, 280–281
early stages, 278
hallucinations, 282
late stage dementia, 282
management, 279
nursing home residents, 279
polypharmacy, 279
screaming, 279
symptoms, 279
transitional patient, 279
Psychological stress models
background context, 216
intrapsychic strains, 216
Pearlin model, 216
primary stressors, 216
secondary role strains, 216
Psychosocial intervention programs, 116,
        211, 286
Psychotropic medications, dose reduction
antidepressant, 283
antiepileptic, 283
antipsychotic, 283–284
benzodiazepines, 283
diphenhydramine, 282
memantine, 284
polypharmacy, 282
quality of life, 284
PT. *See* Polarity therapy (PT)
PTs. *See* Physical therapists (PTs)

Pulmonary disease, 270
Pyridoxine, 15–16, 81

Q
QALY. *See* Quality-adjusted life years (QALY)
Quality-adjusted life years (QALY), 55–56
Quality of life (QOL)
    behavior management, 182
    home interventions, 168
    PwD, 168
Quayhagen, M.P., 178

R
Rantz, M.J.
Reimbursement system, 119
Reminiscence therapy, 67
Residential care/assisted living (RC/AL), 239
Resilience, 151, 156, 160, 163
Resveratrol, 19
Riboflavin, 14, 15
Ringman, J.M., 19
Ritchie, K., 14
Rivastigmine (Exelon)®
    adverse reactions, 76
    Cochrane review, 75
    donepezil, 76
    dosing, 76
    statistically significant correlation, 75
Roadwise Review®, 133
Rowe, M.A., 215–222

S
Sabat, R., 151
Sabat, S.R., 163
Saint Louis University Mental Status (SLUMS), 39, 292
Samala, R.V., 241
Samus, Q.M., 179, 184
SBT. *See* Short blessed test (SBT)
Schulz, R., 221
Screening tests
    AD8, 41
    attributes, 34, 35
    benefits, 33–34
    biomarkers, 35–36
    cognitive disorders, 42
    cultural differences, 34
    environment, healthcare, 42
    incidence, morbidity and mortality rates, 33
    informant-based assessments, 35
    IQCODE, 41
    MCI (*see* Mild cognitive impairment (MCI))
    mental status examination, 36–38
    MMSE, 38
    MoCA, 39–41
    SBT, 38
    SLUMS, 39
Seifan, A., 9–25
Sensory stimulation, 103

Short blessed test (SBT), 38
Silverstein, N.M., 125–147
SLUMS. *See* Saint Louis Unisity Mental Status (SLUMS)
Smith, G.E., 238
Social citizenship, 152
Somme, D., 57
Sommer, B.R., 17
Spiritual support, 257
Ståhl, A., 139
Stanley, M.A., 179
Stapleton, T., 138
Steinberg, M., 179
Stigma, 154, 155, 158, 160
Supporting families, dementia care, 189, 193
Sury, L., 239
Suttanon, P., 179
Swartwood, R.M., 220
Symptom management, 248, 257

T
Tacrine (Cognex)®
    adverse reactions, 74–75
    dosing, 74
Tangles, 79
Tappen, R.M., 179
Tariot, P.N., 87
Tau hyperphosphorylation, 74, 79
Taylor, R., 162
Tchalla, A.E., 179
Teixeira, J., 61–68
Telemedicine, 50, 58
Teri, L., 179, 180
Thalamic processing, pain, 278
Thiamine, 14, 15
Thibault, J.M., 155
Tilly, J., 299–310
Transitional Care Model (TCM), 237
Transitions, PwD
    ACP, 234, 241
    Alzheimer's Association, 234
    care continuum, 234
    cognitive impairment, 233
    decision-making, 233
    HAB-C Monitor, 234
    Hospice Dementia Care, 241
    hospitalization, 235
Trazodone, 87
Tucker, K.L., 16

U
Useful Field of View® (UFOV), 141

V
van Boxtel, M.P., 14
van Gelder, B.M., 14
Vitaliano, P.P., 217
Vitamin B1 (thiamine), 15

Vitamin B2 (riboflavin), 15
Vitamin B6 (pyridoxine), 15–16, 81
Vitamin B12 (cobalamin), 16, 81
Vitamin C and E, 17
Vitamin D deficiency, 82
Vitamin E, 82–83
Vreugdenhil, A., 180

W
Watson, N.M., 155
Wengreen, H.J., 17
White, M.M., 189–211
Williams, I.C., 217

Wolfs, C.A., 56
Wound care, 278

Y
Young-onset dementia (YOD), 160
Yu, F., 220

Z
Zarit, S., 221
Zhang, Y., 78
Zimmerman, S., 207, 238, 240
Zweig, Y.R., 45–58